Hand Therapy

Principles and Practice

Edited by

Maureen Salter MBE MCSP
Former Superintendent Physiotherapist
Joint Services Medical Rehabilitation Unit
Royal Air Force Chessington
Surrey
UK

and

Lynn Cheshire Dip COT SROT
Head Occupational Therapist
Hand and Plastic Surgery Service
St Thomas' Hospital
London
UK

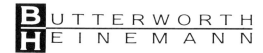

OXFORD AUCKLAND BOSTON JOHANNESBURG MELBOURNE NEW DELHI

Butterworth-Heinemann
Linacre House, Jordan Hill, Oxford OX2 8DP
225 Wildwood Avenue, Woburn, MA 01801-2041
A division of Reed Educational and Professional Publishing Ltd

℞ A member of the Reed Elsevier plc group

First published 2000

British Library Cataloguing in Publication Data
1. Hand – Wounds and injuries   2. Hand – Diseases
I. Salter, Maureen   II. Cheshire, Lynn
617.5'75'06

Library of Congress Cataloguing in Publication Data
Hand therapy: principles and practice/
edited by Maureen Salter and Lynn Cheshire.
  p.;cm.
  Includes bibliographical references and index.
  ISBN 0 7506 1686 5
  1. Hand – Wounds and injuries – Patients – Rehabilitation.
  2. Hand – Diseases – Patients – Rehabilitation.
  3. Physical therapy.   I. Salter, Maureen.   II. Cheshire, Lynn.
  [DNLM: 1. Hand Injuries – therapy.
  2. Hand – physiopathology. WE 830 H2867 2000]
  RD559.H365 2
  617.5'75 – dc21   00–030397

  ISBN 0 7506 1686 5

Composition by Genesis Typesetting, Laser Quay, Rochester, Kent
Printed and bound in Great Britain by The Bath Press, Avon

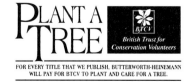

Contents

Acknowledgements

Carole Bexon – to her husband Roy for all his help and support.

Sue Boardman – to her Senior 1 Physiotherapist Nikki Burr for advice and support, and to Jill Shirran for the secretarial help.

Sheila Crowley – as at the end of Chapter 6, page 139.

Alison Davis and **Annette Leveridge** – to those who helped with typing and draft reading, and for all the support and encouragement given.

Sheila Lawton – to Wexham Park Hospital, Slough, Medical Photography Department, for the photographs in Chapter 16.

Lynn Cheshire – to Maureen Salter – for the privilege and pleasure of working with her, (at last!), the Medical Photography Department, St. Thomas' Hospital, London, in particular Mike Messer, for their help in preparing the illustrations for the chapters on splinting.

The companies and their representatives who kindly donated materials and assistance for the preparation of splints for photography, particularly Promedics, Johnson and Johnson, Arthrodax, and Smith and Nephew Homecraft.

Maerian de Jong, Sue Kennedy and Dominique Thomas who made substantial contributions to the text.

Joy Hill, Senior Physiotherapist, Joint Services Medical Rehabilitation Unit, Headley Court, for her help with photography research.

The Victoria and Albert Museum Picture Library and Golley, Slater, Brooker for their kind permission to use the poster illustration of *The Power of The Poster*, V&A Exhibition.

Maureen Salter – to her family for support and help, and also to her co-editor, without whose encouragement this book was unlikely to ever have been finished, and to all the contributors for their hard work and forbearance.

To the medical editors at Butterworth-Heinemann who have provided so much help and support.

To Churchill Livingstone for permission to use material previously published in *Hand Injuries: A Therapeutic Approach*. (Permission has already been granted by Churchill Livingstone.)

All the chapter authors also thank their numerous colleagues, friends and families who typed, read, advised and sacrificed their time and domestic serenity to help and support them.

And the many patients who helped by coming in for extra sessions and by giving permission for photography.

Contributors

Carole Bexon Dip COT
Head Occupational Therapist
Wessex Rehabilitation Centre, Salisbury District
Hospital, UK

Ann Birch BA MCSP SRP
Therapy Department, Wrightington Hospital,
Hall Lane, Wigan, Lancashire, UK

Susan Boardman MCSP SRP
Physiotherapy Department,
Mount Vernon Hospital, Rickmansworth Road,
Northwood, Middlesex, UK

Jeffrey D Boyling MSc BPhty Grad Dep Adv
Manip Ther MAPA MCSP MErgS MMPAA
Director, Jeffrey Boyling Associates, Chartered
Physiotherapists & Ergonomists, Broadway
Chambers, Hammersmith Broadway, London, UK

Lynn Cheshire Dip COT SROT
Head Occupational Therapist,
Hand and Plastic Surgery Service,
St Thomas' Hospital, Lambeth Palace Road,
London, UK

Sheila Crowley MCSP
Superintendent Physiotherapist, Physiotherapy
Department, Adelaide Street Health Centre,
Norwich, Norfolk, UK
Formerly Superintendent Physiotherapist
West Norwich Hospital, Norwich, Norfolk, UK

Alison Davis MCSP SRP
Senior Hand Therapist, King Edward VII
Hospital, Midhurst, West Sussex, UK

Victoria Frampton MCSP SRP
Honorary Fellow of the British Association of
Hand Therapists, Past President of the
International Federation for Societies for Hand
Therapy
Independent hand therapist, 15 Dover Street,
Canterbury, Kent, UK

Lynda Gwilliam BSc (Hons) Dip COT SROT
Therapy Department, Wrightington Hospital,
Hall Lane, Wigan, Lancashire, UK

Sheila Lawton Dip COT SROT
Occupational Therapy Manager,
Wexham Park Hospital, Slough, Berkshire, UK

Annette C Leveridge Dip COT, SROT
Honorary Secretary Education Sub-Committee of
the British Association of Hand Therapy.
Secretary General of the International Federation
for Societies for Hand Therapy
Occupational Therapy Specialist, Burns and
Plastic Surgery and Hand Therapy, Bishopswood
Hospital, Northwood, Middlesex, UK

Maureen Salter MBE MCSP
Former Superintendent Physiotherapist
Joint Services Medical Rehabilitation Unit, Royal
Air Force Chessington, Surrey, UK
Now at: Trees, Houghton Lane, Bury, Pulborough,
West Sussex, UK

Dominique Thomas MCMK (Fr) RPT (USA)
Director, Centre Grenoblois de Rééducation de la
Main, Centre de Rééducation, 1 Bd Clemenceau,
Grenoble, France

Maerian A Van der Heijden-de Jong
Psychosocial Worker, Department of
Rehabilitation, University Hospital, Groningen,
The Netherlands

Dr C. B. Wynn Parry MBE DM FRCP FRCS
Consultant Rheumatologist for the British
Association of the Performing Arts Medicine

Introduction

The principles and practice of hand therapy are integral to all treatment of the hand and upper limb, and the specialism of hand therapy is now recognized worldwide. Development and education are supported by national networks of therapists and globally by the International Federation of Societies of Hand Therapists. This makes the exchange of knowledge and research easily available and specifically focused for our needs.

This book details a myriad of principles and techniques. It is our responsibility as therapists to ensure they are indeed practised and that the key principles of hand therapy are applied; namely:

- Early intervention
- Regular and timely, sometimes highly intensive, interventions
- A holistic, client centred approach in an empathetic environment
- Sound interdisciplinary teamwork
- Effective management and professional education.

EARLY INTERVENTION

This cannot be overemphasized as, without early intervention, many hand conditions rapidly acquire the more chronic problems that result in needless extra hours of therapy and distress to the patient. By 'early' intervention we mean that treatment starts within 24 hours of trauma or surgery. Oedema, pain, stiffness, adhesions – these can all be arrested or prevented by early intervention. Patient education is also essential at this time to keep protective splints and dressings in place and to prepare the patient and their family for any future rehabilitation.

REGULAR AND TIMELY INTERVENTIONS

How much therapy will the patient require and how often? Are there adequate facilities and therapists for a properly evidence-based treatment to be given? The editors of this book have frequent misgivings as to the provision of treatments, particularly intensive treatments. Despite modern knowledge, many patients receive therapy only once a week when outcomes have shown that once a day,

or even several times a day, would be the appropriate frequency for their condition. This is because the patient is fitted to the 'system' and not the system to the patient. More audit and research is still needed to show the false economy of such programming and to evaluate how best to organize hand therapy resources. As hand therapists we must still be prepared to argue the case for the correct treatment for our patients and to consider this a professional responsibility if we are to remain answerable to our clients.

HOLISTIC, CLIENT CENTRED APPROACH

To achieve compliance and therefore satisfactory outcomes we must tailor treatment to the patient's social situation as well as to their condition, and carefully consider all aspects of their case. Many of the chapters in this book emphasize the importance of balance – the essential mix of physical, psychological and social elements – which affect the ultimate results of rehabilitation. To be holistic we know that we often should look further than the hand itself, particularly where pain is the presenting problem (yes, it may indeed originate from the feet). We also need to be holistic in our treatment techniques. Any specialism is in danger of becoming insular, so it is important that we incorporate skills from neurology and psychology in treatment of the hand. For example, developing extension movements in the hand and arm by using balancing patterns and righting reflexes through total body exercise; using colours such as orange and yellow, rather than blue, in hand activities to reinforce a positive, cheerful mood rather than a negative or depressed one.

TEAMWORK, MANAGEMENT AND PROFESSIONAL EDUCATION

Are we united, well organized and up-to-date? We all need adequate time to ensure that we keep our house in order and have time to learn, and teach. If hand therapists do, in fact, supply 80 per cent of any hand patient's total treatment then we have a considerable commitment. For all these elements we require the resources: support staff, efficient record keeping methods, teaching materials and so on. It is not, therefore, a luxury to have such things as electronic assessment tools, clerical assistance, and ready access to medical photography.

We should also feel able to participate in research, without any resulting financial or social burden. For many of us this is not yet the case and is thus retarding the progress of hand therapy and, of course, of our parents.

To conclude, it is obvious that we have still much to do to achieve the standards of hand therapy that we desire. Hopefully this book will go some way to further these aims and to continue the vision of the celebrated surgeons, physicians, anatomists, physiotherapists and occupational therapists who encouraged, demanded, tutored and nurtured the discipline that was to become hand therapy. Some of these founders were our personal 'gurus'. We have often remembered their words while writing these chapters and hope this book is a fitting tribute.

Section 1

1 Function of the hand

Maureen Salter

1. Grasp
2. Support
3. Striking movements
4. Free movements and dexterity
5. Communication and expression
6. Sensory reception
7. Orientation.

> The world can only be grasped by action, not by contemplation . . . The hand is the cutting edge of the mind.
>
> Jacob Bronowski, *The Ascent of Man.*

INTRODUCTION

Man is capable of achieving an extremely wide variety of functions and skills with the hand, and the learning process commences at a very early age. During the first 6 weeks of life, when babies grasp a finger placed in the hand they are not only utilizing reflex activity but also gaining knowledge from the novel sensory input. As the voluntary movements increase, children learn by feeling objects and using all the other sensory modalities – such as watching, listening and testing in the mouth. These stimuli help to ratify the cutaneous sensibility without which children could not build a repertoire of motor activity.

At about 3 months, babies can roll over into the prone position and learn to extend their fingers and support themselves on their forearms (Minett, 1985), acquiring stability of the head on the trunk and the trunk on the hands. This achievement is influenced by the sensory input from the skin and the proprioception of the joints.

At 4–5 months, babies start to reach out independently for toys and to co-ordinate movements, using a primitive pincer grasp to pick up small objects between finger and thumb (Reynolds, 1987). The skill of prehension is acquired during the following months, with gradual improvement in the stability of the upper arm and in hand–eye co-ordination. Encouragement and help from the mother are vital for the normal development of the child. A large part of early life is occupied at play, and much of this time will be spent using the hands for activities. Children who are deprived of these opportunities may be severely affected psychologically for the rest of their lives.

Evolution over many generations has produced anatomical variations, ranging from the squat, muscular hand of the labourer to the long, tapering fingers of the dancer and artist. It is the latter mobile hands that are more vulnerable to severe injury and take longer to rehabilitate.

FUNCTIONS

The main functions of the hand, and those that need to be restored following injury, are:

Grasp

The various types of grip (or prehension) are adjustable according to the size, shape, weight and solidity of the object to be held. Sufficient finger extension must be available for first grasping and then releasing the object. The ability to position the fingers and thumb correctly and without fumbling when initiating grasp is dependent mainly on accurate visual alignment of the thumb, which then provides a post towards which the fingers move.

Power grip
For the power grip, the fingers are flexed around the object with the wrist stabilized in extension. The power in this grip is mainly provided by the strength of the ring and little fingers opposing that of the thumb. The object lies diagonally across the palm, with the metacarpophalangeal joints in ulnar deviation and slight rotation to maintain strong finger contact.

The power grip may be:

- double-handed for activities needing great strength and stability, as in using a shovel or pickaxe, when the whole arm moves and the long flexors of the fingers contract strongly to maintain the grasp (Figure 1.1)

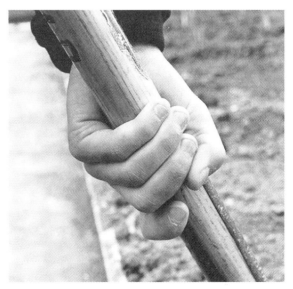

Figure 1.1 Strong grasp. Note power of thumb opposing little and ring fingers, with less strength of index and middle fingers.

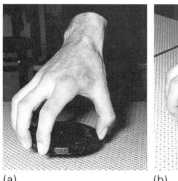
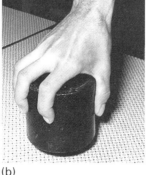

(a)   (b)

Figure 1.2 Span grip: (a) using the tips of the digits for a light weight; (b) using a greater surface area for a heavier object and stronger action of FDP and FPL. Note the altered position of the metacarpophalangeal joints.

- single-handed, as in holding a hammer, with the thumb lying on the shaft directing the hammer head while the movement takes place at the wrist
- a span grip involving all the fingers, with the five digits able to encircle the object due to the arch structure of the hand (Figure1.2a); contact with more of the finger surface may be necessary when a heavier object is grasped (Figure1.2 b), requiring strong activity of the long flexors of fingers and thumb
- an adapted grasp adding some precision, as in holding a knife and fork, where the implements are held firmly by the ring and little fingers with the index finger guiding the line of movement. Full flexion of the little and ring fingers into the palm is necessary to prevent an implement such as a screwdriver, for example, sliding through the hand when pressure is applied.

Precision grip
This is the most frequently used form of grasp. Accurate and precise movements can be achieved by application of the tips of fingers and thumb, utilizing the skin areas with maximum sensory supply. The extent of finger area used will depend on the weight or delicacy of the object being picked up and on the task to be undertaken.
  Precision grips include:

- a pinch or lateral grip, as in holding a key whilst inserting it into a lock (Figure 1.3); this entails opposition of the lateral surface of the index distal phalanx, and there is a strong contraction of the first dorsal interosseous and adductor pollicis muscles, stabilized with lateral support from the middle finger
- an interdigital pinch, such as that used by the smoker when holding a cigarette between the index and middle fingers
- a tip grip, used for small and delicate objects (Figure 1.4); this may utilize the index finger and

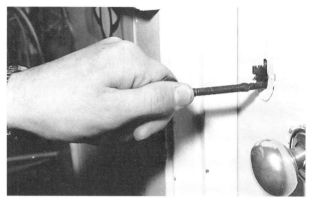

Figure 1.3 Lateral pinch grip. Note activity of first dorsal interosseous.

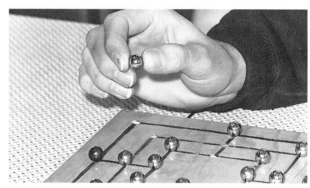

Figure 1.4 Tip grip using finger and thumb only; the smaller the object, the greater the degree of joint flexion required.

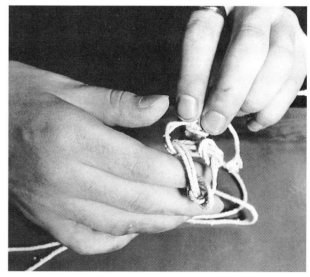

Figure 1.5 Use of nails to unpick string.

thumb only, or the thumb with two or three fingers, depending on the diameter of the object
- use of the nails to pick up minute objects, unpick knots (Figure 1.5) and scrape surfaces – as in removing a sticky label from a jar or adhesive tape from the skin

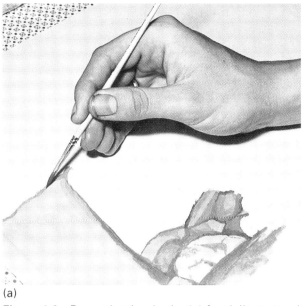

(a)

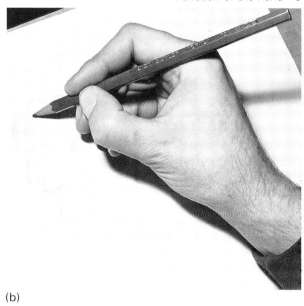

(b)

Figure 1.6 Dynamic tripod grip: (a) for delicate touch; (b) for firmer pressure. Note the altered positions of the joints and the support given by the little finger.

- use of the fingertips for leafing through papers and bank notes; the slight degree of normal skin sweating makes some adherence possible
- a tripod grip (Figure 1.6), with the palmar surfaces of the distal phalanges of thumb, index and middle fingers rotated towards one another and supported laterally by the ring finger; the delicate use of paintbrush and pen and pencil are good examples of this dynamic support (Wynn Parry, 1981).

Awareness of skin and nail use is enhanced by the excellent sensory nerve supply of digit tips and nail beds, and particularly of the dynamic sides of the thumb and index finger.

Extended finger grasp
In the extended finger grasp, the fingers and thumb remain extended at the interphalangeal joints and are opposed when picking up a flat object such as a book or document file.

Hook grip
In the hook grip, the fingers are flexed strongly at the proximal interphalangeal joints and the endurance power of the flexor digitorum superficialis is utilized, as demonstrated when carrying objects such as a bucket or suitcase. The action of holding the handle, mainly by the superficialis muscle, has the effect of flattening the arches (Figure 1.7).

Support
The body weight may be totally or partially supported on the hand. Total hand support, which is a primitive use, should be regained as soon as

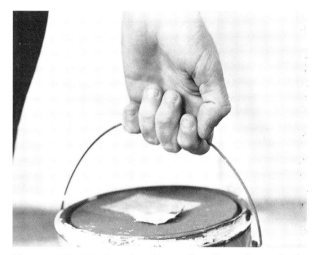

Figure 1.7 Hook grip. Note the flattening of the arches and also that the majority of finger flexion is at the proximal interphalangeal joints.

possible after an injury. The child learns the action early when crawling, and later when performing activities such as handstands and cartwheels. While leaning on the whole hand, the body is supported and balanced by stabilizing the trunk on the arm.

Other types of support include:

- thumb and fingertip support, which steadies the paper or positions a ruler whilst a pen or pencil is used with the other hand (Figure 1.8)
- little finger support, which allows skilled activities to be carried out by thumb, index and middle fingers (e.g. when writing); the hand can be positioned correctly because of the isometric

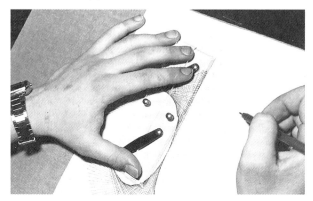

Figure 1.8 Steadying support using fingertips.

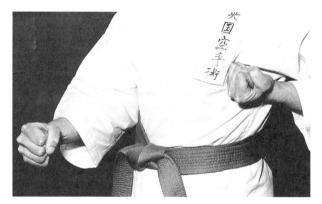

Figure 1.9 Striking power.

contraction of the abductor digiti minimi and other hypothenar muscles, and amputation of a little finger can therefore be a very disabling injury.

Striking movements

These movements are accomplished with fingers either totally flexed as for a punch (Figure 1.9) or extended as in a slap or for karate. The hand, utilizing the strength of the whole arm, can be a powerful weapon for both aggression and protection.

Free movements and dexterity

The simple movements of stroking, caressing and wiping utilize the whole arm, usually with a statically positioned hand. However, fast, intricate movements of the fingers, as in typing and playing musical instruments (Figure1.10), require each hand to be independent of the other. This is possible only when there is suitable posture of the trunk, which provides stability to the upper and lower arm. A large degree of free movement occurs at the metacarpophalangeal joints, and this is monitored closely by proprioceptive feedback, particularly from the numerous sensory endings in the lumbrical muscles. These movements, which are highly skilled and remarkably fast, require a great deal of practice and training, and usually start to develop during childhood. They are dependent on good sensibility of the hand.

Communication and expression

A variety of gestures are used in communication, from simple greetings to the complex sign language of the deaf and dumb. Gestures may be conscious or unconscious, and can denote love and respect or defiance and pure aggression; their use is an integral but individual part of everyone's personality. Dancers of many nations use their hands as a form of cultural expression.

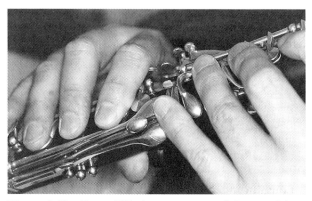

Figure 1.10 Free skilled movements of the musician, the fingers of each hand moving individually (courtesy of Ian Winspur, FRCS).

Sensory reception

Sensibility of the hand is the means by which cutaneous and proprioceptive stimuli are utilized:

- to achieve skilled motor function
- to protect from injury, for awareness of touch and for perception and testing of temperature etc.
- for recognition of objects by gnosis.

Sensory awareness, which we take for granted in our lives, is absolutely essential for normal hand function. It is almost always combined with movement, so any necessary sensory rehabilitation following nerve injury should be undertaken by active means. With specific training, a remarkable degree of sensory awareness can be achieved – for example, the ability to read Braille. If sensation does not recover adequately following a median nerve lesion, the patient is less likely to use the hand efficiently.

PERFORMANCE OF FUNCTIONAL MOVEMENT

In order to execute such a wide variety of movements, certain anatomical and physiological factors must be present. These include stability of the trunk and upper arm, which is necessary for the hand to be able to function at all, and mobility and stability of the hand itself. The hand must be able to change rapidly from a flat support to a dynamic arch, in which position it performs most of its numerous roles.

Frederic Chopin was well aware of the natural posture of the hand for the keyboard, its dexterity and its speed. He was particularly observant of the weakness of the fourth digit, and accordingly wrote his music to accommodate the strengths and weaknesses of the hand.

In the following pages some anatomical aspects affecting functional performance are mentioned which are of particular relevance to therapists. Detailed anatomy of bones, joints and ligaments, muscles, nerves and vascular supply can be found in the relevant anatomy textbooks, and in the numerous articles written by hand specialists (see References).

Arches

The arches play an important role during activity, as it is their adaptability that enables the hand to adjust to such a variety of situations. They can be flattened actively by extension movements, and passively by pressure or weight bearing on to the hand. The main arches are:

1. Longitudinal
2. Transverse
3. Oblique.

Longitudinal arch

The longitudinal arch extends from the proximal row of the carpal bones to the tips of the fingers and thumb (Figure 1.11). It is maintained largely by the tension between the long flexors and extensors of fingers and thumb, together with interaction of the intrinsic muscles.

Transverse arches

These are found proximally through the carpal bones, and distally through the heads of the metacarpals (Figure 1.11). The effect continues to the tips of fingers and thumb, which remain in an arched position even when the hand is relaxed. These transverse arches are maintained by the action of all the small muscles of the hand, and their paralysis produces an arch collapse with resulting deformity and disability. Movements of finger and thumb extension also have the effect of flattening the arches.

Oblique arches

These arise from the thumb when it is positioned in some degree of abduction and opposition, and extend into either the index or little fingers (Figure 1.12). They are maintained largely by the activity of thenar and hypothenar muscles, in conjunction with the extrinsic and intrinsic muscles of the fingers.

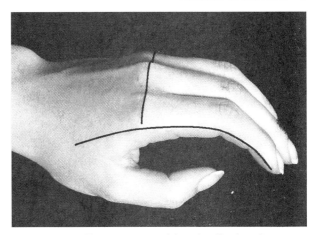

Figure 1.11 Transverse and longitudinal arches.

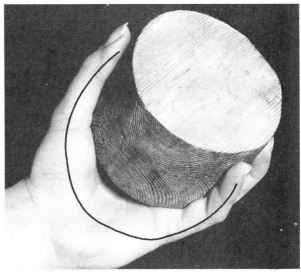

(a)

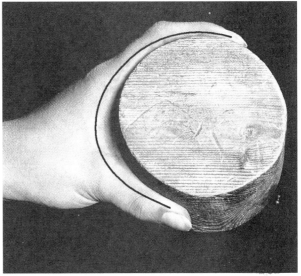

(b)

Figure 1.12 (a) and (b) Oblique arches.

Effect of muscle properties on the arches

When the fingers extend, they automatically abduct and the arches flatten. When the fingers flex, the muscle insertions, together with the transverse arch structure, cause the fingertips to converge towards one another (Figure 1.13). This enables a firm grasp around an object (Figure 1.14). The index finger can additionally rotate towards either the palm or the tip of the thumb (Figure 1.15).

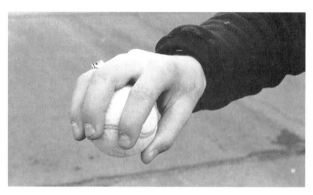

Figure 1.14 The arch formations allow a firm grasp to be made around the object.

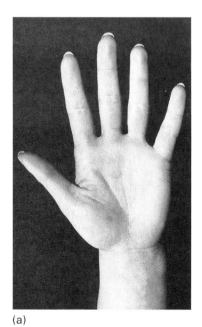

(a)

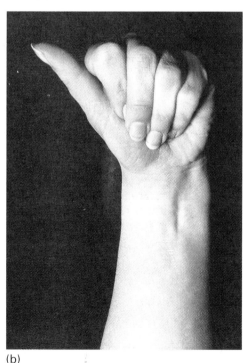

(b)

Figure 1.13 (a) Fingers abduct in extension (b) Tips converge in flexion.

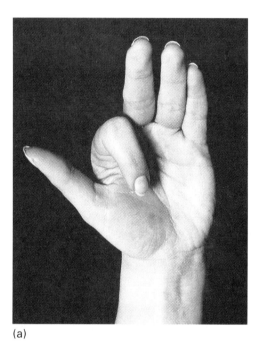

(a)

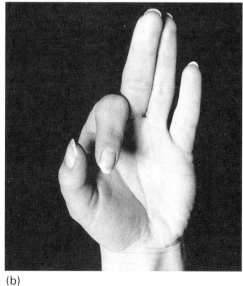

(b)

Figure 1.15 The index finger flexing: (a) towards the palm; (b) towards the thumb.

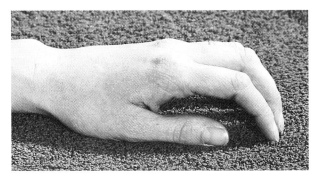

Figure 1.16 The hand in repose illustrates the arch formations always present in the normal hand.

Visco-elastic tension (or tone) causes the normal hand in repose to assume a position with the arches still present (Figure1.16). The wrist is usually slightly extended, the metacarpophangeal joints flexed at about 25°, the proximal interphalangeal joints at about 45° and the distal interphalangeal joints at 15°. The thumb lies anterior to the metacarpal and phalanges of the index finger. This is very similar to the position of function of the hand.

The tone of the long flexors of fingers and thumb is slightly stronger than that of the extensors, which ensures that a strong grasp is possible. A certain degree of finger flexion is therefore maintained at rest.

Clinical notes: It is extremely important to observe any alteration from this normal position of rest when assessing disorders following injury or operative procedure, as it will give clues to the diagnosis. It is also essential that all the arches should be maintained when exercising and splinting the hand, especially when the intrinsic muscles are paralysed.

Spirals of Fibonacci

In 1202 Fibonacci discovered a numerical sequence, each number being the sum of the preceding two numbers, corresponding also to an 'equiangular' spiral. This natural spiral is similar to the biological spirals found in snails, shells and flowers, and also in the flexion movements of the fingers. A finger describes an equiangular spiral during complex flexion (Tubiana, 1989). Littler (1973) observed that the length of metacarpals and phalanges of the same finger resemble the Fibonacci sequence.

JOINT MOVEMENT

The complexity of the movement of the hand and wrist is greatly affected by factors such as the shape of the surfaces of the joints and the position of the ligaments. The resulting close or loose packing of the joints is an issue of particular relevance to therapists.

A discussion of the arthrokinetics of the hand and wrist can be found in Chapter 6, together with indications of the techniques found useful in mobilizing stiff joints.

MUSCLE ACTIVITY

With the many articulations, and particularly the chain formation of the fingers, hand function requires a complex mechanism of muscle control. The combination of extrinsic and intrinsic muscle action enables the variety of movements to be achieved, with the usual interaction of prime mover, antagonist, synergist and fixator.

Broadly speaking, the long muscles produce gross finger movement whilst the small muscles provide power, further control and stability. This is illustrated in the slender hand of the artist or dancer compared with the squat and muscular hand of the labourer.

Flexion movements are the result of a simultaneous shortening contraction of the flexors with a lengthening contraction of the extensors. Extension movements occur when the procedure is reversed. Both must combine with intrinsic activity, however, if the movement is to be normal.

Greater knowledge has been gained from electromyographic studies, which have identified the co-ordinated muscle activity of the hand (Long, 1968; Landsmeer, 1976). A brief description of muscle action follows.

Free flexion at the interphalangeal joints
This is mainly performed by the flexor digitorum profundus (FDP). However, if no flexion is required at the distal interphalangeal joints the flexor digitorum superficialis (FDS) alone contracts, and it does this best with the wrist held in a small degree of flexion as seen in the hook grip (Figure 1.7). Superficialis activity is most pronounced in the index finger, and is sometimes absent or underdeveloped in the little finger.

Flexion followed by extension at the metacarpophalangeal joints with the interphalangeal joints held fully flexed
This is brought about by the long flexors and long extensors, and not by any intrinsic activity. The intrinsics, however, must be capable of being fully stretched to allow this movement to occur.

Interphalangeal joint extension with simultaneous metacarpophalangeal joint flexion
This is mainly performed by the interossei, and not the lumbricals as has been thought in the past. It provides powerful stability in the close-packed position, when necessary, putting ligamentous structures on a stretch.

Full finger flexion followed by full finger extension

This is produced by the long flexors and extensors of the fingers. However, without simultaneous involvement of the lumbricals there is a collapse of the multisegmental finger linkage (Landsmeer, 1963). During movements of extension, the strong visco-elastic property of the flexor digitorum profundus prevents the full extension of the fingers by the extensor digitorum communis (EDC), unless at the same time there is intervention of the lumbricals. This can be seen in the combined median and ulnar nerve lesions at wrist level with resulting clawing, otherwise known as the 'intrinsic minus' deformity (Figure 1.17), when 'rolling' flexion and extension occurs (see Chapter 7).

During normal extension movements it is the action of the lumbricals that slackens the tension of the flexor digitorum profundus distally, thereby allowing the interphalangeal joints to extend. During flexion movements the lumbricals help to keep the fingertips in a functional position away from the palm.

Clinical note: In high median and ulnar nerve lesions, with the FDP and FDS paralysed, the EDC is able to extend all the finger joints efficiently and without a claw deformity.

SKIN AND PAPILLARY RIDGES

The dermis and epidermis of the hand perform a variety of functions, providing:

- a suitable structure for sensory nerve endings and small capillaries
- an attachment for some tendinous insertions
- a tough waterproof and insulated layer for protection of the more delicate underlying tissues.

The papillary dermis of the palm of the hand (and also the sole of the foot) is specially and peculiarly adapted for friction and grip by the presence of papillary ridges. These ridges are arranged in parallel lines and in whorls; these are totally individual and form our fingerprints.

The papillary ridges are arranged differently in the various areas of the hand. They are usually at right angles to the line of friction, thus helping to provide non-slip grip. The crown of each ridge is dotted with sweat glands, and the presence of sweat on the skin surface increases adherence.

The ridges of the skin, together with the subcutaneous tissues, are compressible and conform to the undulations or shape of the object held or touched by the hand. This allows maximum skin contact under full pressure (as in hanging from overhead apparatus), and gives minimum skin contact under light pressure (as in soft sweeping movements). Pressure applied to the fingertips compresses the subcutaneous pulp and the pressure is thus transmitted to the nail bed, which has efficient sensory function.

NEUROMUSCULAR CONTROL

Besides the normal neurophysiological control, there are some specific factors relating to the hand.

Motor units

A great proportion of motor units are of a small innervation ratio with one cell innervating a few muscle fibres only, thus allowing precise movements to be learnt easily. This applies particularly in the small muscles of the hand.

There are mixed types of motor units in the longer muscles. For example, the flexor digitorum superficialis has both small units enabling skilled movements and the larger innervation ratio units, which ensure that the muscle has the stamina needed for the hook grip.

Proprioceptive feedback

This is highly efficient in the normal hand. The lumbricals are sometimes referred to as sensory muscles because they are particularly well supplied with annulospiral nerve endings. They enable specific information to be relayed back to the cortex, including:

- the altering relationship of structures such as muscles and tendons to one another
- the speed of movements.

This feedback assists especially in learning fast skilled movements, such as typing and playing musical instruments.

The plasticity of the nervous system is now recognized, whereby a large degree of adaptation and reorganization may occur if there is damage or

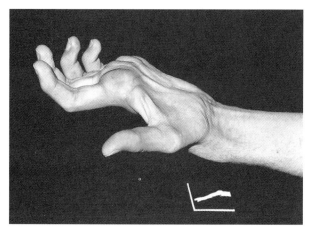

Figure 1.17 The 'intrinsic minus' deformity.

injury to either the central or the peripheral nervous system. This is of particular relevance to therapists, who by selection of appropriate techniques may influence the nervous system during rehabilitation.

SENSATION

Sensibility of the hand is a highly developed function in man, and depends on the ability of the cortex of the brain to interpret the impulses received from both cutaneous and proprioceptive sources. The representation on the sensory homunculus is therefore proportionately higher for the hand than for most other parts of the body.

Sensation must be adequate to enable efficient performance of tasks. Any sensory deficit will reduce performance; conversely, any early difficulty in motor performance is likely to reduce the development of full sensibility. In fact, sensation cannot be divorced from movement. It is therefore essential that assessment and treatment of sensory problems are always considered together with function.

Sensory functions

The main sensory functions are:

1. Sensory feedback from all receptors, which is essential for ensuring a highly skilled and smooth performance of movement; of particular note in the hand is the feedback from the lumbricals
2. Gnosis, or the recognition of objects, combined with palpation and manipulation
3. Protection, which results from excitation of receptors by noxious stimuli
4. Orientation in space.

Sensory modalities

Sensory stimuli are initiated as a result of excitation of sensory nerve endings, and their source may be:

- exteroceptive, which includes the skin, ears, eyes and other internal organs
- proprioceptive, from joint capsules, muscle spindles and Golgi tendon organs.

Cutaneous modalities

The skin of the hand has a particularly prolific supply of sensory nerve endings which act as receptors. Their innervation density increases distally, and especially so on the maximal contact surfaces of the index and middle fingers and the thumb. The brain receives and interprets any differences between the impulses generated by these specific receptors. Anomalies of the cutaneous distribution, especially the radial nerve, occur fairly frequently (Figure 1.18).

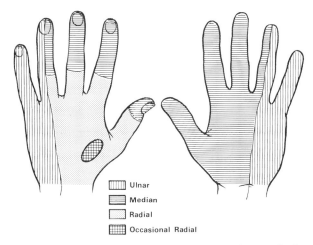

Ulnar
Median
Radial
Occasional Radial

Figure 1.18 Normal sensory distributions of the hand.

The elementary cutaneous modalities are:

- light touch, conveyed by the fast conducting A beta fibres
- pain, heat and cold, conveyed by the A delta fibres.

Pressure incorporates a combination of touch, stretching of skin, slight joint movement, and stretch of muscle fibres and Golgi tendon organs. It is therefore a complex form of judgement.

The vibration sense, tested as the ability to perceive 256 cps and 30 cps, can give a useful indication for commencement of re-education.

Two-point discrimination and localization are developed deductions that can only be made after some years of sensory experience. Both are incorporated together with the cutaneous modalities listed above.

Two-point discrimination is the ability to recognize whether the skin is being touched by one or by two points simultaneously, and is developed to a fine degree in the skin of the tips of the digits. Localization is the ability to recognize the exact position of a stimulus on the skin. Both these parameters are usually tested with moving touch for two reasons: first, the receptors quickly adapt to stationary touch (Dellon, 1984), making judgement more difficult, especially if regeneration has been poor following a nerve lesion; and secondly, more receptors will be stimulated by a moving touch (Marsh, 1990). It is now questioned whether there are receptors for each specific type of stimulus; however, it is considered that the receptors have varying thresholds of sensitivity to the different stimuli (Iggo, 1984). The discharges are then coded in patterns in the spinal cord and central nervous system, and the cortex has the ability to interpret the variations of sensory stimuli received according to factors such as:

- source
- frequency
- intensity
- duration.

Clinical tests can now be performed which are increasingly able to determine the degree to which the sensory nerves are affected and the degree and location of their recovery, and to give an estimate of their probable regeneration. However, results of clinical tests do not always mirror the ability of the patient, and it is essential that the role of assessment and treatment of sensory problems by therapists is considered to be for the functional benefit of the patient.

PSYCHOLOGICAL ASPECTS

The hand plays a very significant role in our normal lives, albeit for many people in a totally subconscious manner. Apart from the physical effects and functional loss that a hand injury may cause, the psychological wellbeing of the patient may also be affected. Serious consideration must be given to the possible adverse social and psychological effects of hand dysfunction, and this is discussed in greater depth in Chapter 3.

REFERENCES

Dellon, A. L. (1984). Touch sensibility in the hand. *J. Hand Surg.*, **9B,** 1.

Iggo, A. (1984). Cutaneous receptors and their sensory functions. *J. Bone Joint Surg.*, **50A,** 5.

Landsmeer, J. M. (1963). Co-ordination of finger-joint motions. J. Bone Joint Surg., **45A,** 1654–62.

Landsmeer, J. M. (1976). *Atlas of the Hand.* Churchill Livingstone.

Littler, J. W. (1973). On the adaptability of the hand. *Hand*, **5,** 187.

Long, C. (1968). Intrinsic–extrinsic muscle control of the fingers. *J. Bone Joint Surg.*, **50A,** 5.

Marsh, D. (1990). The validation of measures of outcome following suture of divided peripheral nerves supplying the hand. *J. Hand Surg.*, **15B,** 25–34.

Minett, P. (1985). *Child Care and Development.* John Murray.

Reynolds, V. (1987). *A Practical Guide to Child Development. Volume 1. The Child.* Stanley Thornes.

Tubiana, R., Thomine, J-M. and Mackin, E. (1989). *Examination of the Hand and Upper Limb.* W.B. Saunders.

Wynn Parry, C. B. (1981). *Rehabilitation of the Hand*, Ch1. Butterworths.

FURTHER READING

Boscheinen-Morrin, J., Davey, V. and Conolly, W. B. (1992). *The Hand: Fundamentals of Therapy.* Butterworth-Heinemann.

Brand, P. and Hollister, A. (1992). *Clinical Mechanics of the Hand.* Mosby Year Book.

Greenspan, J. and Bolanowski, S. (1996). The psychophysics of tactile perception and its physiological basis. In: *Pain and Touch* (L. Kruger, ed.). San Diego Academic Press.

Henderson, A. and Pehoski, C. (eds) (1995). Hand function in the child – foundations for remediation. In: *Development of Hand Skills, Grasp, Release and Bi-manual skills* (Henderson and Pehoski, eds), Ch. 7. C. V. Mosby Co.

Horton, M. E. (1971). The development of movement in young children. *Physiotherapy,* **57,** 155–8.

Kapandji, I. J. (1982). *The Physiology of Joints, Vol. 1: Upper Limb.* Churchill Livingstone.

Katz, D. (1989). *The World of Touch.* Hillsdale, Lawrence Erlbaum Associates.

Kidd, G., Musa, I. and Lawes, N. (1992). *Understanding Neuromuscular Plasticity.* Churchill Livingstone.

Landsmeer, J. M. (1962). Power and precision handling. *Ann. Rheum. Dis.*, **21,** 164–70.

Lister, G. (1993) *The Hand: Diagnosis and Indications*, 3rd edn. Churchill Livingstone.

MacConnaill, M. A. (1964). Joint movement. *Physiotherapy,* **50,** 11.

Merzenich, M. M. and Jenkins, W. M. (1993). Reorganization of cortical representations of the hand following alterations of skin inputs induced by nerve injury, skin island transfers and experience. *J. Hand Ther.*, **6,** 89.

Moberg, E.(1958). Objective methods for determining the functional value of sensitivity in the hand. *J. Bone Joint Surg.*, **40B(3),** 454–76.

Napier, J. (1956). Prehensile movements of the human hand. *J. Anat.*, **89,** 564.

Stevens, J. and Green, B. (1996). History of research on touch. In: *Pain and Touch* (L. Kruger, ed.). San Diego Academic Press.

Tubiana, R. (1989). *Examination of the Hand and Upper Limb.* W. B. Saunders

Tubiana, R. Thomine, J. M. and Mackin, E. J. (1996). *Examination of the Hand and Wrist.* Martin Dunitz.

Voss, D. E., Ionta, M. K. and Myers, B. J. (1985). *Proprioceptive Muscular Facilitation.* Harper & Row.

Williams, P. L. and Warwick, R. (eds) (1989). *Gray's Anatomy.* Churchill Livingstone.

Winspur, I. and Wynn Parry, C. B. (1998). *The Musician's Hand. A Clinical Guide.* Martin Dunitz.

Wynn Parry, C. B. (1981). *Rehabilitation of the Hand.* Butterworths.

2 Assessment

Carole Bexon and Maureen Salter

INTRODUCTION

Loss of function in the hand following injury, surgery and other disorders may result from a wide variety of factors. Immobilization itself can lead to stiffening of the numerous small joints, with adjacent structures becoming contracted and adherent and tissues fibrotic. Two patients with similar diagnoses or apparently identical injuries may have widely differing complications. A thorough initial examination by the hand therapist is therefore essential in order to identify those problems.

An assessment is made by:

- listening to the patient
- observing the hand and its movements
- taking and recording measurements.

AIMS OF ASSESSMENT

The therapist must:

1. Decide on the priorities for treatment in order to devise an appropriate individual programme
2. Monitor progress
3. Retain meticulous records in case of possible litigation.

Reassessment should be either weekly or at suitable intervals, to record progress and enable any changes or additions to be made to the treatment programme.

Close collaboration between the occupational therapist and physiotherapist is desirable, with common methods, systems and tools being used for the assessment. Ideally only one therapist need complete the assessment, saving time for both staff and patient and excluding the possibility of different therapists producing different measurements, which would be confusing for the patient. However, a commonly agreed practice is for each therapist to carry out the different aspects of the assessment, e.g. the physiotherapist measuring range of movement and muscle activity, and the occupational therapist assessing function. By ensuring that there is little or no duplication, the two therapists can share the workload. New staff members joining the team are taught to complete the hand assessments in the agreed manner.

Rehabilitation team

The rehabilitation team comprises:

- a surgeon (and/or physician)
- an occupational therapist
- a physiotherapist
- a nurse
- a social worker
- a clinical psychologist (when required).

Assessments by these team members will identify the patient's current problems, and discussions amongst the whole team are then crucial for a thorough understanding and effective management of the injury or condition.

The assessment and advice of a clinical psychologist can be of great benefit, providing an important insight into patients' attitudes to their problems and suggesting the most suitable approach for each member of the therapy team (see Chapter 3).

Patients need to understand as much as possible about the mechanics of the hand, the effects of the injury, the treatment planned and the support available. They can then become fully involved in their own rehabilitation. Co-operation is essential if a satisfactory outcome is to be achieved. A client-centred approach is to be encouraged, giving patients greater control, dignity and confidence (see Chapter 3).

This chapter gives a general outline of hand assessment. Each case is evaluated and recorded on an individual basis because there are so many variations of hand injury. Not all aspects of assessment will necessarily need to be carried out; only those relevant to the problems that become evident at the initial interview and examination. For example, normal sensation need not be assessed in a patient with no nerve lesion. However, all details should be checked during the initial interview, since the unexpected can frequently arise – for example, a patient who suffered no direct nerve damage during an accident may have median nerve compression caused by oedema.

STANDARDIZATION OF MEASURING AND RECORDING

A choice of measurement techniques and methods is available for the different aspects of hand assessment, the most suitable being selected by the therapist. Standardization of measuring and recording must be agreed and implemented by the therapy team, thereby ensuring a meaningful indicator of progress by allowing comparison and analysis of results. This is essential if any research or clinical audit is being carried out. Meticulous record keeping is also necessary in case of litigation following injury or treatment.

Variables should be eliminated where possible – for example, a standard positioning of the arm should be adopted during assessment. The following factors are prerequisites for standardization of measurements:

1. The assessment must always be performed at the same time of day and early morning is most appropriate if treatment is to follow; however, this may not be a suitable time for the patient with rheumatoid arthritis, who may experience increased pain and stiffness in the mornings (see Chapter 11)
2. The position of the patient must be identical for each measurement
3. The room must be at a comfortable temperature and the patient given long enough for the hand to warm up, especially if coming in from a cold environment
4. The assessor must be the same for each given patient because there will always be a slight discrepancy between therapists' measurements, even though the methods used appear to be the same; if research is being undertaken, the assessor must be independent of the research team
5. Medication must be taken into account, as this can affect the measurements – for example, the introduction of analgesics may improve power grip
6. Calibrated equipment, preferably with normative data established, should be used whenever possible to ensure consistency of readings and their interpretation.

Standardization of records is desirable nationwide and internationally, but is an absolute essential for individual therapy departments and throughout any hospital. Preprinted forms should be designed to meet all aspects of assessment, but should be kept as simple as possible because no single form can cover all types of problem; assessment sheets applicable to the patient's problems can then be selected by the therapist. Desktop publishing now makes it easier to produce assessments that are neat, accurate and professional in appearance. Problem-orientated medical records can provide uniformity and reduce the amount of necessary paperwork.

Results should be presented in a visual format where possible, so that the information can be clearly and quickly understood by the patient and the members of the team. The following points are worth noting:

1. Clarity of charts can be helped by colour coding each assessment diagram in a predetermined sequence, e.g. black (first assessment), blue (second assessment), then red, green, brown, purple and so on
2. A diagram from a computer (Figure 2.1), a commercially produced stamp or a print taken by drawing round the patient's injured or (if necessary) uninjured hand can be used for a

variety of assessment purposes, e.g. recording deformities, amputations and scars
3. Deformities that are three-dimensional and difficult to measure and describe accurately may be recorded on to the handprint, e.g. ulnar deviation of the metacarpophalangeal joints of patients with rheumatoid arthritis
4. Flow charts can be used to record individual measurements (e.g. joint range); the required measurements are listed in a column, with the dates along the top of the sheet and the weekly recordings entered under the appropriate date, thus allowing the progress of each component to be read easily along the row
5. Graphs may also be used to indicate progress of power, daily living activities, etc.

Graphs and forms are automatically printed out during electronic measurement when using computerized measuring programmes.

The terminology used throughout the assessment should be standardized, and the following abbreviations used for joints:

- carpometacarpal – CMC
- metacarpophalangeal – MCP
- interphalangeal – IP
- proximal interphalangeal – PIP
- distal interphalangeal – DIP.

Photography is a useful method of recording, and is very valuable for teaching purposes, for providing case study material and as visual evidence in cases of litigation. The results, however, are not instantly available and are costly, so it is not practical on a day-to-day basis.

Video is also an excellent means of recording, and can fit very practically into the therapy department routine, giving the patient immediate visual feedback. The information can be stored permanently if required for future reference, and can be used for teaching and staff education. Camcorders and

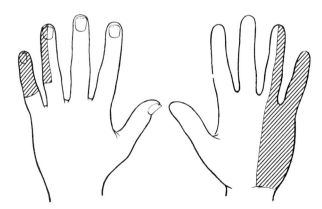

Figure 2.1 A commercial hand stamp or computer print provides a means for recording scars, altered sensation and areas of pain.

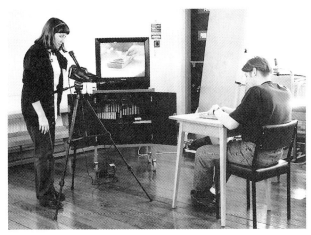

Figure 2.2 A video recorder provides an excellent method to record the state and movements of the hand following injury.

videos are now likely to be familiar to both the patient and the therapist, and ideally all therapists with direct patient care should have easy access to this equipment for both assessment and treatment purposes (Figure 2.2). It is surprising how quickly patient and therapist can forget both the severity of the original injury and its effect on function unless it is visually recorded. Trick movements in particular, which are difficult to describe and record, can be demonstrated effectively when using this equipment.

Problem-orientated medical records (POMR)

These records, which are part of the Problem-Orientated Systems introduced by Dr Weed in 1968 (Bromley, 1978), have provided the means by which medical communication, education and research may be improved. By standardizing documentation it is simpler to carry out concurrent and even retrospective clinical audits for both quality assessment and technique evaluation. Documents that relate to problems only are more precise, more compact and therefore more suitable for standard records.

Ideally, POMR should be used by the whole multidisciplinary team, with each discipline adding its own material. POMR documents can, however, be used effectively by just the therapy department (Richardson, 1979). They provide a system of documentation that is thorough and accurate and also simplifies the transfer of the patient's care from one member of staff to another, because the problems requiring attention are clearly identified.

The four main headings for recording information are database, problem list, plan and progress notes.

Database
This should include patient's:

- name
- sex
- age
- occupation
- employment
- social history
- leisure interests.

It should also give details of:

- the diagnosis
- clinical and/or surgical procedures
- hand dominance (left or right)
- the results of the initial assessment.

Assessment sheets should be filed as part of the database section. Major changes, decisions or actions during treatment should be recorded in the database in chronological order.

Problem list
This numbered list comprises all the identified problems needing therapy or any other treatment and assistance. It might include:

- stiff joints
- functional problems, e.g. eating difficulties
- financial/social concerns.

The date on which each of these problems is resolved is recorded, otherwise problems are considered to be active.

Table 2.1 shows the problem list for a 24-year-old plumber who, on 18 July, lacerated his right (dominant) hand at the wrist, dividing the median nerve, palmaris longus and flexor digitorum superficialis to all fingers. He retained acitivity in the thenar muscles. The structures were repaired and he was immobilized in Kleinert traction, commencing active rehabilitation at 6 weeks (1 September) and returning to work after 18 days of treatment (18 September). He later attended follow-up by the surgeon and therapist (see also Tables 2.8, 2.9).

Plans
This section states the team's long-term aim for the patient, preferably indicating an expected time-scale for its achievement. Short-term plans based on the identified, numbered problems list are drawn up by each therapist treating the patient. The short-term plans outline the detailed management of and therapeutic intervention for each problem, and these plans are explained to, discussed and agreed with the patient.

Progress notes
These are also related to the numbered problem list. They may be recorded diagrammatically as flow charts, with progress plotted weekly, or recorded in

TABLE 2.1
PROBLEM LIST FOR A 24-YEAR-OLD PLUMBER WHO LACERATED HIS RIGHT DOMINANT HAND AT THE WRIST

Date	No.	Problem list	Inactive	Initial
20.07	1.	Oedema	04.09	
	2.	Loss of active ROM – fingers, right hand	01.09	
	3.	Altered sensation		
	4.	Repair requires protection	01.09	
01.09	2.	Lack of complete pull through of flexor tendons	18.09	
	5.	Scar	18.09	
	6.	Loss of strength		
	7.	Function/employment	18.09	

narrative format, either daily or weekly, in the form of SOAP notes:

● S (subjective information) – includes the patient's own account of topics, e.g. improvement of function and reduction of pain
● O (objective information) – includes facts, e.g. results from repeat hand assessments and activities that the patient has performed in therapy sessions
● A (analysis of the present situation and the cause of residual problems)
● P (plan of future treatment) – includes the immediate programme of treatment.

Major plans should be recorded in the plans section rather than the progress notes.

Final discharge summary
This final summary is an essential part of the database, and summarizes the patient's condition on discharge from therapy treatment. It refers back to the problem list, with a record of those problems that have been resolved and any that remain. It should be substantiated by the final hand assessment, which should then be summarized in the database. The final summary should:

● give an account of the ongoing problems
● outline a plan for each problem
● estimate the prognosis.

The therapist should be able to justify why a patient is being discharged with unresolved problems. Any plans and dates for follow-up appointments should be noted.

REFERRAL

The referral from the surgeon or physician should include the following:

1. A diagnosis
2. A brief history of the injury and surgery
3. Reports on relevant investigations, e.g. X-rays
4. The date and the signature of the referring doctor.

The full medical and surgical notes and any X-rays should be available for the therapist to read in detail.

GENERAL OBSERVATION

A recently injured or post-operative patient who requires therapy may still be in bed with the hand elevated or may be ambulant and able to attend the rehabilitation department. The first general observations can be made when the patient is in the ward, or when attending the department. They include:

1. The general posture of hand and arm (Figure 2.3)
2. The patient's attitude, whether cheerful or depressed
3. The use or protection of the hand, when applicable.

The therapist should observe the patient undertaking normal routine daily activities such as dressing or pulling out a chair. In this way, impressions may be formed regarding both the severity of the injury and the patient's attempt to

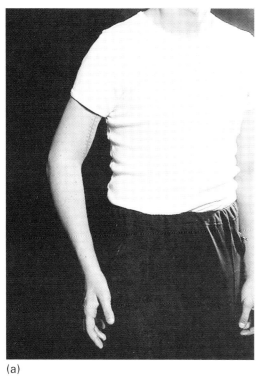
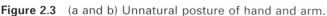
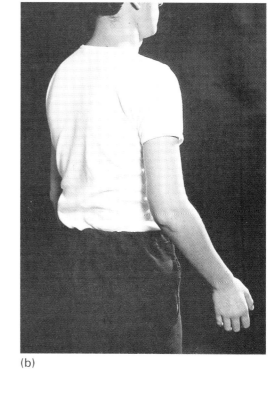

(a)   (b)

Figure 2.3   (a and b) Unnatural posture of hand and arm.

cope with the disability. These observations can give an indication of the patient's probable motivation and therefore help the therapist to decide on the initial treatment.

HISTORY

Information obtained from the patient is mainly subjective, and should include:

1. How, when and where the injury occurred and any background cause or contributing factor; also whether the patient's injury is to the dominant or non-dominant hand. The therapist estimates whether the history is consistent with the injury sustained. Hand injury is not uncommonly associated with other problems such as alcohol, drug abuse, social problems, violence or possible criminal activity, and these may all have a bearing on the rehabilitation needs of the patient. The true cause of the injury may not always become clear until the rehabilitation phase is underway.
2. Details of first aid, surgery and other treatment given.
3. Problems and difficulties as viewed by the patient. Noting their order can be useful at this stage; pain may be mentioned high on the list and it is important for the therapist to know the severity of this problem because it needs speedy assessment and treatment (see Chapter 7). Careful physical handling of the painful limb is very

important. For many hand trauma patients pain may be a significant problem for a few days only; however, chronic pain is likely to be a major feature for patients with rheumatoid arthritis and can be constant, severe and intractable. Pain may also be related to a pre-existing condition. It can be assessed using an analogue scale (see Chapter 4).

4. The patient's employment or occupation, particularly in relation to the hand skills needed (e.g. loads to be lifted), and whether the patient is self-employed or an employee. If applicable, the name and address of the employer should also be recorded. If the accident happened at work, it is important to discover whether the Health and Safety Executive (HSE) has been called in to inspect the workplace, and whether a compensation case is likely, with legal and/or union involvement. Company policy on paid sick leave and compensation should also be established.
5. Hobbies and leisure interests, along with an indication of their level of importance to the patient and the degree of skill required.
6. The social situation. Problems must be identified and solved quickly, as they may distract the patient during treatment – e.g. financial hardship through loss of earnings, or care of dependants such as young children or elderly relatives.
7. The patient's expectations and understanding of the extent of injury or operation, the time necessary for recovery and the probable outcome.

Is the patient satisfied so far, and are his priorities the same as the therapist's?

8. Psychological factors, such as worry about recovery or distress over cosmetic appearance. There may be signs of post-traumatic stress disorder, such as flashbacks and nightmares (see also Chapter 3).

In most cases, the patient history provides all the background information required by the therapist. However, there may be other factors that could affect the patient's attitude and response to treatment, such as criminal proceedings or compensation claims. These may not be immediately apparent.

EXAMINATION

Both patient and therapist should be comfortable during the examination. Good, even lighting is essential, and the patient must be in a position to observe what is happening.

If in bed the patient's hand and arm should be supported on two or three pillows, and if ambulant the patient should sit at a table resting the arm on a pillow or towel. The table must be large enough to support the whole length of the forearm, but small enough so that the therapist can examine the hand without having to reach forward. The chair should be of comfortable height so that hips and knees are at right angles and the feet flat on the floor. If the patient is in a wheelchair, a table with adequate adjustment should be used. The therapist sits next to the patient's injured side.

Observation

Both the patient's hands are rested on the pillow and the affected hand is compared with the normal one (Figure 2.4); the following objective information is then noted and recorded.

Wounds and scars

These may result from the original injury, incisions or skin grafting. Contractures may result because of the scar position and direction. The features can be recorded on an outline print of the hand, and the state of healing should be noted, including:

- whether the wounds are open or closed
- whether sutures have been removed
- any infected areas
- the presence of scar tissue, i.e. the colour and texture, flat or raised, dry or scaly.

Adhesion of scars to underlying tissues such as tendons should be noted, as this can prevent full movement and produce secondary deformity and possible joint stiffness. The adhesions can be seen moving proximally and/or distally on movement.

Oedema

The whole or part of the hand may be affected, and oedema may extend into the forearm (see also Measurements section).

Alterations in size

Following severe injury the affected hand may be enlarged in the early stages due to oedema, or smaller in the later stages due to muscle wasting and loss of subcutaneous tissue, e.g. fingertip bulk (Figure 2.4).

Muscle wasting

Wasting may be noticeable in the:

- forearm
- thenar eminence
- hypothenar eminence
- dorsal and volar interosseous spaces (Figure 2.5)
- thumb web space (Figure 2.5).

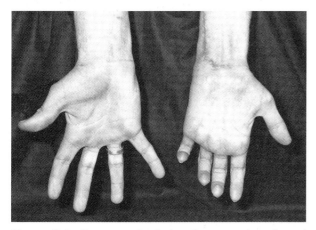

Figure 2.4 Compare both hands: note the altered position of the thumb, the flexed and adducted index, middle and ring fingers, and loss of pulp on the affected side.

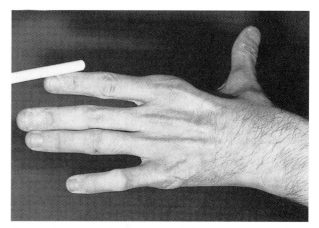

Figure 2.5 Wasting of dorsal interosseous spaces and thumb web space.

Deformity
This may be due to:

- skeletal damage
- an imbalance of muscles
- adherence and contracture of scars
- circulatory damage
- a nerve lesion.

The following sites are observed for specific problems:

- scars – finger movements produce drag on adherent scars
- arches – the arches of the hand may be flattened or reversed
- thumb – this may be positioned flattened alongside the index finger or contracted across the palm
- fingers – the position of the fingers may be abnormal, e.g.
  - a flexion deformity with MCP and IP joints held in more flexion than normal (Figure 2.6)
  - an extension deformity of MCP or IP joints with loss of usual flexor tone in the fingers (see Figures 2.3a, 2.3b)
  - an intrinsic minus or claw hand deformity with MCP joints extended and IP joints flexed (Figure 2.7)
  - an intrinsic plus deformity, with the MCP joints held in flexion and the IP joints extended – there are varying degrees of this deformity, but when it is severe it is usually accompanied by some swan-necking of the fingers with prominence of the bases of the middle phalanges (Figure 2.8)
  - a swan-neck deformity, with the PIP joint in hyperextension and the DIP in some degree of flexion (Figures 2.8 and 2.9)
  - a Boutonnière deformity with the PIP joint flexed and the DIP joint hyperextended (Figure 2.9)
  - a mallet finger deformity with loss of active extension at the DIP joint (Figure 2.10).

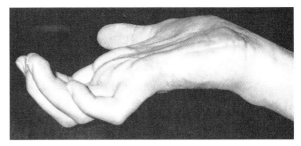

Figure 2.7 Intrinsic minus or claw deformity of a median and ulnar nerve lesion. Note flattening of arches and thenar eminence.

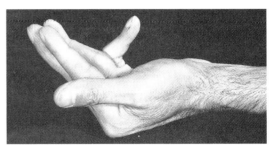

Figure 2.8 Severe intrinsic plus contracture illustrating inability to extend MCP joints. Note some swan-necking of the ring finger in an attempt at extension. The little finger has been affected by a higher Volkmann's ischaemic contracture.

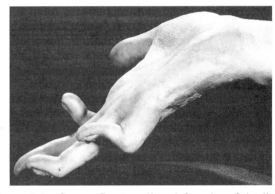

Figure 2.9 Severe Boutonnière deformity of the little finger caused by extensor–expansion damage from burns and a swan-neck deformity of the ring finger.

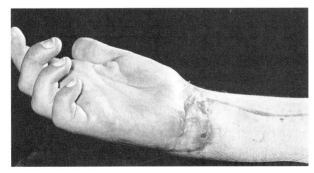

Figure 2.6 Middle, ring and little fingers are held flexed by adhesions at the wrist. Index finger is in normal posture.

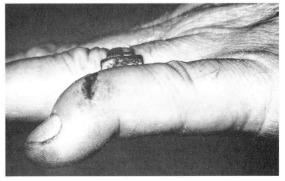

Figure 2.10 Mallet finger deformity with loss of active DIP joint extension.

Condition of skin and nails

Autonomic and nutritional changes in the hand should be noted, as they may follow a peripheral nerve or nerve root pattern. These may include:

- changes in colour, e.g. pinky-purple with mottling (Figure 2.11)
- absent or excessive sweating
- dry and scaly skin surface (Figure 2.12)
- paper-thin and shiny skin texture (Figure 2.13).
- the presence of trophic lesions or burns (Figure 2.14)
- deformed hairs due to follicle changes, or excessive hair growth
- ridged and brittle nails.

These changes can be recorded on a hand outline. X-rays are examined for signs of developing osteoporosis, which is probable after some weeks of disuse of the hand. Patients with complex regional pain syndrome are also likely to show signs of osteoporosis.

Palpation

The therapist assesses, by light touch, the sympathetic changes of the patient's injured hand. Deeper palpation will enable any changes in the underlying tissues to be detected. The area of change may follow a peripheral or nerve root pattern if these structures have been damaged, with the same area affected as in earlier observations (see above). The therapist looks for the following signs.

Skin temperature

The hand may be:

- cool due to poor circulation, which can be caused by injury or a disorder such as Raynaud's disease or complex regional pain syndrome
- cool or warm according to the surroundings
- cold, dusky blue in colour and painful; this is due to cold intolerance and is a common complication following hand injury (particularly when nerve damage has occurred), and patients should be advised of this complication and taught how to manage it (see Chapter 5)
- warmer than normal due to inflammatory or infectious processes.

Sweating

Sweating may be assessed by stroking the skin using the dorsum of the fingers or the shaft of a pen and noting whether the surface of the skin is sticky

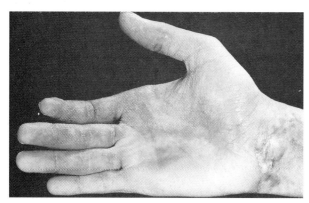

Figure 2.11 Change of skin colour with mottling.

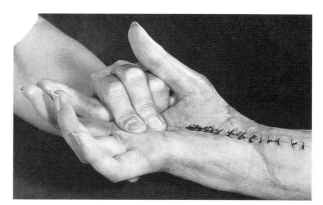

Figure 2.13 Skin may be papery thin and shiny.

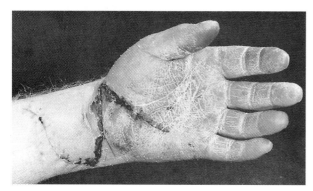

Figure 2.12 Skin surface may become very dry and scaly.

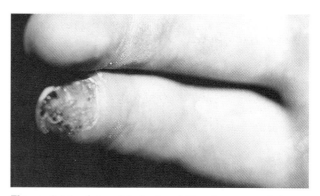

Figure 2.14 A trophic lesion following nerve injury.

or not. Dry and flaky skin following immobilization in a splint may limit the accuracy of this assessment. Loss of sweating is a feature of nerve damage, and increased sweating may occur as a result of anxiety or be one of the signs of complex regional pain syndrome.

Pain

During palpation, particularly sensitive areas will be identified by the painful response of the patient. Pain can be expected following injury or surgery, but this normally resolves within a few days. Following lengthy immobilization or non-use of the hand, pain may become chronic. A patient with complex regional pain syndrome will experience pain that may be acute. Severe intractable pain, when the patient flinches from a touch, may occur following brachial plexus lesions and peripheral nerve damage. It may be preferable to leave palpation until the end of the examination if severe pain is expected. For details on assessment of pain see Chapter 4.

Skin condition

The skin texture may be dry and scaly or very shiny. The skin may become thin and very fragile, and be prone to damage.

Scars, adhesions and the hard induration of tissues

These can be palpated with the fingertips. Depending on the stage of injury or recovery, the adhesions should be palpated on both active and passive movement for signs of scar adherence to the underlying tendons, as this can lead to loss of full movement (see also Observation section). They are recorded descriptively as to size or length, colour, degree of depth or prominence above surface, and whether adherent to other tissues.

Tissue elasticity

Loss of elasticity results in a 'woody' feel to the tissues, which lose their normal flexibility and ability to glide. Active synovitis in the hand, the tissues around joints and the flexor tendon sheaths (particularly in the palm) may feel spongy and 'boggy'. In the swollen hand, oedema causes taut skin which, when pressed, leaves a depression that is slow to disappear.

TYPES OF MEASUREMENT

Assessments made by therapists are either functional or clinical, and both are necessary for good patient management.

Functional measurements

Patients may initially find it impossible to perform functional tests, but the tests are carried out by the therapist as soon as is practicable. Some of the difficulties will already have been noted during the history taking. The therapist must consider the main functional problems carefully, since they will influence the treatment programme. For example, emphasis is placed on increasing the range of any joint identified as limiting functional performance. It is essential that all findings are utilized.

Clinical measurement

Objective clinical measurements are taken as soon as possible after surgery in order to establish a baseline and monitor progress.

Oedema

Oedema, which can be severe following trauma or infection, may:

- effectively splint the hand, making it impossible to flex the fingers
- be a major cause of pain
- possibly cause nerve damage, due to the increased pressure in the carpal tunnel and other compartments
- be followed by fibrosis, with loss of suppleness of soft tissues and flattening of the arches resulting in a stiff, non-functional hand.

It is essential to reduce any oedema in the hand as soon as possible, and therefore it is important to monitor its reduction. A variety of techniques may be used. Hand volume varies depending on the time of day and the recent posture of the hand, and measurements taken early in the morning will minimize the effects of postural variations. They should be taken over a number of days so that a trend can be identified. The techniques include:

1. Circumferential measurement using a tape measure or expanding loop. This is placed around individual fingers at the level of the interphalangeal joints, using ballpoint pen dots marked on the skin to ensure the same site of measurement daily. The palm can be measured in a similar way.
2. Maximum diameter measurement using ring measures and gauges. This method was designed for use with rheumatoid joints, and is the easiest and most reliable method for measuring oedema of the fingers at the level of the PIP joints. The ring measure (Figure 2.15) uses a 0–10 scale (jewellers' ring gauges record on an alphabetic scale). Caution should be taken when measuring patients in the early stages of recovery, particularly those with unhealed tendons; always start with the largest ring measure and work downwards, stopping at the ring size at which any resistance is met.
3. Volume measurement through water displacement. The whole hand is placed in a container already filled with water up to the overflow, and

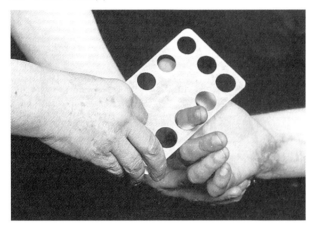

Figure 2.15 Measurement of oedema at the level of the PIP joints using the 0–10 scale of the ring measure.

a support inside the container ensures the identical position of the hand for each measurement. The amount of water that then overflows into a container can be measured accurately. This is not a suitable method if open wounds are still present.

The volume tank (or volumeter) is an accurate piece of equipment when used by the same examiner (Waylett-Rendall and Seibly, 1991). For optimum results it is necessary to ensure that the patient is always measured by the same therapist, and that both hands are measured on each occasion. Hand volume is constantly changing, and therefore measurement of the injured hand volume alone is meaningless.

Van Velze *et al*. (1991) found that only one test was necessary for an accurate measurement. They also determined the difference in volume between normal dominant and non-dominant hands; on average the non-dominant is about 3.4 per cent smaller than the dominant hand. Graphs have been produced that give the predicted volume of one hand when the volume of the other is known, and this relative difference enables the hand therapist to predict the expected volume of the injured hand (prior to injury) from the known volume of the uninjured one. The therapist can then estimate how much oedema needs to be eliminated by subtracting this value from the actual volume of the injured hand.

RANGE OF MOVEMENT

Loss of active and passive movement may occur for a variety of reasons, including:

- joint stiffness as a result of lengthy immobilization
- intra-articular fractures
- joint dislocation
- angulation and rotation of a bone following fracture, leading to a mechanical disadvantage in tendon function

- skin contracture
- adhesions
- inhibition of movement because of pain
- muscle paralysis
- ischaemic contractures involving the long muscles of the forearm or small muscles of the hand
- tendon rupture.

Initially, a single movement of flexion and extension of the fingers followed by opposition of the thumb and little finger will give a quick impression of the problems and identify those measurements needed in more detail. All individual joint movements, the web spaces and the total excursion of fingers and thumb should be examined and recorded.

Individual joint measurements

The shoulder and elbow joints should be checked for full movement and compared to those on the uninjured side, and measurements recorded where necessary. Active, passive and accessory ranges of movement are measured and recorded on charts for the wrist, fingers and thumb.

Active range
A goniometer is used over the dorsum of the fingers, and both flexion and extension are measured (Figure 2.16a). The resting position of the joint may also need to be recorded, for example when adhesions of tendons prevent normal movement. It is essential in deciding treatment strategies to know whether the attempted movement is different from the position of rest.

Finger goniometers are available commercially but a small protractor, modified by riveting a perspex pointer to the central pivot, makes a cheap and suitable alternative (Figure 2.16b). If the hand and fingers are swollen the goniometer should be placed on the line of the shafts of the bones, as measurements over the dorsum of the joints will vary with the oedema.

The individual joint range measurements are described by the American Academy of Orthopaedic Surgery (1974). Flexion and extension must be measured and recorded in order to identify both the specific treatment required and the actual changes that occur. Currently goniometry continues to provide the greatest reliability (Ellis and Bruton, 1998).

Passive range
The passive range of movement should be measured, and recorded if there is a disparity between passive and active ranges. Different coloured ink will help in comparing the two sets of measurements.

Accessory range
The motions of spin, glide and roll should be palpated as appropriate, and the ten movements of

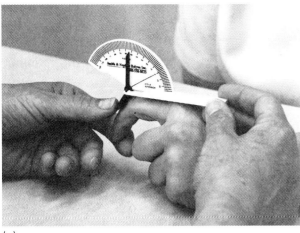

(a)

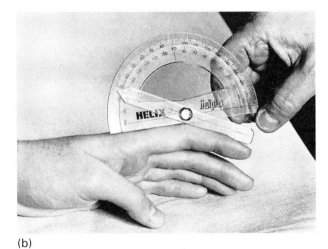

(b)

Figure 2.16 (a) A commercially available finger goniometer (note the facility to measure hyperextension of the MCP joints); (b) A plastic protractor makes a cheap but accurate goniometer.

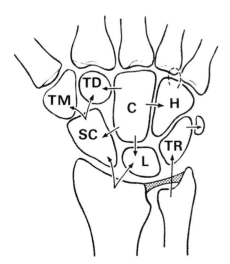

Figure 2.17 Kaltenborn's 10 movements of the wrist.

the wrist described by Kaltenborn (1980) provide a useful reference (Figure 2.17). A record should be made regarding whether accessory movement is full, limited or absent. Alternatively, it could be recorded on the Maitland scale of 0–4 (Maitland 1991; see also Chapter 6).

Total excursion measurements

Odstock wire tracing

Wire tracing is primarily a means of measurement of total excursion of the fingers and thumb, but it can be used to measure individual joint range as an alternative to the goniometer. It is especially useful in the measurement of painful and severely deformed hands, and both active and passive range can be recorded by a simple visual method of wire tracings. An Odstock wire consists of a 17.5 cm length of multicore solder (40/60 tin lead 16 swg) covered with a flexible plastic or rubber sheath such as catheter tubing. The combination of malleable solder and flexible tube allows accurate contouring of the finger without undue pressure. Spring wire is not suitable. The methods for both fingers and thumb are given below.

Fingers

1. Place the wire along the dorsum of the extended finger, with the tip of the wire at the tip of the finger.
2. Gently adjust the shape of the wire until it exactly matches the contour of the finger (Figure 2.18a). If the finger is painful to touch, bend the wire without making skin contact, then place it on the finger and check for accuracy. Repeat this procedure until the correct contour is achieved.
3. Place the wire horizontally on to a piece of paper, ensuring that the MCP joint is to the left of the PIP joint. Carefully trace the underside using a solid line; this indicates extension (Figure 2.18b).
4. Mark the MCP, PIP and DIP joints with a dash and label them.
5. Repeat the steps (1) and (2) above, but with the finger in flexion.
6. Superimpose the wire onto the extension wire tracing using the MCP–PIP line as a baseline (the apparent lengthening of this line is due to the shape of the joints); the centres of the two MCP–PIP lines should be made to coincide. Using dotted lines to indicate flexion, trace the underside of the wire except for the MCP–PIP baseline. Using the proximal phalanx as a baseline allows changes at both the MCP and PIP joint to be seen clearly, and subsequent tracings can be superimposed in different colours. All the fingers from one hand can be represented on one side of A4 paper, and the thumb will require a separate sheet of paper.

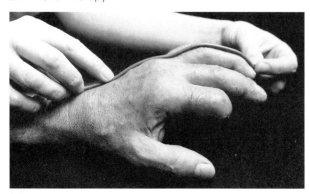

(a)

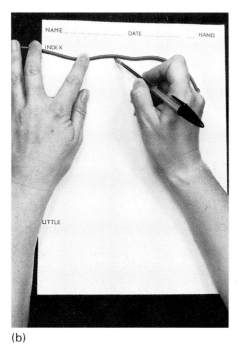

(b)

Figure 2.18 The Odstock wire measurement. (a) The wire is adjusted to the contour of the finger. (b) The outline is traced onto the paper, superimposing it onto any existing outline.

Thumb Measuring flexion and extension of the thumb using Odstock wire tracings is more difficult because there is no simple baseline. The tracings are best recorded on to a handprint as follows:

1. Place the patient's hand on a sheet of paper, ensuring that there is enough room for the extended thumb and checking that forearm, third metacarpal and middle finger are all in a straight line.
2. Keeping these points static, ask the patient to extend the thumb. Draw round the hand, ensuring that the position of the finger webs is noted. This records the thumb extension and marks the reference points needed to record thumb flexion.

3. Remove the patient's hand from the paper and position in supination, asking the patient to flex the thumb as far as possible into the palm.
4. Use the Odstock wire to trace along the dorsum of the thumb and the side of the radius over the CMC joint. The tip of the wire should be on the tip of the thumb. The therapist must note accurately the point to which the thumb flexes in the palm in relation to the fingers, the web spaces and the distal palmar crease. This point and the CMC joint are the two reference points used to record thumb flexion.
5. Hold the wire at the level of the CMC joint and transfer it on to the handprint, positioning the thumb end of the wire at the reference point identified in the palm. Trace along the underside of the wire, using a dotted line to indicate flexion. Subsequent readings can be superimposed in different colours as for finger wire tracings. The therapist must be very careful to make accurate observations and recordings, because this method is open to error.

Ruler measurements
Each individual joint may be fully mobile, but total excursion of thumb and fingers from full flexion to full extension may be limited by weakness or restriction of the soft tissues. A ruler or tape that starts at zero can be used to measure the following:

1. The distance from the fingertips to the distal palmar crease with the fingers in flexion, and a further measurement in extension (Figure 2.19a). The wrist crease or a scar may provide a more suitable line for measurements in the early stages when movement is severely restricted. These reference points of measurement must be clearly noted.
2. The distance of each fingertip from the tabletop when the hand is resting on the table with the palm uppermost, i.e. extension deficit (Figure 2.20). It is not possible to measure a gross flexion deformity by this method.
3. The distance of the tip of the thumb from the tip of each finger and from the base of the little finger. Pulp-to-pulp pinch should be recorded as achieved (tick) or as a deficit (e.g. minus x mm). Contact achieved only by using a lateral pinch should be noted. This records any increasing ulnar deviation deformity, especially in patients with rheumatoid arthritis.
4. The web spaces:
   • the thumb web (and thumb abduction) should be measured between the inner surfaces of the MCP joint of the index finger and IP joint of the thumb (Figure 2.21), so avoiding inaccuracies due to varying mobility at the joints; the position of the thumb (extension or abduction) must be recorded

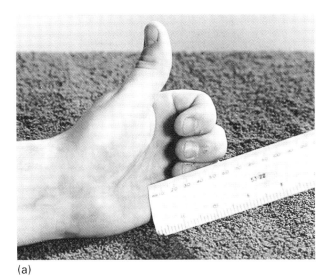

(a)

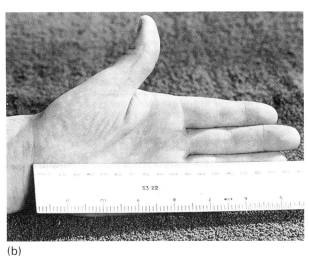

(b)

Figure 2.19 Distance of fingertips (a) towards palmar crease and (b) away from wrist crease.

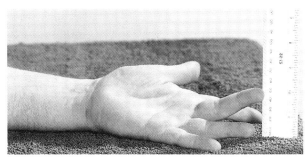

Figure 2.20 Finger extension deficit measure.

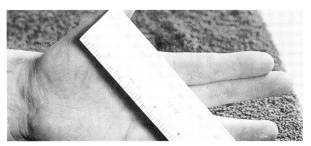

Figure 2.21 Ruler measure of thumb web space.

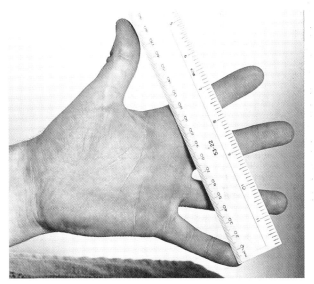

Figure 2.22 Total span.

- individual finger webs can be measured between the middle of each fingertip
- total span between the middle of the tips of the thumb and little finger can also be recorded (Figure 2.22).

An alternative method for recording the web spaces in finger abduction is by using a hand print. The forearm, third metacarpal and middle finger should be aligned and maintained as a baseline; this method is not possible when flexion contractures are present. Subsequent readings can be superimposed on the baseline using a different colour.

Salter measure

An L-shaped measure with a scale on the short arm can be used to measure muscle recovery following a radial nerve lesion by recording the deficit of active movement against gravity. The passive range of movement should be full.

1. The forearm is supported on the table with the wrist held in the neutral position. The measure is placed in position over the arm, with the fingertips close to the scale (Figure 2.23a), and the patient is asked to extend the fingers up the scale as far as possible. Each fingertip is recorded separately, as a negative reading.
2. If the patient is able to extend the fingers to or beyond the neutral position, the measure is turned over and the forearm rested on the top of it (Figure 2.23b). The patient is again asked to extend the fingers, but with the wrist actively extending also. Each finger is again recorded individually, but with a positive reading.

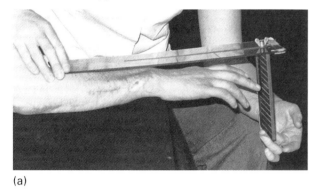
(a)

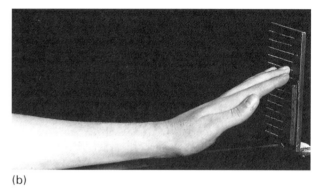
(b)

Figure 2.23 Salter measure for indicating motor recovery following a radial nerve lesion: (a) showing some wrist extension and early activity in extensor indicis, (b) nearly full finger and thumb extension after a posterior interosseous nerve lesion (passive range was full in both patients).

Kapandji measurement of thumb range of movement

This technique (Kapandji, 1992) is a simple, practical measurement of thumb opposition and counter-opposition based on observation of the movement of the thumb. For assessment of opposition, Kapandji defined 11 stages through which the normal thumb can be expected to travel and noted the stage to which the thumb can currently reach. The first three stages describe a lateral pinch, not opposition. The sequence of stages is as follows:

Stage 0   Tip of thumb to lateral aspect of index finger proximal phalanx
Stage 1   Tip of thumb to lateral aspect of index finger middle phalanx
Stage 2   Tip of thumb to lateral aspect of index finger distal phalanx
Stage 3   Tip of thumb to tip (or pulp) of index finger; this is the first and minimum stage of opposition
Stage 4   Tip of thumb to tip of middle finger
Stage 5   Tip of thumb to tip of ring finger
Stage 6   Tip of thumb to tip of little finger
Stage 7   Tip of thumb to distal interphalangeal joint crease of little finger
Stage 8   Tip of thumb to proximal interphalangeal joint crease of little finger
Stage 9   Tip of thumb to proximal crease at the base of the little finger, over the base of the proximal phalanx
Stage 10 Tip of the thumb to the distal palmar crease of the little finger, over the MCP joint

It must be possible to pass a cylinder (e.g. a pencil) through the opposition arch formed by the thumb in order to describe this movement as opposition; if the thumb lies flat in the palm, this is a movement of flexion and not opposition. Some people may be unable to reach all the stages of opposition due to the natural shape and bulk of their hand.

It only takes a few minutes to learn this numbering system, e.g. by inking the numbers on ones own hand and practising the sequence. The patient should be observed while completing the sequence and the furthest stage reached recorded, e.g. 'Thumb opposition: Kapandji 4'. Always note the patient's normal range of movement in the uninjured hand. This method cannot be used where there is a very poor range of finger movement.

Counter-opposition or reposition is the inverse motion to opposition, and this is measured using the uninjured hand as the reference. The injured hand needs to be placed with the palm flat on a table, and the uninjured hand rests on its ulnar border adjacent to the thumb of the injured hand. The patient then extends the thumb on the injured hand, lifting it up from the table as high as possible whilst keeping the remainder of the hand pressed firmly on the table. The height achieved is measured against the MCP joints of the other hand using the following points:

Stage 0   The thumb cannot be lifted off the table
Stage 1   Thumb tip to the MCP joint of the little finger
Stage 2   Thumb tip to the MCP joint of the ring finger
Stage 3   Thumb tip to the MCP joint of the middle finger
Stage 4   Thumb tip to the MCP joint of the index finger (this is an exceptional range of movement)

As in the case of opposition, the results can be scored easily, e.g. 'Counter-opposition: Kapandji 1'.

Special notes for measurements

1. Care should be taken to ensure that any proximal soft tissue involvement does not produce a variable distal measurement. Standardized positioning of the wrist is therefore necessary when measuring total movement of fingers.

2. Scarring and adhesions of skin, tendons and subcutaneous tissue proximal to the wrist may limit the simultaneous extension of wrist, metacarpophalangeal and interphalangeal joints. However, if the wrist joint is flexed, the extension may be full in the other joints.
3. Direct injury to the arteries or constriction from a tight plaster may cause ischaemic damage, which can lead to muscle contracture and the inability of the muscles to contract through their full range.

Volkmann's ischaemia of the forearm prevents combined extension of the wrist and fingers. As the wrist extends, the fingers are pulled into a greater degree of flexion; conversely, the wrist has to flex to allow the fingers to extend. Occasionally the extensors may also be affected, making it impossible to flex the fingers and thumb due to the contracture of the extensor muscles. These contractures are difficult to measure, and the proximal joints need to be stabilized in a standard position while a measurement is made. For example, the wrist should be held in a neutral position.

Intrinsic contractures of the small muscles of the hand are also difficult to measure. They may easily go undiagnosed, since they are not as obvious as a Volkmann's contracture. Nevertheless, they can be extremely disabling, probably due to the additional proprioceptive loss.

If the intrinsic 'plus' contracture is really severe, it is possible that the patient will not be able to extend the MCP joints or flex the fingers. To determine this, the MCP joints should be extended into a neutral position and the IP joints fully flexed, thus putting the small muscles on a stretch. A measurement of the distance of each fingertip towards the proximal finger crease is made while the MCP joints are held in maximal extension.

If the thenar muscles are affected by an ischaemic contracture, the thumb may be held in flexion across the palm. When this occurs it will severely interfere with function by preventing flexion of the index and middle fingers into the palm. The thumb web should be measured in both abduction and extension.

Suggested sequence for measurement of joint range

Not all of the previous measurements need to be recorded. When full active range is not possible, the passive physiological movements of the wrist and each joint of the thumb and fingers are examined, taking care to relax any skin or tendon tension.

The following sequences should help in the selection of appropriate measurements.

When passive physiological movement is limited:

1. Measure and record active movement
2. Measure passive movement, and record only when it differs considerably from active range

3. Examine accessory movement, and record only if limited by either pain or stiffness
4. Measure and record excursion of the fingers and thumb from flexion to extension
5. Measure the web spaces and record if less than on unaffected side.

When passive physiological movement is full:

1. Measure and record the excursion of the fingers and thumb from flexion to extension
2. Measure the web spaces and record if reduced from normal.

Measurement of individual active joint range may not be necessary when the passive movement is full, except following tendon surgery if adhesions in the flexor sheath are limiting finger movement. Progress can then be monitored by measuring the range at the interphalangeal joints.

Outcome measures

There are several methods of using outcome measures to analyse joint range of movement. These may have particular use in clinical audit, and may only need to be used on admission and discharge. They include total active movement (TAM) and total passive movement in a single finger and outcome of flexor tendon repairs (Strickland, 1980, 1989 or Kleinert *et al.*, 1973).

Strickland method
In this method,

$$\frac{(\text{active PIP+DIP flexion}) - \text{extension lag of PIP and DIP})}{175} \times 100\%$$

= % of normal active PIP and DIP joint motion

The results are graded as follows:

Percentage	75–100	50–74	25–49	0–24
Grade	Excellent	Good	Fair	Poor

It should be noted that the Strickland assessment takes no account of movement at the MCP joint.

Kleinert method
The therapist measures the distance from the fingertip to the distal palmar crease (cm) and the loss of extension at the MCP, PIP and DIP joints, and the results are graded as follows:

Tip to distal palmar crease (cm)	Extension deficit (°)	Grade
0–1	0–15	Excellent
1–1.5	16–30	Good
1.5–3.0	31–50	Fair
>3.0	<50	Poor

Ratings are established for flexion and for extension, and the overall result is determined by the lowest rating.

MUSCLE POWER

The normal interaction of agonist or prime mover with antagonist, synergist and fixator may be altered following injury, especially when nerve lesions are involved. To test muscle activity accurately the therapist must be familiar with the anatomy of the hand and arm, particularly the following:

- the origins, insertions and small slip attachments of muscles
- the general direction and line of pull of each muscle
- the position of the muscle or tendon relative to the axis of the joint over which it passes
- the relative positions of muscles and tendons
- the nerve supply and possible anomalies
- the possible presence of trick movements.

TYPES OF MUSCLE POWER ASSESSMENT

The three types of tests for muscle power are:

1. Manual tests of muscle groups
2. Manual tests of individual muscles
3. Objective tests of grip and pinch grip strength.

The first two tests provide only a subjective assessment of muscle power, and it is therefore essential that objective tests using calibrated equipment are performed as soon as possible. Points to note include that:

- group activity testing is relevant where muscles are expected to be weak from disuse but are otherwise normal
- individual muscle testing is essential to help diagnose and to monitor recovery following a nerve lesion and also for the selection of suitable muscles for tendon transfer surgery (see Chapter 7)
- objective tests of grip and pinch are of greatest value when function is limited due to weakness.

The results of the tests are considered together with those gained from functional testing.

Group action of muscles

All proximal muscles are tested, followed by the distal ones. The patient is first asked to perform all neck, shoulder and shoulder girdle movements through full range, with resistance applied where suitable. The procedure is then repeated for the distal joints. Movements are graded as normal, slightly weak or extremely weak, and the results recorded. Only those muscles that are weak need to be retested.

Individual muscle testing

Individual muscle tests can be used to determine the power of each of the muscles acting on the hand and arm. The tests described in detail are of those muscles acting distally to the elbow, shown in Table 2.2.

After a suspected or confirmed nerve lesion, the following tests are undertaken (Table 2.3):

1. Assessment of the muscles proximal to the lesion including shoulder and upper arm
   - normal innervation is expected in these muscles
   - weakness caused by disuse may be identified and can be recorded by terms such as 'slightly weak', 'very weak' etc; this type of weakness should improve rapidly with exercise
   - if there is a lack of muscle activity where some is expected, the cause must be investigated.
2. Assessment of the muscles distal to the lesion, including
   - muscles expected to be unaffected by the nerve damage, having an alternative and intact nerve supply
   - muscles normally supplied by the nerve which has been damaged.

Anomalies may be present due to natural diversity from textbook anatomy.

TABLE 2.2
MUSCLE CHART (SHOULDER, UPPER ARM AND ELBOW)

Supinator	Flexor carpi radialis	Abductor pollicis brevis
Brachioradialis	Palmaris longus	Flexor pollicis brevis
Extensor carpi radialis longus	Flexor digitorum profundus to index	Opponens pollicis
Extensor carpi radialis brevis	and middle fingers	Lumbricals 1 and 2
Extensor carpi ulnaris	Flexor digitorum superficialis	Abductor digiti minimi
Extensor digitorum	Flexor pollicis longus	Flexor digiti minimi
Extensor indicis	Pronator teres	Opponens digiti minimi
Extensor digiti minimi	Pronator quadratus	Adductor pollicis
Extensor pollicis longus	Flexor carpi ulnaris	Lumbricals 3 and 4
Extensor pollicis brevis	Flexor digitorum profundus to ring	Interossei dorsal
Abductor pollicis longus	and little fingers	Interossei volar

TABLE 2.3
JOINT MOVEMENT AND MUSCLE ACTIONS CHART

Movements	Prime movers	Secondary action by:
Wrist		
Wrist flexion	FCR, FCU, PL	FDP, FDS, FPL, APL, EPB
Wrist extension	ECRL, ECRB, ECU	EDC, EDM, EI, EPL
Ulnar deviation	ECU, FCU	
Radial deviation	FCR, ECRL, (ECRB)	APL, EPB
Fingers		
MCP flexion	Interossei	
Lumbricals	FDS, FDP	
MCP extension	EDC, EI, EDM	
MCP abduction	Interossei – dorsal	EDC
MCP adduction	Interossei – palmar	FDP
PIP flexion	FDS	FDP
PIP extension	Intrinsic muscles and EDC	
DIP flexion	FDP	
DIP extension	Intrinsic muscles and EDC	
Thumb		
CMC		
Palmar abduction	APB	OPP with APL
Adduction	Add P	EPL with FPL
Radial abduction	APL, EPB	
Extension	EPL	
Opposition	OPP with APB, FPB and Add P	
MCP flexion	FPB	FPL
MCP extension	EPB	EPL
IP flexion	FPL	
IP extension	EPL	APB, FPB

Add P, adductor pollicis; APB, abductor pollicis brevis APL, abductor pollicis longus; ECRB, extensor carpi radialis brevis; ECRL, extensor carpi radialis longus; ECU, extensor carpi ulnaris; EDC, extensor digitorum communis; EDM, extensor digiti minimi; EI, extensor indicis; EPB, extensor pollicus brevis; EPL, extensor pollicis longus; FCR, flexor carpi radialis; FCU, flexor carpi ulnaris; FDP, flexor digitorum profundus; FDS, flexor digitorum superficialis; FPB, flexor pollicis brevis; FPL, flexor pollicis longus; OPP, opponens pollicis; PL, palmaris longus.

Method of testing

Ensure that the patient is warm, comfortably positioned and supported, can see what is happening and understands the purpose of testing.

1. Select the muscle and the joint movement required:
   - check that the muscle and joint have the expected passive range of movement
   - describe and demonstrate the movement to the patient on both the affected and unaffected sides using clear, simple commands.
2. Observe:
   - any movement at the selected joint, checking for any unwanted movement of joints not involved in the testing
   - any contraction of the muscle belly and tendon.
3. Palpate, if possible:
   - any contraction of the muscle belly
   - any movement of the tendon close to its insertion.

4. Utilize the following types of muscle activity:
   - isotonic prime mover action – use outer to middle range, as this is usually the first to recover
   - isometric contraction – this muscle action is sometimes easier to teach to the patient, e.g. in the intrinsic muscles; again use outer to middle range first
   - synergic action – this may occasionally be identified, during early muscle re-innervation, before prime mover activity (for example, the abductor digit minimi may be felt to contract when the patient opposes the thumb to the little finger, before a prime mover contraction of ADM is identified).
5. Facilitate the desired muscle activity by using proprioceptive neuromuscular facilitation techniques (PNF); after a nerve lesion the threshold of nerve conduction is raised, and muscle activity can be improved by bombarding the recovering nerve using some of the following techniques:

- muscle stretch
- joint approximation
- joint traction
- application of resistance
- encouragement of the patient
- practising the required movement on the uninjured side simultaneously.

6. Record the muscle power using the Oxford scale of muscle grading on a 0–5 scale (Medical Research Council, 1976).

Oxford scale of muscle grading

0 No contraction
1 A flicker of movement
2 Movement with gravity eliminated
3 Movement against gravity
4 A full range of movement against gravity and some resistance
5 Normal movement and power as compared with the unaffected side

A comprehensive anatomy book in the department is essential. A note of caution is also warranted at this point; tissue structures should not be stretched or put under resistance in the early stages following damage or surgical repair. The use of PNF techniques and these stronger grades of muscle testing are therefore delayed.

Problems in muscle testing and their solutions

1. Scars and adhesions may prevent full excursion of the tendon:
   - check the contraction proximal to the level of the injury
   - palpate and observe the scar when the patient is attempting movement.
2. Muscles may contract unexpectedly:
   - check for anomalies in the nerve supply by using electrical stimulation
   - stimulate the unaffected nerve directly, both at the wrist and the elbow
   - observe if the muscle contracts.
3. Deformities may change the angle of pull, making muscles inefficient:
   - check the X-rays to analyse the effect that the deformity may have on muscle function.
4. Sensory loss may make it difficult for a patient to feel what he or she is trying to do:
   - check that the patient can see the activity
   - check with the contralateral limb that the correct movement is being performed
   - ensure that the patient makes several attempts to produce the best action.
5. Trick movements following peripheral nerve lesions occur when the patient compensates in an attempt to produce movement:
   - therapists must critically analyse all movements to ensure that trick patterns are not being used.

6. Severe pain may totally inhibit muscle contraction:
   - the cause of pain must be treated first in these cases.
7. Total absence of movement is very unusual:
   - the patient will usually be able to make some sort of movement in the limb, even if it is simply a withdrawal motion of the arm on the shoulder girdle
   - the therapist should eliminate the possibility of a severe brachial plexus lesion or an hysterical response to trauma; if an hysterical problem is suspected, the clinical psychologist should be asked to complete an assessment and recommend an approach to treatment.

Trick movements

Therapists can anticipate which movements will be lost as the result of a peripheral nerve lesion, but frequently the patient can produce more joint movements than expected because of trick or compensatory movements. These are classified in detail by Wynn Parry (1981), but can be divided broadly into four categories:

1. Normal secondary muscle action
2. Anomalous nerve supply
3. Pathological processes and surgical procedures
4. Deceptive (or trick) movements.

Normal secondary muscle action Detailed anatomical knowledge is needed of the origins and insertions of the multiarthrodal muscles, the direction in which they lie and their relationship to the fulcrum of the joints over which they pass.

For example:

1. The slip from abductor pollicis brevis (APB) which inserts into the dorsal expansion of the thumb enables the APB to extend the distal joint of the thumb when the extensor pollicis longus is paralysed in a radial nerve lesion.
2. In the forearm, wrist and finger flexors and extensors frequently provide a small amount of elbow flexion when the biceps is paralysed. This is because the origins of the common flexor and common extensor tendons are attached to the epicondyles of the humerus and are thus proximal to the elbow joint. This is known as Steindler action, and can be utilized in transfer procedures.
3. The position of the abductor pollicis longus (APL), as it passes over the wrist joint, lies anterior to the fulcrum of the joint. Although it is grouped with the forearm extensors and abducts the thumb radially, it also flexes the wrist. In a combined high lesion of median and ulnar nerves, wrist flexion will therefore remain, produced by the APL.

More details will be given of the expected trick movements due to secondary muscle activities with individual nerve lesions.

Anomalous nerve supply Anomalies of nerve supply can be misleading, as they are present in about 15 per cent of patients and therefore make diagnosis more difficult. Stimulation of an unaffected nerve may identify a possible anomaly, and this is important for correct diagnosis.

Pathological processes and surgical procedures Denervation or ischaemia may frequently lead to a contracture of muscles. Functionally this can sometimes be used to advantage when the antagonists are graded 4 or 5 on the Oxford scale. Although the joints may be independently mobile, the contracture will prevent full passive movement of all joints simultaneously and the antagonist is therefore unable to move all joints through the full range simultaneously. As the proximal joint is moved in one direction the distal joint will be moved passively in the opposite direction and *vice versa*, and this is known as a tenodesis action. For example:

1. With a high median and ulnar nerve or brachial plexus lesion, the fingers will flex passively when the patient actively extends his wrist (Figure 2.24), especially if the flexors are contracted.
2. With a radial nerve lesion, active movement is present in the wrist and finger flexors but absent in the extensors. Finger flexion may produce passive wrist extension if the extensors have shortened adaptively.

Trick movements can improve the function of the hand and appear normal. They can be facilitated by a surgical tenodesis (or tendon shortening procedure) in patients who are unlikely to gain further muscle re-innervation. Tendon transfers can improve function by repositioning muscles together with their neurovascular bundles (see Chapter 6).

Deceptive (or trick) movements Patients may use the effect of gravity to achieve movement, but this is unlikely to be functional. For example, wrist flexion may appear to be present if gravity is not eliminated, or elbow flexion and extension may appear present although the biceps and triceps are paralysed. The movement is produced by rotating the shoulder, first internally then externally.

Stabilizing the distal joints and contracting the proximal muscles may give the appearance of activity at the middle joints. For example, with the therapist supporting the hand the patient will be able to extend the elbow, even though the triceps is paralysed, by strong contraction of pectoralis major.

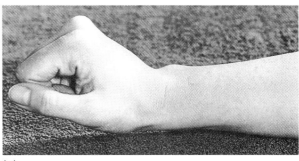
(a)

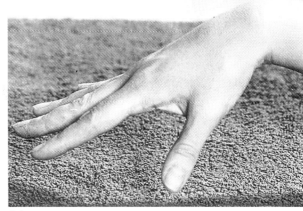
(b)

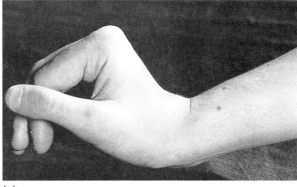
(c)

Figure 2.24 (a) and (b) Finger flexion followed by extension of a normal hand. (c) Attempted finger flexion in a high median nerve lesion: note extreme wrist extension, utilizing the tenodesis effect to produce passive finger flexion.

Rebound can result from relaxation of the antagonist muscles following their strong contraction. It may look deceptively like a small contraction of the agonists. For example, in the patient attempting flexion of the DIP joint, the extension of the DIP joint followed by its relaxation can appear to be a small movement of flexion.

The paradox of trick movements is twofold: a different action occurs from that which is required, and there is movement at joints other than the one selected.

For example:

1. If a patient with a radial nerve lesion is asked to extend the MCP joints, the wrist is flexed to achieve this.
2. If a patient with an ulnar nerve lesion is asked to abduct and adduct the MCP joint of the middle finger, the whole hand is moved laterally on the fixed tips of the other fingers. Abduction and adduction occur passively at the MCP joints of the other fingers but there is no movement at the required joint.

Reduction of trick movements is usually the first sign of early muscle recovery.

Anterior antebrachial muscles

These anterior forearm muscles may give slight assistance to elbow flexion because the common flexor origin is attached to the epicondyle of the humerus, and thus is proximal to the elbow joint. They have a mildly pronating effect when contracting as a group, and mostly assist in wrist flexion.

Nerve supply The ulnar nerve supplies:

- flexor carpi ulnaris
- medial (ulnar) portion of flexor digitorum profundus – this is usually to the ring and little fingers, but is occasionally to the middle finger also.

The median nerve supplies the remaining muscles:

- pronator teres
- flexor carpi radialis
- palmaris longus
- flexor digitorum profundus
- flexor digitorum superficialis
- flexor pollicis longus.

Testing position
The patient should sit with the forearm resting on a table, palm upwards.

Flexor carpi ulnaris (FCU)

1. Ask the patient to flex the wrist and deviate in an ulnar direction.
2. Rest the patient's hand, with the wrist in some extension, over a pillow.
3. Palpate the tendon immediately proximal to the pisiform (Figure 2.25).
4. Add resistance when suitable.

Action: Flexes the wrist in combination with flexor carpi radialis, and ulnar deviates the wrist with extensor carpi ulnaris. In isolation, FCU produces a diagonal movement of flexion combined with ulnar deviation. It contracts strongly as a synergist when opposing the thumb to the little finger.

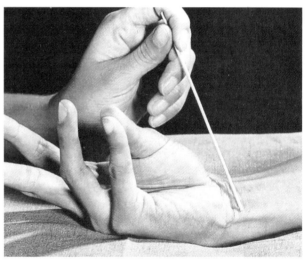

Figure 2.25 Flexor carpi ulnaris contracts strongly as a synergist when opposing thumb to little finger.

Pronator teres (PT)

1. Rest the patient's hand in full supination over a pillow.
2. Ask the patient to turn the palm downwards.
3. Palpate the muscle and observe the movement.
4. Add resistance when suitable.

Action: Pronates the forearm from full supination to full pronation. It can become a strong elbow flexor, especially in the absence of the biceps.

Flexor carpi radialis (FCR)

1. Rest the patient's hand over a pillow, with the wrist in some extension and the forearm supinated.
2. Ask the patient to flex the hand at the wrist.
3. Palpate the tendon immediately proximal to the scaphoid and lateral to the tendon of the palmaris longus (Figure 2.26).
4. Add resistance when suitable.

Action: Flexes the wrist in combination with FCU and assists in radial deviation of the wrist together with the extensor carpi radialis longus

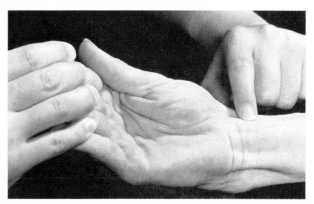

Figure 2.26 Flexor carpi radialis.

and abductor pollicis longus. In isolation, it produces an oblique movement of flexion combined with radial deviation and some pronation.

Palmaris longus (PL)

1. Rest the patient's hand over a pillow, with the wrist in a neutral position and the forearm supinated.
2. Ask the patient to flex the wrist and, while holding this position, to oppose the thumb and little finger.
3. The tendon of PL will be seen to stand out (Figure 2.27).
4. This procedure may be reversed, by first opposing and then flexing the wrist.

Action: Contracts the palmar fascia and assists in flexing the wrist. PL is used as a donor in both tendon transfers and grafts, so assessment of its presence is important. It is absent in a small percentage of the population.

Flexor digitorum profundus (FDP)

1. Rest the patient's hand over a pillow with the wrist in some extension and the forearm supinated.
2. Test each finger independently.
3. Support the middle phalanx.
4. Ask patient to flex the fingertip at the DIP joint (Figure 2.28).
5. Observe movement at the DIP joint.
6. Add resistance when suitable.

Action: Flexes the DIP joints of the fingers and assists in flexing the PIP joints, MCP joints and the wrist.

Flexor digitorum superficialis (FDS)

1. Rest the patient's hand over a pillow with the wrist in the neutral position, the fingers extended and the forearm supinated.
2. Hold three of the patient's fingertips in full extension.
3. Ask the patient to flex the free finger; the PIP joint will flex without any activity at the DIP joint if the FDS is contracting (Figure 2.29).
4. Gradually add resistance over the middle phalanx to test power and check that there is no action occurring of FDP at the distal joint.
5. Test each finger similarly.

Action: Flexes PIP joints of the fingers and assists in flexing the MCP joints and the wrist. FDS to the little finger is congenitally absent in a small percentage of the population.

Flexor pollicis longus (FPL)

1. Rest the patient's hand over a pillow with the wrist in some extension, the thumb fully extended and the forearm supinated.
2. Support the proximal phalanx.
3. Ask the patient to flex the tip of the thumb.

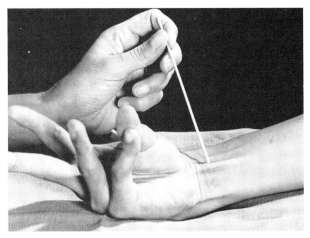

Figure 2.27   Palmaris longus contracts when first the thumb and little finger are opposed, and second the wrist is flexed.

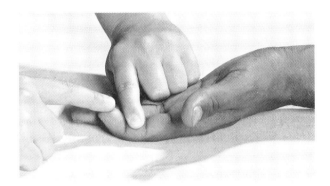

Figure 2.28   Flexor digitorum profundus tested with resistance.

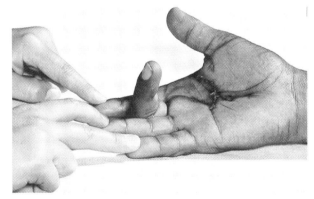

Figure 2.29   Flexor digitorum superficialis. Strength may be tested by resisting the muscle when the finger is already flexed.

4. Observe movement at the IP joint and palpate the tendon at its insertion and over the proximal phalanx (Figure 2.30).
5. Add resistance when suitable.

Action: Flexes the IP joint of the thumb and assists in flexing the MCP joint and the wrist. In the absence

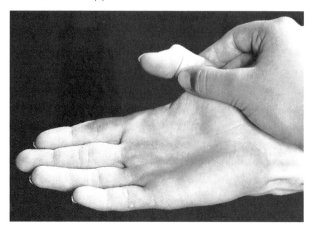

Figure 2.30 Flexor pollicis longus.

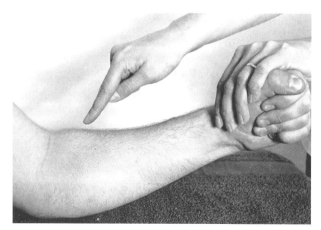

Figure 2.31 Brachioradialis.

of adductor pollicis action, FPL combines with extensor pollicis longus to produce adduction from the abducted position due to its diagonal direction over the wrist and the CMC joint.

Posterior antebrachial muscles

These forearm muscles share a common extensor tendon origin at the lateral epicondyle of the humerus, and can also give slight assistance to elbow flexion in the same manner as the forearm flexors. This is called the Steindler action, and may be observed in patients with no activity in the biceps muscle. It may be used for tendon transfer procedures, to restore some functional flexion to the elbow by proximally repositioning the common tendon origins. These posterior antebrachial muscles also have a mildly supinating effect.

Nerve supply The radial nerve supplies:

- brachioradialis
- extensor carpi radialis longus.

The posterior interosseous branch supplies:

- supinator
- all other extensor muscles in this group.

Testing position The patient sits with the forearm resting on a table and in the pronated position except when testing the brachioradialis.

Brachioradialis

1. Rest the forearm in the mid-position on a pillow.
2. Ask the patient to flex the elbow.
3. Palpate the muscle belly distal to the elbow joint (Figure 2.31).
4. Add resistance when suitable.

   Action: Flexes the elbow in the mid-position and assists both supination and pronation to the mid-position.

Extensor carpi radialis longus (ECRL) and brevis (ECRB)

1. Rest the patient's hand over a pillow with the wrist in some flexion.
2. Ask the patient to extend the wrist.
3. Palpate ECRL on the thenar side of the base of the second metacarpal; the ECRL is easier to palpate when the thumb is flexed across the palm (Figure 2.32).

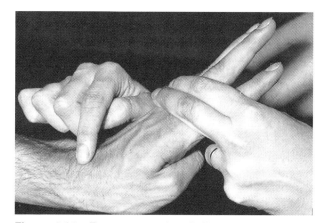

Figure 2.32 Extensor carpi radialis longus, palpated while the thumb is flexed across the palm.

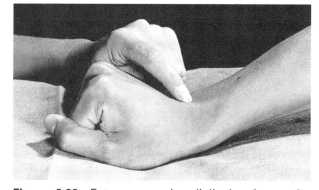

Figure 2.33 Extensor carpi radialis brevis can be palpated most easily when a strong fist is made.

4. Palpate ECRB on the thenar side of the base of the third metacarpal with the fingers in flexion.

Action: ECRL extends the wrist with radial deviation, and the ECRB provides straight extension of the wrist. It stabilizes the wrist during gripping movements and can be palpated easily when a strong fist is made (Figure 2.33).

Extensor carpi ulnaris (ECU)

1. Rest the patient's hand over a pillow with the wrist in some flexion.
2. Ask the patient first to extend and ulnar deviate the wrist and then to abduct the fingers and thumb.
3. Palpate the tendon immediately distal to the ulnar styloid.

Action: ECU extends the wrist with ulnar deviation and contracts strongly as a synergist when the fingers and thumb are abducted (Figure 2.34).

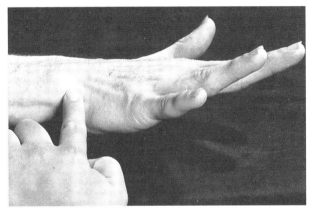

Figure 2.34 Extensor carpi ulnaris contracts strongly when abducting all digits.

Extensor digitorum communis (EDC)

1. Rest the patient's hand over a pillow, with the wrist in a neutral position and the MCP joints in some flexion.
2. Ask the patient to extend the MCP joints whilst keeping the IP joints flexed (Figure 2.35a), and prevent wrist flexion when the patient is attempting to extend the MCP joints.
3. Ask the patient to extend the fingers simultaneously at the MCP and IP joints (Figure 2.35b).
4. Palpate the tendon at the level of the wrist joint and observe for both extension of the MCP joints and contraction of the tendons over the metacarpals.

Action: EDC primarily extends the MCP joints. It extends the IP joints only in conjunction with the intrinsic muscles (Figure 2.35b), and it also assists in extension of the wrist.

Extensor indicis (EI)

1. Rest the patient's hand over a pillow with the index MCP joint in slight flexion and the middle and ring fingers in total flexion.
2. Ask the patient to extend the index finger, keeping the other fingers flexed; this excludes the activity of EDC.
3. Palpate the tendon of EI (Figure 2.36).

Action: EI extends the MCP joint of the index finger.

Extensor digiti minimi (EDM)

1. Rest the patient's hand over a pillow with the little finger in slight flexion and middle and ring fingers in total flexion.
2. Ask the patient to extend the little finger, keeping the other fingers flexed; this excludes the activity of the EDC.
3. Palpate the tendon of the EDM (Figure 2.37).

Action: EDM extends the MCP joint of the little finger.

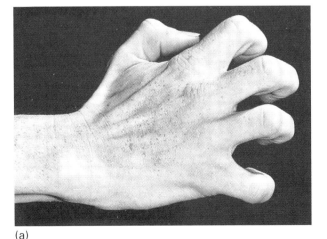

(a)

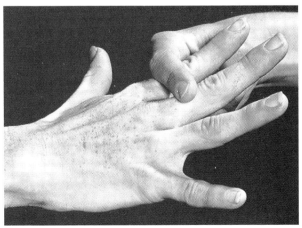

(b)

Figure 2.35 Extensor digitorum contracting with interphalangeal joints: (a) flexed and (b) extended.

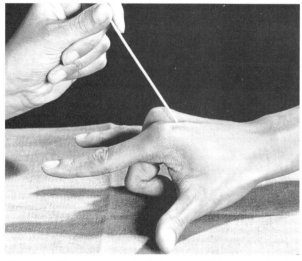

Figure 2.36 Extensor indicis should be tested with middle and ring fingers flexed.

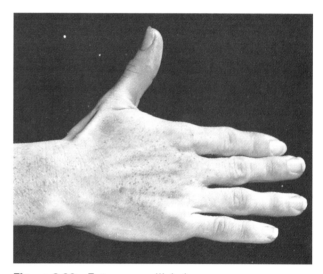

Figure 2.38 Extensor pollicis longus.

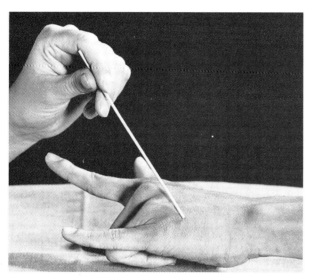

Figure 2.37 Extensor digiti minimi should be tested with middle and ring fingers flexed.

Extensor pollicis longus (EPL)

1. Rest the ulnar border of the patient's hand on the pillow.
2. Ask the patient to extend the distal interphalangeal joint and extend the whole thumb, keeping it in the same plane as the index finger.
3. Add resistance when suitable.
4. Palpate the tendon and observe the contraction of the EPL on the ulnar border of the anatomical snuffbox (Figure 2.38).

(As an alternative to points 1 and 2 above, ask the patient to place the hand flat on the table with the palm downwards and the forearm pronated, and to lift the thumb up off the table whilst keeping the rest of the hand still.)

Action: EPL extends the IP joint of the thumb, assists in extension of the MCP, CMC and wrist joints, and adducts and externally rotates the thumb column into supination. Do not support the thumb during this test, as this may conceal a trick movement.

NB: Interphalangeal joint extension of the thumb may be produced in a radial nerve lesion by the abductor pollicis brevis (see Chapter 6). However, the APB will, at the same time, pull the whole thumb into palmar abduction with medial rotation.

Abductor pollicis longus (APL)

1. Rest the patient's hand over a pillow.
2. Ask the patient to abduct the thumb.
3. Palpate the tendon on the radial border of the anatomical snuffbox, volar to the extensor pollicis brevis tendon (Figure 2.39).

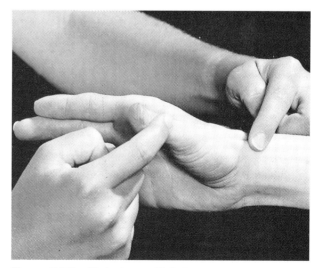

Figure 2.39 Abductor pollicis longus.

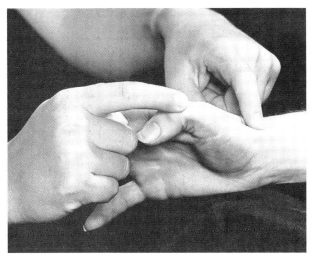

Figure 2.40 Extensor pollicis brevis.

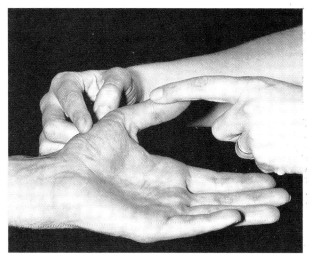

Figure 2.41 Abductor pollicis brevis abducts the thumb in a plane at 90° to the palm.

Action: APL abducts the thumb and radially deviates the wrist joint. It also assists in flexion of the wrist due to its slightly anterior position to the fulcrum of the joint. This action is evident with high combined lesions of median and ulnar nerves, when patients can unexpectedly flex the wrist. Frequently there is a slip insertion into the origin of abductor pollicis brevis.

Extensor pollicis brevis (EPB)
1. Rest the patient's hand over a pillow.
2. Place the thumb in a position of IP joint flexion and MCP joint extension.
3. Ask the patient to hold this position (Figure 2.40).
4. Palpate the tendon on the radial border of the anatomical snuffbox immediately dorsal to the APL tendon.

Action: EPB extends the MCP joint of the thumb, and assists in CMC extension.

Small muscles of the hand

These muscles take their origin distal to the wrist joint.

Nerve supply The nerve supply is from the median and ulnar nerves, and there are frequent anomalies between the two.
    The median nerve usually supplies:

- abductor pollicis brevis
- flexor pollicis brevis
- opponens pollicis
- two radial lumbricals.

The ulnar nerve usually supplies:

- the two ulnar lumbricals
- all interossei
- abductor digiti minimi

- flexor digiti minimi
- opponens digiti minimi
- deep head of flexor pollicis brevis
- adductor pollicis.

Abductor pollicis brevis (APB)
1. Rest the patient's hand on a pillow with the palm upwards and the thumb resting anterior to the index finger.
2. Ask the patient to abduct the thumb at right angles to the plane of the palm; the thumb must not drift into radial abduction.
3. Palpate the muscle bulk close to the shaft of the first metacarpal (Figure 2.41); the ability to hold the thumb away from close proximity to the palm suggests some activity in the muscle.

Action: APB produces palmar abduction of the thumb at the CMC joint. It assists extension of the IP joint of the thumb because of its slip insertion into the dorsal expansion, and acts as a strong stabilizer of the thumb.

    APB has been found on testing to contract more strongly with the wrist in the extended position. This is probably because frequently there is a slip from the APL into the origin of the APB. The extended wrist puts the APL on a stretch, thus providing a more stable origin for the APB.

Flexor pollicis brevis (FPB)
FPB arises from two heads, the deep being supplied by the ulnar nerve and the superficial by the median nerve.

1. Rest the patient's hand on the pillow with the palm upwards.
2. Position the thumb with a flexed MCP joint and extended IP joint (Figure 2.42).
3. Ask the patient to hold this position against slight resistance.

4. Palpate the muscle belly immediately proximal to the MCP joint.

Action: FPB flexes the MCP joint, and assists in abduction and internal rotation of the thumb.

Opponens pollicis (OP)
1. Rest the patient's hand on the ulnar border with the thumb in radial abduction.
2. Ask the patient to touch the tip of the index finger with the tip of the thumb and to rotate the thumb to achieve a pulp–pulp contact (Figure 2.43).

Action: OP rotates the column of the thumb into pronation.

NB: Combined palmar abduction and MCP flexion, e.g. when touching the tip of little finger with the tip of the thumb, automatically produces a conjunct rotation of the thumb. This can be misleading when assessing the opponens muscle.

Abductor digiti minimi (ADM)
1. Rest the patient's hand on a pillow with the palm upwards.

2. Ask the patient to abduct the little finger with the MCP joint in slight flexion (Figure 2.44).
3. Palpate the muscle belly.
4. Ask the patient to oppose little finger towards the thumb.
5. Palpate the muscle belly again.

Action: ADM abducts the little finger and assists in flexing the MCP joint from full extension to slight flexion. It acts as a synergist during opposition of the little finger towards the thumb.

Flexor digiti minimi (FDM)
This muscle assists in MCP joint flexion of the little finger and in raising the fifth metacarpal head during opposition. It acts in conjunction with the other hypothenar muscles, and cannot be tested specifically.

Opponens digiti minimi (ODM)
1. Rest the patient's hand on a pillow with palm upwards.
2. Ask the patient to lift the little finger towards the thumb (Figure 2.45).
3. Palpate the muscle belly volar to ADM.

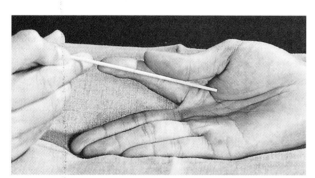

Figure 2.42 Flexor pollicis brevis. Note that the interphalangeal joint is extended.

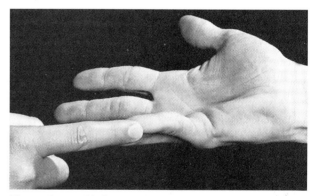

Figure 2.44 Abductor digiti minimi.

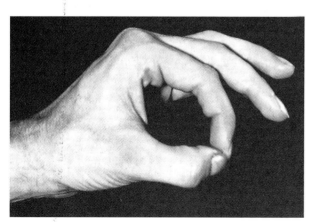

Figure 2.43 Opponens pollicis rotates the thumb so that pulp of index finger and thumb contact one another. Opponens pollicis should not be tested with the little finger, as conjunct rotation of the thumb automatically occurs and is deceptive.

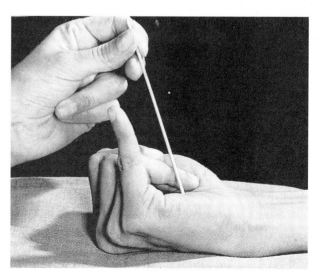

Figure 2.45 Opponens digiti minimi.

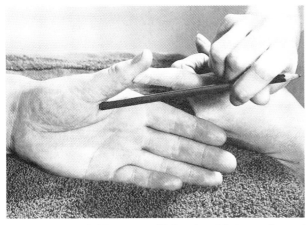

Figure 2.46 Adductor pollicis should be palpated deep in the thumb web from the volar aspect.

Action: ODM helps to raise and medially rotate the fifth metacarpal head for opposition of the little finger towards the thumb.

Adductor pollicis (Add P)
1. Rest the ulnar border of the patient's hand on a pillow, with the thumb in palmar abduction.
2. Ask the patient to adduct the thumb to a position anterior to the index finger, and look for a smooth movement of adduction without pronounced thumb IP joint extension or flexion.
3. Palpate the muscle belly deep in the thumb web from the volar aspect (Figure 2.46).

Action: Add P adducts the thumb at the carpometacarpal joint.

Interossei: dorsal (DI) and palmar (PI)
The two actions of the interossei should be tested separately.

Action 1: flexion of the MCP joints with extension of the IP joints
1. Rest the patient's hand on a pillow with palm upwards and the MCP and IP joints in extension.
2. Ask the patient to flex the MCP joints while keeping the IP joints in extension (Figure 2.47a). It may be easier for the patient if the fingers are placed in the required position and he is asked to keep them there. A quick approximation of the joints will facilitate the desired activity.

Figure 2.47 (a) Interossei maintaining flexion of the MCP joints together with extension of the IP joints. This is a position of power. (b) and (c) Normal abduction by the interossei of the middle finger in both directions. Note the finger is held in slight extension while performing this movement. (d) First dorsal interosseous is essential for pinch grip.

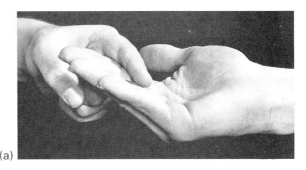
(a)

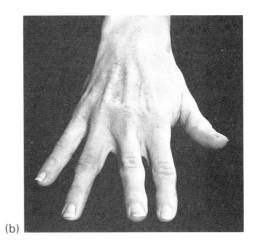
(b)

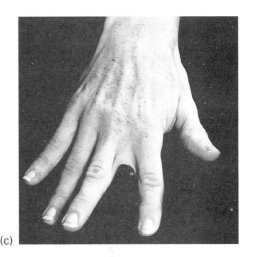
(c)

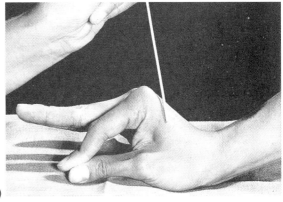
(d)

Action: When the dorsal and palmar muscles contract simultaneously, they flex the MCP joints and extend the IP joints.

Action 2: abduction and adduction of the fingers

1. Rest the patient's hand palm downwards on a pillow, with the MCP joints in extension and slight abduction.
2. Ask the patient to extend the middle finger, and then move it from side to side (Figures 2.47b, 2.47c); note that movement takes place only at the MCP joint of the finger being tested.
3. Resistance may be added when suitable.
4. Repeat step 2 for the ring finger.

Abduction and adduction of the index and little fingers can be misleading. When the interossei are totally paralysed, some movement may be produced by a rapid alternating contraction of EI and EDC to the index finger. Similarly, abduction and adduction of the little finger may be produced by an alternating contraction of first EDM followed by EDC to the little finger. It is usually possible to observe these alternating contractions of the tendons at the MCP joint level of the index and little fingers.

The first DI should be palpated during testing (Figure 2.47d). Its activity is essential in providing stability for a pinch grip and for holding objects such as a pencil or a knife.

Action: The interossei cause abduction and adduction of the MCP joints when these joints are in extension. They are strong stabilizers of the fingers when the MCP joints are in flexion, and particularly so of the index finger during pinch grip.

Lumbricals

These muscles should be tested in conjunction with the long flexors and long extensors of the fingers, as they normally act as a composite group.

1. Rest the patient's pronated forearm on a pillow with the hand over the edge and the wrist in some flexion.
2. Ask the patient first to extend all the joints of the fingers (Figure 2.48) and then to flex them.
3. Look for normal movement (i.e. that the fingers extend with no clawing, that they flex with simultaneous movement at all joints, and that the fingertips are kept away from the palm).

Action: The lumbricals act as the controlling mechanism between the long flexors and the long extensors of the fingers. By releasing the strong pull of the flexors, they prevent clawing and enable the fingertips to be held away from the palm in movements of flexion and extension. They are also very important in providing proprioceptive information such as speed of movement.

The lumbricals have both their origin and insertion into tendons, and consequently they cannot

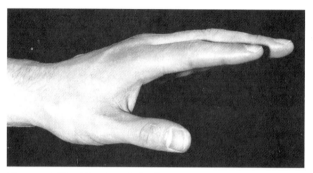

Figure 2.48 The lumbricals are active in this photograph, as without them the fingers claw and it is impossible to hold the tips away from the palm during flexion and extension movements.

provide strength and stability but have an adaptive and proprioceptive function. The lumbricals assist the interossei in producing combined MCP joint flexion and IP joint extension, but it is not their main action.

The median nerve supplies the lumbricals to the index and middle finger. Following an ulnar nerve lesion, the index and middle fingers can hold a position of MCP joint flexion and IP joint extension. However, this movement is very weak and collapses if given slight resistance, which is a further indication that it is not one of the main actions of the lumbricals (see further details in the Nerve lesions section of Chapter 6).

Objective power assessment

Power is a good indicator of hand function, and its measurement must form part of any hand assessment. The most commonly measured aspects include:

- grasp
- lateral pinch
- opposition pinch.

It is important to measure the type of grip relevant to the patient and, when possible, to use standardized procedures. Power grip is not usually assessed during the early stages of hand trauma, or before there is full tendon and bone healing – i.e. not until approximately 6 weeks post-surgery.

Grip strength

There are several pieces of commercial equipment available for this measurement, including rigid dynamometers, rubber bulb dynamometers, and pressure bags.

Rigid dynamometers:

- provide the most meaningful and consistent means available for recording power
- may have a pointer, which remains in the maximum position for easy reading

- may produce discomfort because of their hardness and rigidity, with resultant muscle inhibition
- may lack sensitivity at low readings.

Rubber bulb dynamometers:

- have selectable bulb sizes
- are comfortable to hold
- can partially adjust to hand deformities and deficiencies of grip
- produce extremely variable results, and can therefore only be used to illustrate a trend in progress.

The Jamar dynamometer The Jamar dynamometer:

- measures cylinder grip
- is widely available to hand therapists
- has a standardized method of use
- has normative values established for its use (Mathiowetz *et al.*, 1985)
- is widely accepted by hand therapists.

The normative values are particularly useful when it is necessary to compare the patient against norms, for example when assessing the patient before preparing a legal report (Gilbertson and Barber Lomax, 1994).

Jamar suggested the following standard procedure for using the dynamometer:

1. The patient can be tested in a sitting or standing position
2. The shoulder must be held in adduction and neutral rotation, i.e. with the elbow tucked in to the side
3. The elbow should be flexed to 90° and the forearm and wrist must be in the neutral position
4. The handle should be adjusted to fit comfortably in the hand when in a cylinder grip (Figure 2.49a), and the patient asked to squeeze the handle smoothly to the maximum strength and then relax
5. The peak reading should be noted
6. Each test should be repeated three times and the average taken.

In addition:

- the patient may be allowed a recovery period after each measurement by assessing alternate hands
- the position of the adjustable handle should be noted to ensure standardization for that patient on repeat measurements
- Jamar identified a positive correlation between grip strength and the patient's weight, hand width, height and mesomorphy.

Pressure bag Power grip can also be assessed using a pressure bag as follows (Figure 2.49b):

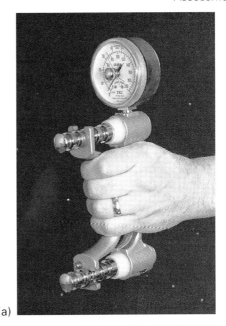
(a)

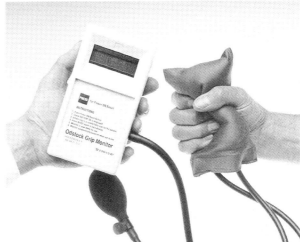
(b)

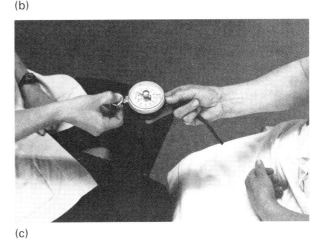
(c)

Figure 2.49 (a) The Jamar dynamometer, which measures cylinder grip, has a standardized method of use with normative values established. (b) The pressure bag (by permission of Polytronics Design Ltd). (c) Measurement of pinch grip.

1. The bag should be inflated to a pressure of 10 mmHg to make it easier to grip.
2. The patient is then asked to rest the elbow on the table and, with the wrist in the neutral position (or up to 15° extension), to squeeze the bag as hard as possible.
3. Each test should be repeated three times for each hand, and the maximum reading recorded to measure change.

Some commercial versions of this equipment (such as the Odstock Grip Meter; Polytronics Design Ltd, Emsworth, Hants) automatically record the peak reading, giving improved accuracy. Normal adult grip strength ranges from 200–900 mmHg, and ideally the equipment should measure the whole range. This design of equipment is comfortable for the patient to hold and is particularly suitable for assessing patients suffering from rheumatoid arthritis, who usually score values well below 300 mmHg.

Pinch grip There are three types of pinch grip:

1. Lateral
2. Opposition
3. Tripod.

The therapist must state clearly which type is being assessed, and ensure that the technique used is reproducible.

Pinch grip can be measured using a bulb dynamometer, a mercury sphygmomanometer or a pinch gauge (hydraulic and digital models; Figure 2.49c). Commercial equipment has been specifically developed for this assessment, and provides the most accurate method of measurement.

Variables affecting power measurement
Accurate readings are essential, but may be difficult to obtain from some types of equipment. It is therefore preferable to use equipment that has a maximum hold facility, with the readings on a digital display. The assessor can then concentrate entirely on the patient, checking for abnormal and compensatory movements.

Several variables affect the measurement of power, including:

- the patient's age, sex and posture
- the position of the hand, its size and the direction of forces during gripping
- the time of day and the environment
- the patient's occupation and hobbies, which may affect strength levels
- the psychological and general physical fitness of the patient
- fatigue
- pain levels
- the method of administration of the test.

Studies have shown a very wide variation between normal subjects, and comparison of a patient's score with an average is therefore of limited value. Similarly, judgements should not be made from a single reading; it is essential to look at trends rather than absolute values.

The strength of the unaffected hand should serve as the most accurate reference in the evaluation of the impaired hand. Some studies of hand dominance have shown the dominant hand to be generally the strongest, whilst others have indicated no significant difference. The latter appears to be the most commonly found conclusion, and therefore supports the use of the unaffected hand as a control whenever possible.

SENSATION

The topic of sensory evaluation is a complex one, and a wide variety of tests is needed to identify the degree to which the different modalities of sensation have been affected. The main considerations for the therapist are:

- to discover whether sensation is lost, reduced or recovering
- to appreciate that this will seriously affect the patient's functional ability
- to provide thorough, ongoing and reliable assessments, which are vital for informed management of a sensory disability
- to identify when the appropriate degree of recovery has occurred so that re-education of sensory function can be commenced and monitored.

This section discusses the sensory assessments that are useful, and the stages of recovery at which they are applicable. Careful examination can achieve an acceptably accurate picture of nerve involvement and recovery, although there are relatively few objective forms of measurement. Procedures (including both clinical and functional tests) should be kept to the minimum essential for each stage, otherwise evaluation can be very time consuming and frustrating for both patient and therapist. Details of each test will be found following the three main stages described below.

Early stage following nerve injury/surgery
Following diagnosis of peripheral nerve disorders such as axonotmesis, neurotmesis or entrapment, the knowledge that sensation is normal, absent or altered and in which distribution it occurs will help in:

- confirming a diagnosis
- recognizing the degree to which reduced sensibility will be affecting the patient's hand function
- providing data for medico-legal reasons.

The most useful assessments to include at this stage are:

- observation
- light touch (Von Frey hair, cotton wool or fingertip), to identify the areas of anaesthesia or altered sensation
- Semmes–Weinstein monofilaments, for assessing the threshold of touch and pressure.

Intermediate stages
During the intermediate stages (patient assessed 6–8 weeks after the initial problem and reassessed at 8-week intervals), any changes that occur following the initial assessment may indicate that:

- nerve regeneration is progressing satisfactorily
- no nerve regeneration (or possibly further nerve degeneration) is occurring; this may need investigation and even possible surgery, and the surgeon should be made aware of these circumstances
- the stage may have been reached when sensory re-education should be commenced.

The tests included are:

- light touch
- monofilaments
- the Tinel test to indicate that regeneration is occurring
- a tuning fork to test vibration sense, one of the earliest sensory modalities to return.

Later stages
The timing of this assessment is dependant on factors such as:

- the distance of the injury from the fingertip
- the age of the patient
- tissue nutrition.

The rate of axon regeneration in a young adult is approximately 1 mm per day, but is faster in children and slower in older people. Normal sensibility is unlikely to return automatically following nerve division due to:

- the inability of axons to regenerate to their original end organs
- the likely formation of a neuroma at a suture line
- the state of the nerve at surgery, the number of suture lines, the degree of stretch applied to the suture, etc.

When there has been some nerve regeneration and sensory return to the tips of the fingers and thumb, it is important to discover how much the quality of sensation (and therefore the function of the hand) has been affected by utilizing:

- timed pick-up tests
- stereognosis tests

- the patient's own subjective test of sensory recovery
- dexterity tests, which are dependant on good sensation (see Dexterity section).

Depending on the above results and on the special sensory needs of the patient (i.e. in the home, at work and for leisure activities), additional sensations may need to be tested and selected for retraining if found particularly deficient. Testing may include:

- two point discrimination
- localization
- vibration sense
- heat and cold
- proprioception
- sweating
- pain as a response to a noxious stimulus such as a pinprick (the concept of pain is discussed in Chapter 3).

Assessment methods
Patients should be masked during testing, as they might be tempted to take a quick look unless prevented from doing so. A screen with a hole for the arms can be used for research purposes, but psychologically this tends to detach the patient from the task. For most practical purposes, a mask or a folded triangular sling will make a suitable and comfortable blindfold.

The following factors should be considered when testing:

1. Noises when handling some objects may give the patient clues as to their nature; this can be eliminated by working on towels
2. The smell of an object, such as soap, may help to reveal its identity; such objects should be excluded from assessments
3. The use of fingers with normal sensation needs to be prevented by strapping them in to the palm or by wearing surgical gloves over those particular fingers.

Sensory assessments are not easy procedures for either patient or therapist, and both must:

- understand the objectives
- be clear on the method of assessment
- be willing to co-operate
- sit in a quiet place for good concentration.

Light touch
This tactile test is used to identify whether the skin is:

- normal
- anaesthetic
- hyperaesthetic
- hypoaesthetic.

The therapist can perform the test quickly and easily by using the light touch of a fingertip, cotton wool or a Von Frey hair to gain a basic sensory picture. It provides an indication of both degree of nerve involvement and stage of recovery. Careful support must be provided under the patient's hand so that the touch does not produce any joint movement. The patient is asked:

- whether or not the touch is normal compared to the equivalent location on the uninjured hand
- if it differs, to describe how – e.g. pins and needles, cotton wool sensation.

The variations in sensation of both the dorsal and volar surfaces are drawn onto a printed outline of a hand using different colours to define anaesthesia, hyperaesthesia, hypoaesthesia and acute hypersensitivity. Areas where light touch is experienced as pain may occur following nerve injury (particularly with brachial plexus involvement); this is known as hyperpathia (see Chapter 8). A legend must be included for this sensory map (Figure 2.50).

Semmes–Weinstein monofilaments

This discrimination test assesses the threshold stimulus necessary for the perception of touch, from light touch to deep pressure (Stanley and Tribuzi, 1992). The filaments were developed in 1962, and consist of a rod or handle onto which is attached a nylon filament at right angles to one end of the rod. The filament will bend at a certain force when applied against the skin. Monofilaments were designed to provide specific measurable thresholds

of force or stress relative to a range of progressive pressures, and are used to assess the threshold stimulus necessary for touch perception from light touch to deep pressure. This allows the course of nerve recovery after injury, or the deterioration of nerve function in compression, to be followed. Much of the research translating the test for use in the hand therapy arena was conducted by Judith Bell-Krotoski, and the original use of 20 filaments has been fine-tuned to the five filaments (the 'mini-kit') that are most predictive of change in functional discrimination (Bell-Krotoski *et al.*, 1995).

The test is performed in a quiet area away from noise and other distractions to allow both therapist and patient to concentrate. The patient should be comfortable with the hand supported, but unable to see the test procedure. By starting in an area of normal sensation, the patient can understand the test and how it will proceed. The therapist works in a distal to proximal direction for assessing the hand.

It is considered correct practice to stabilize the hand on a bed of therapeutic putty. This prevents muscle and joint proprioception and sensation from skin and any other areas of the hand from confusing the test.

Commencing with the lightest, the filament:

- is applied to the skin until it bends into a crescent shape
- is kept perpendicular to the skin
- is held in position for 1.5 seconds
- is not allowed to skid.

The first filament (green – 2.83) correlates to normal sensation. Because it is very light, the filament

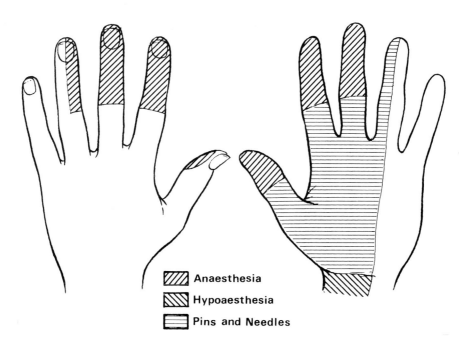

Anaesthesia

Hypoaesthesia

Pins and Needles

Figure 2.50 Progression of sensory recovery following a median nerve lesion at just above wrist level. A legend is used, with different colours denoting the different recovery stages.

should be applied three times to each area before a negative response is recorded. If not felt over the whole area it may be necessary to check the responses of the uninjured hand, as people with thick and callused skin may not feel the green filament but will identify the next (blue – 3.61) as their starting point.

The thicker filaments may be applied once only to each area; however, in practice the therapist will often need to repeat some areas to establish an accurate result, especially around the borders between reduced and intact sensation. Areas not detected with one filament are tested with the next, working from the finest to the thickest and establishing the level at which threshold sensibility is intact. A map is drawn for each filament, shading the response area with the colour matching the filament used, and the sequence of maps gives a clear record of progression. To shorten the time taken over the test, a few precise areas may be selected for testing – for example, following a median nerve lesion the tips of thumb, index and middle fingers together with the base of index finger and the base of thumb may be tested.

The 'mini-kit' found to provide an adequate sensory picture in most circumstances consists of the following sequence of filaments:

Green (2.83)	Normal	Light touch and deep pressure cutaneous sensation within normal limits
Blue (3.61)	Diminished light touch	The patient may have diminished but not absent texture discrimination; this may be indicative of early nerve compression
Purple (4.31)	Diminished protective sensation	At this level the patient may be liable to injury, and is likely to demonstrate absent texture discrimination, impaired stereognosis, impaired temperature discrimination and a tendency to drop things
Red (4.56)	Loss of protective sensation	The patient is liable to injury and will have absent stereognosis, but deep pressure sensation should be present
Red (6.65)	Deep pressure sensation	The patient has deep pressure sensation but only limited deep cutaneous peripheral nerve response, and is unable to feel the 4.56 filament but should be aware of a pinprick
	Untestable	The patient is unable to feel any of the filaments

Care must be taken to avoid giving the patient proprioceptive clues by moving the finger during testing, especially with the larger filaments.

More recently the WEST (Weinstein Enhanced Sensory Test) has been introduced; this is based on the 'mini-kit' and used in the same way. It's filaments are less liable to damage or to slip on the skin, and the kit can be carried in a pocket. When used systematically, the technique gives a clear map of progression of nerve recovery or deterioration, and assists the team in planning therapy or surgical and medical intervention.

Hot and cold discrimination
For patients who work close to heat sources or in cold storage units, it is necessary to assess this function following nerve involvement. Awareness can be assessed using commercially available insulated metal tubes.

For this test:

- water is prepared in insulated mugs at 4.5°C (40°F) and 43°C (110°F)
- two tubes, each with a thermometer on top for monitoring, are placed in each mug and allowed to equilibrate
- the whole hand is assessed randomly
- the patient should be able to identify hot or cold within a few seconds
- the results for heat and cold are recorded on to separate pre-printed sheets with designated testing points.

The response, recorded immediately, can be indicated as present (tick), absent (cross) or inconclusive (?). Use of the same reference locations as for the 0–10 subjective scale (see below) is helpful.

0–10 subjective scale
This scale can be used for self-rating of sensation by the patient, and although subjective can still identify change. The patient rates the sensation in comparison with the unaffected hand on a scale of 0–10, where 0 is no sensation and 10 is normal.

For this test:

- a sensory input is applied by the therapist touching the patient's fingers along the longitudinal axis of the digit, ensuring that only one digital nerve is stimulated at a time
- each finger is tested in six places – along both radial and ulnar borders of the proximal, middle and distal phalanges
- the scores are recorded on a pre-printed hand plan, with a description of the sensation (e.g. pins and needles, woolly, distant, vague, oversensitive, etc.).

Subsequent recordings will indicate a trend, but should not be over-analysed.

Proprioception
Total proprioceptive loss is extremely disabling. It is usually experienced following high combined

median and radial nerve lesions, and patients complain frequently of dropping articles. An ulnar nerve lesion with intrinsic muscle involvement may also severely reduce proprioception. Joint position sense is tested:

- with the patient's eyes closed or blindfolded
- with the patient's finger held on both sides so that there is no increase of pressure in the direction of movement
- using a minimal amount of movement into either flexion or extension
- by asking the patient to state in which direction the movement is occurring.

Proprioception can be tested functionally by using several blocks of wood (or other material) of slightly varying degrees of thickness. The patient should grade these blocks in increasing order of thickness (Figure 2.51).

Tuning fork

This test is suitable for deciding when to commence sensory re-education. It tests vibration sense at 30 cps and 256 cps, and the results at each frequency should be recorded on a hand chart:

- awareness of 30 cps indicates Meissner corpuscle function
- awareness of 256 cps indicates function of the Pacinian corpuscles.

Vibration sense at 30 cps will return before that at 256 cps, and Dellon (1981) suggests that sensory re-education should not be started until the patient has awareness of vibration at 256 cps.

Sweating (skin resistance)

Sweating is a function of the sympathetic nerve supply, and assessment is therefore a useful measure of sympathetic nerve function. Additionally it may offer an indication of the recovery of sensation,

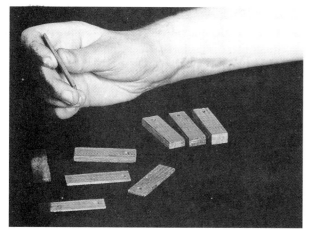

Figure 2.51 Joint position sense may be tested functionally by putting different wooden blocks in order of thickness.

since sweating usually increases as nerve recovery occurs. The electrical resistance of the skin (which depends on its moisture content) can be measured using a commercially available skin resistance meter.

The assessment is quick and objective:

- 28 predetermined points on the volar aspect of the hand are assessed; these are on the radial and ulnar borders of each digit, over each phalanx
- the uninjured hand must always be assessed for comparison
- the results can be easily compared by establishing the ratio of skin resistance values for the injured and uninjured hands.

Sensory recovery is most likely to mirror the sympathetic nerve recovery; however, it is well recorded that this is not always the situation, and in certain case studies there has been full recovery of sweating function without any return of sensation. Recovery of sympathetic and sensory nerve functions have frequently been found not to correlate with one another. Normative data exist (Moberg, 1958; Swain *et al.*, 1985; Wilson, 1985).

Tinel test

The level of sensory nerve regeneration and the site of the injury following a peripheral nerve injury can be estimated by using the Tinel test (Henderson, 1948), but this should be considered only as a most probable and not an infallible indicator.

First, the therapist taps a finger along the course of the nerve in the distal to proximal direction; this is known as the positive or advancing Tinel:

- pins and needles may be experienced by the patient in the sensory distribution of the nerve (often in the tips of the fingers) when the tapping reaches the site of nerve regeneration
- if continued proximally, the tapping may produce an increased discharge of sensation when reaching the site of maximum nerve regeneration
- both distal sites should be measured in millimetres from a suitable bony point or skin crease.

The therapist then taps along the course of the nerve, starting proximal to the estimated site of the lesion and continuing in a distal direction towards the lesion; this is known as the static or negative Tinel:

- the exact site of the lesion is likely to be identified by the intense degree of paraesthesia experienced by the patient, which is caused by some of the sprouting neurones forming a neuroma
- the lesion should be sited and recorded by reference to landmarks in the hand.

The Tinel test must be carried out in the order suggested due to the carry-over of the sensations experienced. The distance between the advancing and static Tinel points and the comparison of strength of the discharges will indicate the degree and rate of nerve regeneration. It should be re-tested every 1–2 months to identify nerve regen-eration. Once the advancing Tinel reaches the fingers, it becomes difficult to locate. It is a test that, if advancing, provides good encouragement for the patient in showing that progress is being made.

Secondary modalities of sensation

Following the recovery of primary sensation the quality of sensation may improve over a period of time, with the return of some degree of sensations such as:

- two point discrimination
- localization
- gnosis.

These modalities should only be tested when primary sensation is present. As in childhood, the acquisition of these judgements involves a learning process. Following nerve injury and regeneration, a furthering of this process is required to remodel the sensory maps in the patient's brain. It is an essential for improvement in the function of the hand, and must therefore be encouraged.

Two point discrimination

This test is used to evaluate the perception of either one or two points of touch. It will indicate recovery in the large myelinated A beta fibres responsible for functional sensibility (Tubiana, 1984; Moberg, 1991). It is sufficient to assess two point discrimination either moving (i.e. the prongs are moved slightly along the skin) or static (i.e. the prongs remain in one place). Dellon (1981) recommends the use of a moving touch. The test has been described by a wide variety of authors.

The therapist should have clear reasons for undertaking this test because:

- it can be time consuming
- it demands considerable concentration from both therapist and patient
- it is open to considerable error and is therefore of no value if precise assessment techniques are not used
- it does not necessarily correlate with functional ability.

Two point discrimination is assessed using a small tool which has prongs at fixed spacings from 2 mm up to 15 mm. The ends of the prongs should be rounded – paperclips should not be used because of the sharp burrs. Only skin known to have light touch perception should be tested.

In this test:

- the patient is not allowed to see the hand
- the prongs should be applied with a constant but minimal force so as not to blanch the skin, and the therapist must ensure that the patient's hand is firmly supported in order to avoid unwanted motion or vibration
- testing should begin with the prongs at a separa-tion of 15 mm or 10 mm
- either one or both prongs are used randomly, and are applied in a longitudinal axis of the digit, along the radial or ulnar border of each phalanx
- the patient is asked whether one or two points has been felt.

The use of either one or two prongs at random increases the reliability of interpretation of the patient's answers.

One of three possible responses is recorded immediately on to a pre-printed sheet:

- a correct response (tick)
- an incorrect response (cross)
- a 'don't know' (?).

The American Society for Surgery of the Hand (1990) recommends that, for the given area under test, seven correct answers out of ten tests are necessary before two point discrimination can be recorded as intact and further testing continued.

Finer discrimination is assessed by progressive reduction of the distance between the prongs. Normal two point discrimination for each location on the hand should be known (Dellon, 1981), and the spacings should not be less than this threshold for each site. For example, only the finger and thumb tips are normally able to discriminate two points at a distance of 2–3 mm; therefore only the tips should be tested at these thresholds. If time is limited, the test can be restricted to flexor tendon zones 1 and 2 of the hand (see Chapter 7). Results should be presented in a clear summary.

Discrimination of 7 mm in the tips of the fingers and thumb indicates that there should be a return of some sensation useful for retraining and for coping with functional activities. The technique indicates change and improvement in the quality of sensa-tion of a patient who has some sensory awareness, and can be valuable where detailed information is needed (e.g. in assessment for research or litigation purposes).

Localization

Localization may be altered following nerve suture, due to crossed re-innervation, when the sensory neurones have been unable to regenerate to their correct end organs. This test is used to discover whether the patient can correctly identify the exact position of touch, and to indicate any need for sensory re-education.

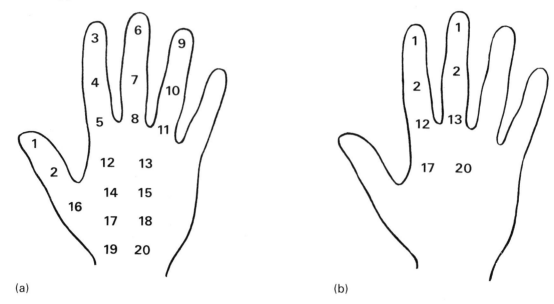

Figure 2.52 (a and b) Localization. Areas are numbered in sequence on the left hand chart. The position of touch that the patient indicates, if incorrect, is referenced from the left hand chart and recorded onto the right hand chart at the therapist's actual point of touch.

Testing can only be carried out in the areas where some sensation has returned. Two identical outline prints of the hand are used. The first is numbered in sequence over the affected sensory area, and the second has any incorrect localization recorded on it using the corresponding numbers (Figure 2.52).

In this test:

- with the patient's eyes closed, a small area of skin is touched briefly but with slight movement; this prevents adaptation of the nerve endings
- the patient is then asked to open the eyes and point to the exact spot that was touched; this is done to prevent any searching around for the spot
- the position indicated, if incorrect, is referenced from the first print and that number is recorded onto the second print (using a different colour of ink) at the point of the therapist's touch (Wynn Parry, 1981)
- many recorded numbers will indicate poor localization, and as it improves the numbers will decrease.

An alternative method of recording localization is as follows:

- using a hand print, a dot is made on the print corresponding to where the patient's hand has been touched
- an arrow is drawn from the dot to the point where the patient feels the stimulus.

In the early stages the patient's hand print may contain many arrows indicating poor localization, but the number of arrows should reduce as local-ization improves. Later, the length of time taken by the patient to localize correctly is recorded on the chart, until recognition time is instantaneous.

Moberg pick-up test

The Moberg pick-up test (Moberg, 1991) is a valuable test that measures the function of a hand with sensory loss (Dellon, 1990). It is quick to perform, and gives both patient and therapist a clear demonstration of functional ability. However, it can only be performed if there is a reasonable return of normal sensation to the fingertips. Fingers with intact sensation should be excluded by strapping them into the palm or holding them in extension.

Test equipment includes:

- 10 small objects that require a precision grip (e.g. coin, paper clip, screw, safety pin etc.)
- a container
- a stop watch.

The objects should be placed alongside the container on the side corresponding to the hand being tested, i.e. on the right side for the right hand.

In this test:

- the patient, watching what he or she is doing, is timed whilst using the uninjured hand to pick up the objects one at a time and place them in the container
- the patient is then timed using the injured hand
- the therapist should record if the thumb has normal sensation and how well the test has been performed, in order to ensure repeatability

- the test is then repeated blindfolded for each hand.

Using the uninjured hand, the patient will normally take twice as long to complete the test when blindfolded. However, the task will take considerably longer for the patient with sensory loss and should be stopped after 5 minutes, making a note of how many objects have been correctly placed. A comparison between the two hands can be obtained for assessments with and without sight.

Where s = standard time (i.e. using the uninjured hand) and t = test time (i.e. using the injured hand),

$$t/s \times 100 = \% \text{ standard time}$$

Using this percentage value for 'with' and 'without sight', it is easy to compare subsequent results; if these percentages are tabulated it is also possible to monitor recovery. The 'with sight' data provide a baseline and show change through improved dexterity, whereas the 'without sight' data should improve as sensation returns. The ratio of the test time without sight to test time with sight should reduce to about 2:1 as recovery takes place.

Moberg said, 'without sensation the hand is blind'. This test clearly demonstrates the functional significance of that statement for the patient.

Stereognosis

This gnosis testing, used for determining whether and how quickly patients can identify objects and materials, should be performed only when the patient has some normal sensation present in the fingertips. If hyperaesthesia is strong, it will be much more difficult to differentiate between objects. The patient should be blindfolded during testing.

In this test:

- a selection of 30 everyday articles (Figure 2.53) is divided into three equal groups of 10 according to size (Table 2.4); the selection can be different for men and women
- the group of larger size objects is used first, and each object is passed for identification
- the patient is asked for as rapid an answer as possible
- the time for correct recognition of each object is recorded in seconds; an incorrect response is noted using a cross, and 'don't knows' by a dash or a question mark
- 30 seconds is allowed per object.
- the patient is not told whether the answer is correct or not
- all the objects in the group must be examined once commenced
- the articles are not shown to the patient at the end of the test, in order to prevent memorizing.

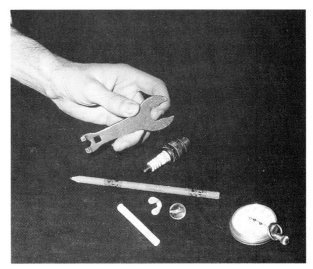

Figure 2.53 Recognition of articles should be timed in seconds.

TABLE 2.4
STEREOGNOSIS IS TESTED USING LARGE, MEDIUM AND SMALL OBJECTS

Large	Medium	Small
Beer mat	Ballpoint pen	Button
Bottle	Bulldog clip	Cork
Electric plug	Can opener	Drawing pin
Handlebar grip	Match box	Key
Nailbrush	Nut and bolt	Marble
Scissors	Pencil	Paper clip
Screw top	Playing card	Eraser
Shuttlecock	Sparking plug	Rubber band
Tennis ball	Spanner	Safety pin
Pocket comb	Tape measure	Screw hook

If successful in identifying most (70 per cent) of the large objects, the patient is next tested with the medium articles; if successful again, with the small articles. If, however, the therapist quickly realizes that the patient is able to name none or only a few of the objects, the test should be delayed. The large number of objects included reduces the patient's opportunity to memorize them. For the same reason, testing should be repeated at not less than 4–6 weekly intervals.

Sensory evaluation of activity

Sensory feedback in the hand is essential for efficient function, so some test of function is an important part of sensory evaluation (Jerosch-Herold, 1993). The test should include selected bilateral activities of daily living that can be timed and also performed without looking (or in the dark). Suitable activities include:

• tying and untying shoe laces
• putting on and taking off a pair of gloves
• tying a tie
• doing up and undoing the buttons on a shirt
• screwing and unscrewing the lid of a jar
• taking coins out of a purse.

The tests should be standardized as far as possible. In this test:

• the patient first performs the test with sight to ensure that he or she is familiar with the task and is capable of performing it
• the task is timed
• the patient is then asked to repeat the test without looking, and is again timed.

The results can be analysed to see the trend in recovery.

This type of functional assessment will help to highlight the problems faced by patients whose jobs involve working in situations where they are unable to see their hands, e.g. car mechanics.

DEXTERITY

Dexterity is the ability to manoeuvre and manipulate objects easily using a variety of types and sequences of grip. The normal hand is able to move smoothly from one pattern of grip to another, e.g. from lateral pinch to pulp-to-pulp pinch. Objects can be manipulated, rotated and aligned into position without being dropped or needing to be put down and picked up again. Dexterity is also the ability to pick up or collect a number of objects and specifically sort and select them one at a time whilst still managing to hold the remainder in the hand. Normal sensation and normal function of the intrinsic muscles are essential for good dexterity, which can show considerable variation between individuals.

It may be necessary to assess dexterity following hand trauma, but it is not usually appropriate to do so in the early stages of rehabilitation when hand function is poor; this could be a frustrating and demoralizing experience for the patient. In the later stages of rehabilitation it can help to measure progress, particularly when assessed in relation to speed. It should not be measured more frequently than every 3–4 weeks, as improvement is unlikely to occur more rapidly.

Assessment of dexterity, measured against standardized norms, may be valuable:

• in pre- and post-operative assessments of tendon transfers in the hand
• for work assessment
• in the preparation of legal reports.

There are a number of commercially available dexterity tests including some designed for candidate selection in the electronics industry, which may be difficult to complete within the standardized times even by an uninjured person. All tests are timed and must be executed exactly as described, including the standardized verbal instructions to the patient. Unless procedures are followed accurately, these norms cannot be used to analyse the patient's results.

Useful tests for the assessment of dexterity include the following.

1. The Rolyan nine-hole peg test. This simple test involves placing nine smooth pegs one at a time into a board whilst being timed. It is widely used in hand therapy research for evaluating outcomes.
2. The grooved peg test. This task demands dexterity, but is possible for most patients to complete following hand injury. Twenty-five grooved pegs are fitted into a board with randomly positioned slots, and each peg (with a round and a flat side) must be manipulated and rotated into correct alignment. The patient is timed, and the number of dropped pegs is noted. This test is of value for dexterity assessment in a wide range of patients.
3. The Minnesota manual dexterity test. This test measures hand–eye co-ordination, and is a simple and rapid procedure. There is no need for complex dexterity and precision. Two independent aspects of the test use the same equipment, i.e. blocks (approximately the size of large draughts pieces) and a slotted board.
   • The placing test is for the affected hand, and involves moving blocks from a designated space into the slotted board; four timed attempts are needed to complete the test.
   • The turning test is performed bilaterally, and involves taking the pieces out of the slots one at a time and turning them over using one hand only. They are replaced in to the board with the other hand. The dominant and non-dominant hands lead alternately, and four timed attempts are needed to complete the test.
4. The O'Connor finger dexterity test. This test utilizes a board with 100 holes, each large enough to hold three pins. The patient, using one hand only, picks up three pins at a time and places them in a hole until the whole board is filled. A pre-determined sequence is used and the test is timed. A high level of dexterity and speed is demanded in order to achieve acceptable test results, measured against the standardized norms. It is suitable:
   • for patients in the late stage of rehabilitation
   • when specific detailed assessment of sensation is needed, e.g. for a legal report.

5. The O'Connor tweezer dexterity test. This test has similar uses to that mentioned above. It involves filling a board of 100 holes, each large enough to hold one pin. The patient picks up one pin at a time from a tray, lightly using the tweezers and allowing the pin to swing into the vertical position ready to place in to the hole. The patient is timed on filling the board completely. Normal administration time for the test totals 8–10 minutes.

FUNCTIONAL ASSESSMENT

The climax of the hand assessment is the test of function – the ability to use the hand and the impact that the injury may have on lifestyle are both vital factors for the patient. Aspects such as range of movement, power and sensation do not in themselves reflect true functional ability, since deformity does not always lead to dysfunction. For example, a fused joint, although having total loss of movement, may provide power through its painless stability.

Hand function chart

The function chart forms the basis for analysing how the patient uses the hand and identifies his or her own priority problems. It contains a list of everyday activities (Table 2.5), and the patient is required to rate these tasks for both right and left

TABLE 2.5
Hand function assessment chart (hand trauma)

Patient name: A. N. Other
Date: xx/xx/xx (1 year post-repair)
R = right, L = left

Difficulties list   Reason

Daily activities	E	F	D	I	1	2	3	4	5	6	7	8	9	10	11
Buttons			R			✓	✓								
Zips (e.g. trousers, coat)		R					✓								
Shoelaces			R			✓	✓								
Socks	R														
Tie		R						✓							
Using the toilet	R														
Taps	R														
Wringing out flannel	R														
Using soap/washing	R														
Cleaning teeth	R														
Getting in/out bath	R														
Using cutlery		R				✓									
Cutting bread/meat			R			✓	✓								
Unscrewing lids		R				✓									
Tin opener		R				✓									
Lifting saucepan		R				✓									
Lifting/pouring kettle	R														
Opening packets/cartons		R				✓	✓	✓							
Electric plugs	R														
Using door key	R														
Using car key	R														
Car hand brake	*	*	*	*											
Driving	R														
Handling money			R				✓	✓							
Scissors		R				✓									
Other (specify)															
Total	12	8	4	0	–	9	6	3	–	–	–	–	–	–	–

E = easy, F = fair, D = difficult, I = impossible
Not applicable – LH activity,

TABLE 2.6
PROBLEM INDEX AND AND DIFFICULTIES LIST

1   Loss of active range of movement
2   Decreased strength
3   Altered sensation
4   Loss of dexterity
5   Cold intolerance
6   Loss of digit length
7   Scarring
8   Pain
9   Machine phobia
10 Oedema
11 Other – loss of speed

TABLE 2.7
PRIORITY PROBLEM LIST

1   Loss of strength
2   Loss of sensation in median nerve distribution
3   Loss of dexterity due to poor sensation

hands as easy, fair, difficult or impossible. R and L denote the hands used, and the results are recorded in the appropriate score box.

Any tasks that are difficult or impossible are analysed by patient and therapist together. The reason for the difficulty is identified from a standard index (Table 2.6) and indicated by a tick in the numbered 'reasons' boxes. Some activities may be difficult for a single reason, but often the causes are multiple and each cause should be ticked.

The therapist totals the number of activities that are graded easy, fair, difficult, or impossible. The 'reasons' chart is also totalled, adding the number of ticks in each column. Reasons for difficulty are then placed in priority order on a report sheet separate to the hand function chart, listing the reasons in descending order with the highest score first. This creates the priority problem list (Table 2.7).

Particular points may need clarification, and the therapist should make specific comments. If the verbal rating appears not to give an accurate account of the activity, a written observation is also necessary.

Two different hand function charts should be available for patients who have rheumatoid arthritis (see Chapters 13–15) and those who have suffered trauma or other disorders. Charts for activities and the 'reasons' for difficulties need to be different for both patient groups. The employment needs and specific work tasks (Tables 2.8, 2.9) must also be considered when assessing the trauma patient, besides activities of daily living.

The hand function chart should also be used for evaluating outcomes of medication, surgery and therapy.

Functional ability remains for the patient the most important measure of the outcome of the treatment process.

Case history
With regard to the right-handed 24-year-old plumber referred to earlier (Tables 2.1, 2.8 and 2.9):

- he had divided his median nerve, palmaris longus and flexor digitorum superficialis tendons to all fingers, but retained function of the thenar muscles
- all the divided structures were repaired and he underwent rehabilitation
- at 1 year post-repair, he returned for re-assessment with the therapist and surgeon
- he had regained full tendon function.

At 1 year:

- all left-hand activities were of normal efficiency (not recorded)
- of the right-hand tasks, 12 were easy, eight were fair, four were difficult and none were impossible.

The tasks graded difficult and impossible were analysed (some having multiple reasons) and the reasons summed up by column. Of these tasks:

- eight were difficult due to reason 2 (decreased strength)
- six were difficult due to reason 3 (altered sensation)
- three were difficult due to reason 4 (loss of dexterity).

The ranking of these reasons formed the priority problem list (Table 2.9) and led to the conclusions below. Other supporting information should be included in the analysis; i.e. loss of speed and cold intolerance both contributed to problems with employment.

Assessment conclusion:

- the chart highlighted the functional problems, mostly relating to sensory loss and weakness (not severe)
- the patient was encouraged to begin sensory re-education
- no further treatment was indicated
- clinic follow-up with surgeon and therapist was organized for 6 months' time.

The hand function chart described above is illustrative only, and must be tailored broadly to the clinical condition but on an individual basis. A patient with rheumatoid arthritis will require a different chart from one who has suffered trauma, as 'activities' and 'reasons' will be different.

TABLE 2.8
EMPLOYMENT ASSESSMENT CHART

Patient name: A. N. Other

Date: xx/xx/xx (1 year post-repair)

Job description: Plumber/heating engineer. Fitting heating systems; using ladders; lifting (e.g. boilers); use of spanners and screwdrivers; needs to work in awkward positions without seeing the task.

	E	F	D	I	1	2	3	4	5	6	7	8	9	10	11
Lifting (specify type of load and weight															
Boiler @ 50 kg			R			✓									
Carrying (specify) ladders		R				✓									
Tools:															
Hammer			R			✓									
Screwdriver			R			✓	✓	✓							✓
Saw															
Spanners			R			✓	✓	✓							✓
Blowlamp			R			✓									
Use of machinery (specify)															
Climbing ladders		R				✓	✓								
Working at speed			R			✓	✓	✓							
Working in a cold environment.			R						✓						
Writing (note quality and speed)		R				✓	✓								
Keyboard skills															
Other:															
Working blind				R		✓									
Hobbies (specify):															
Golf			R			✓									

TABLE 2.9
PRIORITY PROBLEM LIST

1 Loss of strength
2 Loss of sensation in median nerve distribution
3 Loss of dexterity due to poor sensation
4 Loss of speed
5 Cold intolerance

The ADL page will probably be suitable for most patients, but the employment form must be designed specifically. The scores from the ADL chart must only be used to measure improvement in a given patient and not for inter-patient comparison.

Hand function tests

Hand function may also be tested by asking the patient to undertake a series of practical tasks. These differ from dexterity tests, as the selection of activities is orientated to everyday functions rather than abstract tasks. The hand function tests are often timed and used to analyse patterns of grip and form a problem index (Figure 2.58 b). They are particularly useful in assessment situations where the therapist has not had the opportunity to observe the patient using the hand – for example, in the case of an outpatient assessment to decide on further medical and surgical management of the hand. The hand function test may be used to analyse problems and evaluate treatment outcomes.

There are many versions of hand function tests. Some of these are commercially available, but many have to be constructed to match the description in the literature. It is helpful for the therapist to have test material commercially prepared, particularly if it is available with standardized times against which to analyse the performance of the patient; this saves valuable time. Two tests, the Jebsen and the Sollerman, are described below.

The Jebsen hand function test consists of seven sub-tests:

1. Writing
2. Card turning
3. Picking up small objects (paper clips, bottle caps and coins)
4. Simulated feeding – picking up kidney beans with a teaspoon
5. Picking up wooden draughts pieces
6. Picking up empty tin cans
7. Picking up full tin cans.

Each test is timed, and there are published standardized times against which to evaluate the performance of the patient (Jebsen *et al.*, 1969). The Jebsen hand function test has been widely used to evaluate hand function in a number of medical and surgical conditions.

The Sollerman hand function test consists of 20 tasks covering activities of daily living, such as turning a key and a door handle; undoing zips, nuts and bolts and buttons; and handling a knife and fork and water jug. The test enables the therapist to analyse the patterns of hand grip through structured observation as well as to record the time taken, with the results utilized to give a score. The test is available commercially but currently is not supplied with standardized times.

PSYCHOLOGICAL ASSESSMENT

The psychological effects of hand impairment are considerable and must therefore be given serious consideration in both assessment and treatment. There are a number of useful psychological assessments which can be used by therapists, e.g. the Hospital and Anxiety Depression Scale (HAD) and the Revised Impact of Event Scale. The assessment of phobias following injury is of particular importance, as the phobia is likely to be focused around the tool that caused the injury (e.g. circular saw, industrial machinery, knife, etc.). If the problem is not recognized and treated at an early stage, it can become a genuine barrier to re-employment.

It has been suggested that patients with a compensation claim pending may be slow to respond to treatment in order to substantiate their claim. Whilst this may occur in a few isolated cases, there is no evidence to support it generally. The therapist should therefore be extremely cautious in making any comment of this nature until clear evidence of this behaviour is available.

Psychological assessment is dealt with further in Chapter 3.

WORK ASSESSMENT

Hand trauma can have a severe impact on the patient's employability, resulting in considerable financial and psychological problems. It is very important to enable the patient to return to work as soon as possible, as prolonged time off work may lead to redundancy, especially during a period of high unemployment and consequent job insecurity. For those already unemployed there is the added worry that a serious hand condition may exclude them from the open employment market.

The therapist should obtain details concerning:

- the patient's job
- the name and address of the employer
- whether or not the job is still available
- the terms and conditions of the employment (e.g. sickness payment, sick leave allowed, etc.).

If the injury occurred at work, it should be determined whether the Health and Safety Executive (HSE) have been called in to investigate the circumstances.

The job description

A comprehensive job description should be obtained from the patient at the start of the rehabilitation phase. This not only assists in the planning of treatment, but also reinforces to the patient that eventual re-employment is the long-term aim. The following details about employment should be obtained.

1. General details:
   - job title and basic description of job; whether the work is unskilled, semi-skilled or skilled; whether it is repetitive or flexible
   - name, address and telephone number of the employer, and a named point of contact (e.g. foreman)
   - conditions of employment, including wages, bonus schemes, seasonal variations in pay
   - the financial situation, benefits being received, special insurances
   - length of service with current employer
   - hours of working, e.g. shift work, rosters, overtime requirements, rest periods, whether singleton or member of a team
   - patient's qualifications and any special skills
   - specific skills and requirements of the job, including the need to drive
   - environment of the job, e.g. working in a cold store, all weather working, substances to which the patient is exposed

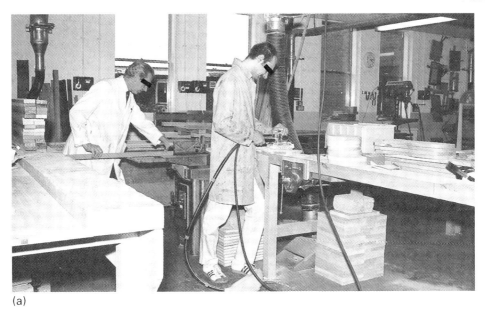

(a)

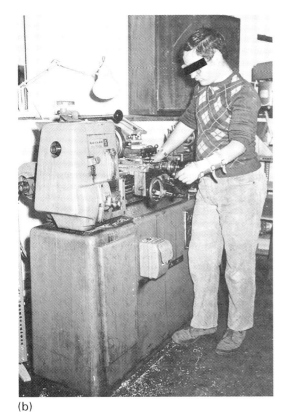

(b)

Figure 2.54 Work assessments in a rehabilitation workshop.

- Health and Safety information about the working environment, e.g. company policy, accident record, protective equipment provided
- level of supervision received; any systems for quality assurance
- Trades Union affiliation, advice and involvement.

2. Physical details:
   - specific movements and muscle power required, e.g. lifting, bending, crawling, working in awkward postures
   - dexterity and hand–eye co-ordination requirements
   - sensory requirements, e.g. need to work with the hand blind
   - speed and accuracy
   - tools, machinery and materials to be used (Figure 2.54).

It should be possible in the majority of cases to simulate both the physical and cognitive demands of the patient's job within the occupational therapy and rehabilitation workshop areas. However, if it is not possible or too difficult to appreciate fully what the job involves, it will be necessary for therapist and patient to undertake a work visit. A work visit may also be necessary towards the end of the rehabilitation period if the job needs to be adapted or changed. The therapist then acts as a mediator between patient and employer to negotiate a return to some satisfactory form of employment.

A work visit must always be organized with the full consent of:

- the patient
- the employer
- the direct line manager
- the Trades Union representative if relevant.

In the event of impending or actual court action from the Health and Safety Executive, the therapist should consider carefully whether a work visit is appropriate. Any visit should be thoroughly documented and filed as part of the POMR database, with copies of any report and action plan being given to both patient and employer.

If the patient is unlikely or unable to return to his original employment, the work assessment will need to be extended to include the following information about the patient:

- an in-depth educational and employment work history in chronological order
- cognitive abilities, e.g. numeracy, literacy, level of intelligence, reasoning abilities, use of initiative and problem-solving skills
- leadership qualities
- social skills
- potential to learn, e.g. scope for retraining.

Disability Employment Advisor (DEA)

The rehabilitation team should decide whether it is necessary to request the services of the advisor, who is based at the local Job Centre and will accept a referral either directly from the patient or from the rehabilitation team. The advisor may be able to help the patient to return to work in the original job by:

- funding the special equipment now necessary for the patient to perform the job
- offering the employer help and financial incentives, in the form of a grant, to compensate for any shortfall in performance
- offering the patient access to further assessment and retraining schemes.

ESTABLISHING A PROBLEM LIST

A comprehensive assessment of the patient and the hand injury enables the therapist and rehabilitation team to establish the patient's problem list using:

- background medical information
- all the assessments considered in this chapter, including the problem index (see Table 2.6)
- a psychological assessment (if considered advantageous).

The priority problem list (Table 2.7) will be the basis upon which treatment is planned. Each problem should be numbered and recorded in the patient's POMR along with the date on which it is identified. The date on which each problem is then resolved should also be noted (see Table 2.1).

The list is likely to change during the rehabilitation period, some problems being resolved and new ones being identified. Ongoing assessment will ensure accurate evaluation of the treatment programme and allow timely modification of treatment aims.

The therapist has the following considerations and options in treatment planning once the list has been determined:

1. Begin (or continue) to treat each problem through appropriate and specific occupational therapy and physiotherapy. Priority should be given to:
   - reduction of oedema
   - management of pain
   - improvement in hand function.
2. Attempt to find practical solutions to the patient's functional problems.
3. Refer the patient, if necessary, for treatment of any psychological problems.
4. Remediate social and employment problems – involving social work colleagues as appropriate.
5. Contact medical/surgical colleagues if their intervention is indicated.
6. Continue to monitor the problems through re-assessment, if therapy intervention is not indicated for any specific problem.
7. Discharge the patient from treatment if further intervention is not required.

Intensive early treatment over a short period of time can be more effective than brief treatment over a much longer time span, and this must be taken into account when planning the treatment programme. Full-time rehabilitation may make all the difference between a poor result and an efficiently functioning hand.

REFERENCES

American Academy of Orthopaedic Surgeons (1974). *Joint Measurement and Recording.* Churchill Livingstone.
American Society for Surgery of the Hand (1990). *The Hand, Examination and Diagnosis,* 3rd edn, pp. 43. Churchill Livingstone.
Bell-Krotoski, J., Fess, E., Figarola, J. *et al.* (1995). Threshold detection and Semmes–Weinstein monofilaments. *J. Hand Ther.,* **8(2)**, 155–62.
Bromley, A. I. (1978). The patient care audit. *Physio,* **69**, 270–1.
Dellon, A. L. (1981). *Evaluation of Sensibility and Re-education of Sensation in the Hand.* Williams & Wilkins.
Dellon, A. L. (1990). The sensational contribution of Erik Moberg. *J. Hand Surg.,* **15B(1)**, 14–24.
Ellis, B. and Bruton, A. (1998).Clinical assessment of the hand – a review of joint angle measures. *J. Hand Ther.,* **3B**, 5–8.
Gilbertson, L. and Barber-Lomax, S. (1994). Power and pinch grip strength recorded using the hand-held Jamar Dynamometer and B+L Hydraulic Pinch Gauge. British normative data for adults. *Br. J. Occ. Ther.,* **57(12)**, 483–8.
Henderson, W. R. (1948). Clinical assessment of peripheral nerve injuries. Tinel's test. *Lancet,* **2**, 801.
Jebsen, R. H., Taylor, N., Triegchmann, R. B. *et al.* (1969). An objective and standardised test of hand function. *Arch. Phys. Med. Rehabil.,* **50**, 311.
Jerosch-Herold, C. (1993). Measuring outcome in median nerve injuries. *J. Hand Surg.,* **18B(5)**, 624–8.
Kaltenborn, F. M. (1980). *Mobilisation of the Extremity Joints.* Olaf Norlis.

Kapandji, I. A. (1992).Clinical evaluation of the thumb's opposition. *J. Hand Ther.*, **2,** 102–6.

Kleinert, H. E., Kutz, J. E., Atasoy, E. *et al.* (1973). Primary repair of flexor tendons. *Orth. Clin. North Am.*, **4(4)**.

Maitland, G. D. (1991). *Peripheral Manipulation*, 3rd edn. Butterworth Heinemann.

Mathiowetz, V., Kashman, N., Volland, G. *et al.* (1985). Grip and pinch strength: normative data for adults. *Arch. Phys. Med. Rehabil.*, **66,** 69–74.

Medical Research Council (1976). *Aids to the Examination of the Peripheral Nervous System*. HMSO.

Moberg, E. (1958). Objective methods for determining the functional value of sensibility in the hand. *J. Bone Joint Surg.*, **40B(3)**, 454–76.

Moberg, E. (1991) The unsolved problem – how to test functional value of hand sensibility. *J. Hand Ther.*, **4(3)**, 105–110.

Richardson, J. (1979). Problem-orientated medical records and care in North America. *Physio*, **65**, 184–5.

Strickland, J. W. (1980). Digital function following tendon repair in zone 2: a comparison of immobilisation and controlled passive motion techniques. *J. Hand Surg.*, **5(6)**, 537–43.

Strickland, J. W. (1989). Biological rationale, clinical application and results of early motion following flexor tendon repair. *J. Hand Ther.*, **2(2)**, 71–82.

Swain, I. D., Wilson, G. R. and Crook, S. C. (1985). A simple method of measuring the electrical resistance of the skin. *J. Hand Surg.*, **10B(3)**, 319–23.

Tann, A. M. (1992). Sensibility testing. In: *Concepts in Hand Rehabilitation* (B. Stanley and S. Tribuzi, eds.), pp. 104–5. F. A. Davis.

Tubiana, R. (1984). Sensibility evaluation. In: *Examination of the Hand and Upper Limb* (R. Tubiana, ed.), pp. 177–9. W.B. Saunders.

van Velze, C. A., Kleuver, I., van der Merwe, C. A. and Mennen, U. (1991). The difference in volume of dominant and nondominant hand. *J. Hand Ther.*, **4(1)**, 6–9.

Waylett-Rendall, J. and Seibly, D. S. (1991). A study of the accuracy of a commercially availably volumeter. *J. Hand Ther.*, **4(1)**, 10–13.

Wilson, G. R. (1985). A simple device for the objective evaluation of peripheral nerve injuries. *J. Hand Surg.*, **10B(3)**, 324–30.

Wynn Parry, C. B. (1981). *Rehabilitation of the Hand*. Butterworths.

FURTHER READING

Barr, N. and Swan, D. (1988). *The Hand: Principles and Techniques of Splinting*. Butterworths.

Bell-Krotoski, J. (1999). Research in clinical testing – a personal journey. *Br. J. Hand Ther.*, **4(1),** 13–22.

Boscheinen-Morrin, J., Davey, V. and Connolly, W. B. (1992). *The Hand: Fundamentals of Therapy*. Butterworth-Heinemann.

Curtin, M. (1994) Development of a tetraplegic hand assessment and splinting protocol. *Paraplegia*, **32,** 159–69.

Jacobson, C. and Sperling, L. (1976). Classification of the hand grip. *J. Occ. Med.*, **18(6),** 395–8.

Jones, L. A. (1989). The assessment of hand function: a critical review of techniques. *J. Hand Surg.*, **14A(2)**.

Kapandji, I. A. (1982). *The Physiology of the Joints: Upper Limb*, Vol.1., 2nd edn. Churchill Livingstone.

Lacote, M. (1987). *Clinical Evaluation of Muscle Function*. Churchill Livingstone.

Macey, A. C. and Burke, F. D. (1995). Outcome of hand surgery. *J. Hand Surg.*, **20B(6)**.

Mathiowetz, V. (1990). Effects of three trials of grip and pinch strength measurements. *J. Hand Ther.*, **3,** 195.

Melvin, J. L. (1995). *Rheumatic Disease in Occupational Therapy*. F. A. Davis.

O'Neill, G. (1995). The development of a standardised assessment of hand function. *Br. J. Occ. Ther.*, **58(11),** 477–80.

Palmer, P. J. (1989). Sensory re-education in the hand following nerve repair using guidelines based on neurophysiological function. *Br. J. Occ. Ther.*, **52(11),** 421–8.

Sollerman, C. and Sperling, L. (1978). Evaluation of ADL function – especially hand function. *Scand. J. Rehabil. Med.*, **10,** 139–45.

Sperling, L. and Sollerman, C. (1977). The grip pattern of the healthy hand during eating. *Scand. J. Rehabil. Med.*, **9,** 115–21.

Tubiana, R. (1989) *Examination of the Hand and Upper Limb*. W. B. Saunders.

Tubiana, R., Thomine, J. M. and Mackin, E. (1996). *Examination of the Hand and Wrist*. Martin Dunitz.

Waylett-Rendall, J. (1998). Sensibility evaluation and rehabilitation. *Orth. Clin. North Am.*, **19(1)**.

Weinstein, S. (1993). Fifty years of somatosensory research. *J. Hand Ther.*, **6(1),** 11–22.

3 Psychosocial aspects of hand therapy

Lynn Cheshire with Maerian A. van der Heijden-de Jong

The author is most grateful for substantial help with this chapter from Maerian A. van der Heijden-de Jong, whose contributions appear on a tinted background.

INTRODUCTION

Because hand therapists have frequent and sometimes prolonged contact with the patient, they may take on the responsibility of 'case managers' and are in a position to ensure that patients are receiving the necessary care and services. They must therefore understand the relevant psychosocial factors inherent in hand rehabilitation in general, as well as in their specific interventions as hand therapists.

Hand trauma, as opposed to other conditions of the hand, is the main focus of this chapter. However, it should not be forgotten that surgery, despite the patient's consent, is also an insult to the human organism, and can cause many of the elements of shock that occur following a traumatic accident. Until the 1980s, little was written or researched concerning the psychosocial aspects of hand injury; however, there is now more evidence on which to base assessment and treatment. This chapter attempts to present a salient selection of considerations for the practice of hand therapy and for further study, with particular emphasis on the importance of multidisciplinary teamwork and the involvement of the clinical psychologist.

THE FUNCTIONS, VALUES AND SIGNIFICANCE OF THE HUMAN HAND

Apart from its physical function, the psychological significance of the hand and its meaning to the human being is more the subject of philosophy, literature and art than of scientific psychological investigation. Much work has been done in anthropology, because the type of hand was pivotal to the classification of the hominid or prehistoric man. More precisely, it can be stated that the two things that elevate humans above the ape are the size and complexity of the brain, and the ability to perform a fine manipulative pinch. The hand is therefore peculiarly and outstandingly human. It is also dependent on the brain, and conversely the brain is dependent upon the hand. The human hand has been aptly described as 'the servant of the brain' (Napier, 1966) and 'the cutting edge of the mind'

(Bronowski, 1973). Neurologically, the brain and the hand have a vast and highly developed network of connections – literally a human 'cyber-highway' of their own.

The hand is both a receptor and an executor. Sight, hearing and sensory appreciation from the hand form the major trio of reception; with speech, the hand forms the duo of expression. Upper limb function and speech are the human being's most powerful executive 'tools'. The hand is also the main organ of gesture, and gesture is important not only in communication but also in the development of speech and intellectual function. Tubiana (1984) wrote that:

> Gestures with the hand have helped shape language by contributing a rhythm, by mimicking the oratorical action. The hand, along with speech, mirrors our emotions.

The hand is so many things. It is a feeler, shaper, sculptor, gripper, stabilizer, manipulator, giver, taker, caresser, soother, welcomer, protector, aggressor, expresser and signaller. Each of these words conveys a combination of physical, psychological and social values, and graphically illustrates the hand's significance and its many roles.

The hand is a strong component of a person's self-image, supposedly stronger than that of the face. The rationale supporting this hypothesis begins with the development of hand–eye coordination. The baby gradually comes to recognize that the little hand that is so frequently present in his field of vision is a part of himself, part of his identity and self-concept. This hand can feel, grasp, and begin to exercise the power of manipulation on his small world. In conjunction with the baby's other primary touch receptor, the mouth, his hand is busy building a personal bank of perceptual information in a unique combination of intimate personal and emotional detail (Figure 3.1).

That part of our self-image that is embodied by the hand is largely subconscious. Although the hand is constantly in our field of vision, it is not actually the focus of our sight and our attention as we touch, grasp or feel. This therefore makes it difficult for us to understand that it is present in the psyche and is integral to our self-concept and image. Interestingly, however, we use the phrase 'I know it like the back of my hand'.

A large proportion of the cortex of the brain is dedicated to the hands, and 80 per cent of the motor cortex is devoted to the function of the upper limb and the mouth (Tubiana, 1984). When injury or dysfunction of the hand occurs it affects a large proportion of the patient's neurological activity and, consequently, their psychological state. The human being is essentially an excitable organism, and has a considerable need for input from a multitude of stimuli to maintain healthy vivacity of the nervous system and, reciprocally, the health of

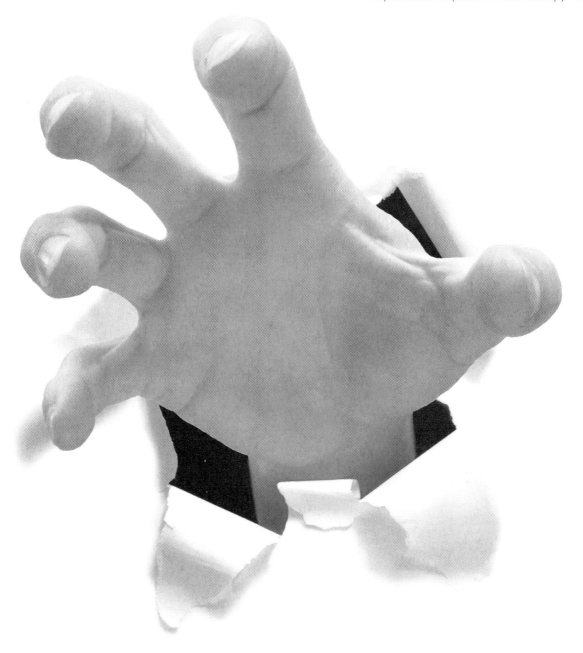

THE POWER OF THE
POSTER
2 APRIL TO 26 JULY 1998

The Victoria and Albert Museum

0800 801 964

Exhibition sponsored by The Maiden Group, JCDecaux, Mills & Allen and More Group

Figure 3.1   The power of the poster – or is it the power of the hand? (With kind permission from the V&A Picture Library and Golley Slater Brooker.)

the other systems and organs. It is well known that isolation, lack of human or animal contact and lack of sound and light soon have serious detrimental effects. The hand is a major receptor and activator of stimuli, and when it is out of action the normal level of stimulus is greatly reduced. The patient then suffers neurological and psychological deprivation, which may lead to depression, anxiety and varying psychosomatic symptoms.

HAND DYSFUNCTION – THE PSYCHOLOGICAL EFFECTS

The human equilibrium consists of a somatic, a social and a psychological component. A disruption of any one of these components will upset their dynamic balance and therefore have consequences for the other components. Losing one's job may lead to somatic complaints, like a headache or high blood pressure, but also to psychological complaints such as depression. The term 'psychosomatic complaint' clearly indicates the link between psychological and somatic components. In the case of a traumatic hand injury (an assault on the somatic component), psychological and social assessment should be included as well as the obvious physical, somatic diagnosis. The treatment of hand injury should therefore consist of a multidisciplinary approach if the aim is to restore all the affected components of the individual patient.

Some aspects of hand dysfunction

The way in which a person copes with the disruption of a hand injury varies between individuals. It depends on a number of aspects, and the most important of these will be discussed here.

The severity of the injury
A relatively mild injury with good prognosis and the expectation of early recovery, will be easier to cope with than a serious injury in which hand function is severely compromised and therapy and reconstructive surgery may be prolonged. In general, it can be said that the greater the degree of function lost, the more likely it is that there will be a loss of equilibrium. Losing the tip of the little finger may be relatively insignificant to a schoolteacher, but insuperable to a professional pianist.

Many patients suffer doubts and anxieties because they feel they are making too much fuss. The disruption to their life appears to be out of proportion to the size of their hand injury, particularly to the size of the exterior wound. 'It's only your little finger' is the kind of remark they find upsetting and diminishing, as their level of distress and disability has not been recognized. Had the same size of wound been on their face (a part of our more conscious self-image), they would have received much greater sympathy. Some patients find it helpful to see a diagrammatic representation (a 'homunculus' is useful) of the large proportion of the cortex of the brain that is dedicated to the hand and to this so-called 'little' finger (Figure 3.2). Perceived severity, however, is not always proportional to the physical extent of the injury, and is often highly subjective. It is important therefore to assess the patient's perception of severity, and to take appropriate consideration and action.

Personality traits
A well developed, adequately functioning person, who has a wide repertoire of adaptabilities, will be more able to handle the disruption of trauma than someone who is less resilient and does not possess these qualities. Flexibility and adaptability are required when changes in life occur.

Previous traumatic experiences
Somatic, psychological and social traumas may have seriously undermined the patient's resilience. The trauma that led to the current hand injury may be one too many, 'the last straw'. The person who has met the fewest setbacks in life seems better off and at an advantage. It has been shown that hand injury patients who have suffered fewer previous problems experience a lower rate of difficulty and consequently need less support. Complications in treatment may therefore be avoided by assessment of the previous history of adverse events in the patient's life (Johnson, 1993).

Coping skills
What are the patient's skills in coping with setbacks and traumas in general? If the patient is emotionally unable to assimilate a trauma, in particular the current trauma, then their rehabilitation may be seriously hampered. An emotionally unassimilated trauma produces a chronic stress situation, and this may ultimately lead to post-traumatic stress disorder requiring intensive psychotherapy. The emotional impact of the current trauma may also rise dramatically because previously unassimilated traumas are being reactivated.

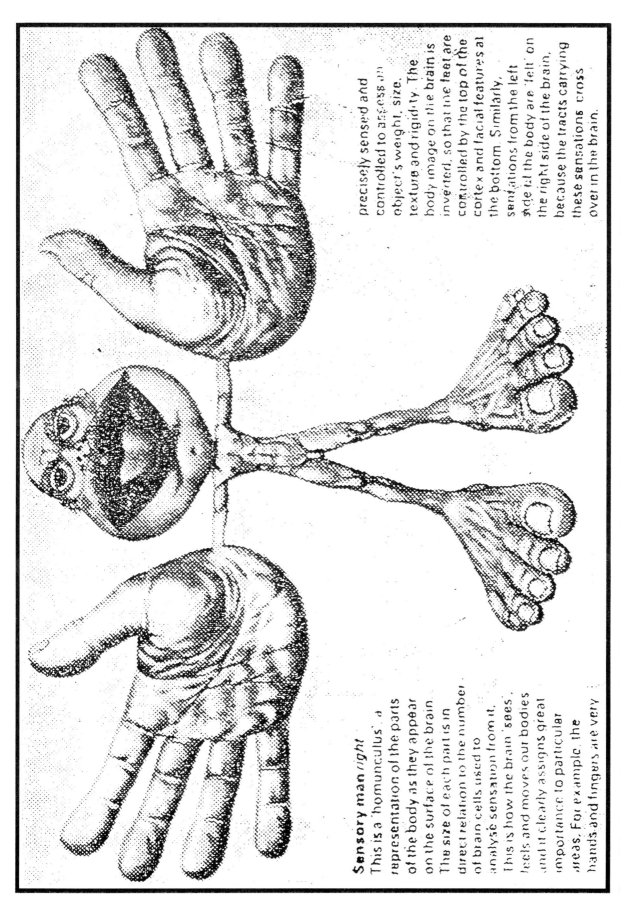

Sensory man *right*
This is a 'homunculus', a representation of the parts of the body as they appear on the surface of the brain. The size of each part is in direct relation to the number of brain cells used to analyse sensation from it. This is how the brain 'sees', feels and moves our bodies and it clearly assigns great importance to particular areas. For example, the hands and fingers are very

precisely sensed and controlled to assess an object's weight, size, texture and rigidity. The body image on the brain is inverted, so that the feet are controlled by the top of the cortex and facial features at the bottom. Similarly, sensations from the left side of the body are 'felt' on the right side of the brain, because the tracts carrying these sensations cross over in the brain.

Figure 3.2 Homunculus representation of the sensory cortex of the brain demonstrating the relative significance of the hand.

Loss of hand function, whether complete or partial, temporary or permanent, will in most cases lead to a mourning process in which various stages have to be worked through (see Loss, below). Most people have their own coping strategies, whether 'talking it out' or going away quietly and processing a problem mentally. It is normal to have crises in life, and it is also normal to be able to cope in some way.

Counselling may therefore be inappropriate. In the last few years there has been much re-examination of crisis intervention, particularly for 'disasters' involving a number of people. It is now thought that support should be offered rather than given, and that the 'victim' should be allowed more control of the situation. This would seem to be a much more client-centred, respectful and un-intrusive approach. However, it raises the question of how help should be offered, and in which way it is most likely to be utilized by the patient who has a real need (or desire) for support. It also has indications for the care of patients who expect to be self-reliant and to cope without help. This can be particularly true of patients who work in 'coping' professions, such as nurses and police officers (Pratt *et al.*, 1997).

Timing is another factor. The patient may not feel – or recognize – the need for support at the time that it is offered. For instance, it is not unknown for a counselling request to be made as much as 2 years after the trauma. This is indicative of the individual's assimilation and coping abilities, and therefore any offer of support should include information regarding its long-term availability, preferably in writing and with contact details.

Again, it must be stressed that any form of counselling should only be undertaken by properly trained personnel or with the supervision of a psychologist. Methods of counselling should also be current and evidence-based, particularly in the light of modern debate on this subject.

The social situation
A sound social environment, i.e. a family that is understanding and supportive, will affect recovery in a positive way and make it considerably easier for the patient to cope. However, even if the family environment has been unproblematic to date, it may be unable to cope with the particular stresses of a new set of circumstances.

The work situation
Work usually plays an important role in the patient's life, finance being just one of the relevant aspects. An employer who guarantees a return to work gives the patient hope for the future and a goal to pursue. If the injury is due to an industrial accident and/or someone else is at fault, legal proceedings can be anticipated. Lawsuits may have a negative influence on the patient's recovery, but there is evidence to show that this must not be assumed (see Compensation and litigation section; also References).

Pre-existing psychosocial problems
At the time of the accident, the patient's equilibrium may already be disturbed. Awareness of such problems, when possible, is important in making a proper assessment of the patient's needs. These may include marital problems, coping with illness in the family, facing redundancy and so on. The injury itself may be the direct result of psychosocial problems. It is well known that distraction and lack of concentration are a significant cause of accidents, and that preoccupation with a psychosocial problem is a predisposing factor for injury (Sims, 1985). Some 20 per cent of the population is considered to experience psychological or social problems of some kind, and this will be no less relevant for people with hand injuries.

Psychosocial problems and far-reaching life events also seem to increase the possibility of developing complex regional pain syndrome, and psychological intervention is again strongly indicated in these cases to prevent chronic disability (Johnson, 1993).

Loss
The response to loss is described (Cone and Hueston, 1981) as:

> Three stages – namely denial and disbelief, grief and disorganisation, and finally restitution and rehabilitation.

It may also include anger, regret and euphoria, and any mixture of these producing emotional confusion. Murray-Parkes (1996) organizes the processes following loss into the 'stages of grief' and the 'tasks of mourning'. The hand therapist must understand all aspects of loss, as it is essential to appreciate the patient's progress and to be able to detect when problems and lack of progress are hindering overall rehabilitation.

Understandably, loss of function is frequently an outstanding feature of hand injury. Patients express the frustration they experience when bathing and dressing, and the fatigue produced by the awkwardness and tedious time needed for the simplest tasks. Loss of function is evident as an important issue in Haese's study (Haese, 1985). She interviewed hand injury patients during treatment to compare their views with those reported in the literature. She found that 'inability to use the hand' and 'desire to return to work' were given the most emphasis in questioning on the aspects of injury, and that these two factors were ranked as more important than either disfigurement or fear of returning to the scene of the accident.

Sexual dysfunction
There is a high reporting of sexual problems in hand injury patients, due, it is thought, to the fact that the hand is bound with body image, sexuality and human contact, and is seen as a sexual organ. Grunert et al. (1988a) wrote that sexual dysfunction was reported in 49 per cent of severe hand injury cases during the initial 2 months post-trauma, and in 19 per cent of cases at 6 months. They concluded that early psychological assessment and therapy are required to prevent persistent problems.

Vocational aspects

Financial considerations/motivation
Haese (1985) found that 'financial loss' was rated of low importance by patients. In a study on a group of patients in Hong Kong, the medical rating of loss of earning capacity was not predictive of overall occupational or psychosocial adjustment (Lee et al., 1985). In Bear-Lehmann's (1983) study to assess the influence of life work tasks in the hand-injured wage-earner population, 'financial need' and 'level of activities of daily living and participation in occupational therapy' were found to be directly related to return to work.

Occupational hand injuries
Severe work-related hand trauma is frequently followed by post-traumatic stress disorder (Grunert et al., 1990). Various degrees of exposure to the work site were shown to be an effective form of treatment depending on the type and severity of psychological symptoms: early return to the work site for patients with milder avoidance; graded work exposure for those with moderate reactions (Grunert et al., 1992a); and on-site job evaluation for those with severe avoidance reactions.

Early return to work, as distinct from early worksite exposure, has been found to be a significant factor in the prevention of chronic problems, depression and disruption of the patient's personal relationships.

On-site work evaluations were also used as a method of psychological desensitization (Grunert et al., 1989), and were found to be particularly valuable for patients who had failed to respond to traditional psychological strategies.

Compensation and litigation
Hand injury patients who are involved in litigation may exhibit attitude and compliance behaviour that is detrimental to recovery. Education, advice and support from properly informed professionals, including legal advisers, are essential if the patient is to have a realistic and constructive attitude to treatment. The patient's symptoms must also be correctly assessed so that they are not mislabelled as malingering or 'accident neurotic'. Grunert et al. (1991a) concluded that post-traumatic stress disorder was not significantly potentiated or sustained by concomitant litigation if the patient received early psychological intervention.

PROFESSIONAL PSYCHOLOGICAL INTERVENTION

It goes without saying that the hand therapist should be able to recognize the emotional effects of trauma and offer opportunities for expression of these feelings. However, psychological and social problems are often hard for the somatically trained therapist to identify, and their impact is often difficult to assess. Professional psychological diagnostics and, if necessary, treatment are therefore correct practice. The efficiency and cost-effectiveness of the patient's total treatment should also be borne in mind. There is little point in pursuing lengthy physical treatments when the element that is preventing progress is psychological.

Professional psychological assessment should be carried out at an early stage of treatment. Various authors (Johnson, 1986, 1989, 1993; Grunert et al., 1988b, 1992b, 1992c) support and have demonstrated the effects of early interventions. They have shown that early psychological evaluation and treatment can:

- prevent conditions such as post-traumatic stress disorder, avoidance behaviour and body-image disturbance from becoming chronic
- facilitate the successful assimilation of the experience of trauma, thus allowing full participation in rehabilitation (see also Rusch, 1998)
- restore patients' control of their life
- provide appropriate therapy for sexual dysfunction and prevent persistent problems (Grunert et al., 1988a)
- achieve an earlier return to work.

If it becomes apparent to the hand therapist that psychosocial factors have a major role in a patient's recovery, referral to a psychologist may be seen by the patient as loss of face; this must be sensitively overcome if treatment is to be adequate. A hand therapist who merely focuses on the somatic aspect may thereby cause a somatic fixation in which a change of focus to the psychosocial context becomes almost impossible, and certainly much less effective than earlier refocusing. The effort and time that the psychologist must then expend to correct this situation is considerable.

COPING WITHOUT A PSYCHOLOGIST

For various reasons, a psychologist is not always involved in the treatment of hand injuries – the psychology department may be understaffed, there may be no policy or protocol for referral, or there may simply be a lack of funding. In this case, additional psychosocial knowledge and skills will be expected from the hand therapist. As approximately half of an occupational therapist's undergraduate studies concern psychosocial subjects, this task largely falls to this member of the team; however, all staff must be alert to the signs or verbal cues that may signal problems. It is encouraging to see that the recognition of psychosocial elements in physical trauma is being emphasized by the nursing profession, in particular by plastics specialist nurses (Rusch, 1998).

Hand therapist interventions

Some practical considerations/assessment
When starting hand therapy, the initial assessment should include some evaluation of the patient's psychosocial situation and any factors that may affect the total intervention. It is important to find out whether the patient makes an accurate assessment of the severity and the nature of the injury, the time the treatment will take and the expected outcome. If the patient's view is not in keeping with the treatment team, this will need correction in a gradual, simple and unambiguous way, bearing in mind that all the team should be consistent when giving the patient information. Over the course of time, the therapist should check what the patient remembers. If long and intensive therapy is expected, the patient may need help to adjust to this expectation. The patient temporarily has a 'new job' that will use most of his or her time and energy: that of being a hand patient. The patient's history and previous coping skills should also be assessed. Suitable questions to ask include:

1. Have you been able to keep a job for some time?
2. Do you have a long-standing relationship?
3. Have you ever seen a psychologist or psychiatrist for emotional problems (e.g. depression)?
4. Have you experienced an episode of addiction or criminal behaviour?
5. What are your leisure activities, interests or sports?
6. What education and employment skills have you acquired?
7. What are your intellectual and cognitive capacities, such as attention and concentration? (This relates to the comprehension of treatment aims and compliance with instructions, and ability to take the therapist's advice.)
8. Have you suffered any serious physical trauma or disease before and if so, how did you cope with that? Concerning previous traumas and the present one, do you still experience nightmares or flashbacks and do you avoid things that remind you of the trauma? (Avoidance behaviour is frequently seen after major traumas.)
9. How are your partner, children and relatives responding to the situation? (As the patient is unable to perform all the usual domestic tasks, the partner is taking the extra load. How supportive and understanding is the partner? It is helpful to meet the partner, and invite him or her to accompany the patient to a treatment session. This gives a feeling of inclusion and fosters understanding for both patient and partner.)
10. What is the work situation, and the employer's attitude? Does the patient expect to fulfil normal activities, and does the therapist judge this to be realistic? Have there been any signs of support or sympathy from work colleagues or employer? If the injury is due to an industrial accident, does the patient receive legal assistance or does fear of losing the job make the patient reluctant to seek legal help?

If the findings from this set of questions reveal significant problems, including denial of any difficulties and avoidance of honest answers, it is essential to seek professional psychological help. This will not only prevent considerable suffering for the patient, but may also avoid such dangers as marital breakdown, severe anxiety, depression or suicide.

The patient's experience and emotions related to the traumatic accident are the specialized field of the psychologist, so it is necessary for liaison between the psychologist and the hand therapist to be clearly defined, with full understanding of each other's roles and the establishment of proper teamwork. The patient should be encouraged to talk about the accident and the events that followed, but this may trigger emotional reactions. For example, the patient may burst into tears and not be able to say what happened; may tell a very condensed version of the event due to having 'forgotten most of it'; or may describe the accident in a very distant and detached manner.

The patient's emotional state and feelings concerning the trauma can be assessed by tests administered by the psychologist, such as the Symptom Check List, the Hospital Anxiety and Depression Scale and the Revised Impact of Events Scale (see Psychological assessments, p.68). Repetition of the tests at an appropriate time offers the means of comparative measure.

Therapist approach

A listening, understanding, non-judgmental attitude is fundamental to trust and rapport and to the creation of a sound patient–therapist relationship. It is also important for the patient to feel that the hand therapist understands the non-somatic aspects of the situation. The offer of professional psychological counselling can be clearly made, with emphasis that this is a normal treatment for people who have experienced a similar trauma. If the patient is adamant in refusing to see a 'shrink', or if counselling is unavailable, then psychological support for the hand therapist may be a satisfactory option. In this case the therapist will have the security and supervision required to create an appropriate approach, and can help the patient to work through the necessary processes of recovery.

Most patients are happy (and often eager) to express their feelings and anxieties, but questioning may present awkwardness or difficulties. It is helpful to have practical methods that facilitate the expression of problems, and these strategies include:

- sitting side by side rather than face to face – this can be less confrontational
- discussion while doing something else – this creates a more natural atmosphere of having a talk rather than of being 'interviewed'

- self-appraisal – a list of printed questions can be offered to the patient to allow more privacy; assurance of confidentiality must also be given
- cueing or detecting cues – opening the subject by intentional but indirect reference to patients' feelings, and being receptive to patients' remarks when they verbally 'touch' on a problem; patients may offer the cue in a very casual manner, testing the interest or ability of the therapist to pursue a sensitive discussion
- finding or constructing the 'appropriate moment'
- patient group discussion and support – this may be within the hand therapy activity session, over a cup of tea, or in a more formal and structured situation
- offering help objectively, for example by saying: 'most patients with your kind of injury have found it helpful to discuss any problems and perhaps to have some support from our specialist counsellor'.

Cosmesis, acceptability and disfigurement

Patients may be anxious that a disfigured hand is unacceptable to others, both to look at and to touch. The hand therapist can be instrumental in correcting this problem, which will inevitably be connected with feelings of sexual acceptability. During examination and treatment the therapist must take care to hold the patient's hand in an accepting and empathetic manner. Handling the patient must be neither overdone nor avoided, as the therapist's reactions to any disfigurement will be carefully watched by the patient and can give the first social cues as to the physical acceptability of the hand. Scarring and loss of normal appearance must not be denied, but a positive attitude shown to restoration and emphasis of those features of the hand that are preserved (e.g. elegant fingers, good skin texture) should be stressed. A second step in the process can be made with other patients in group treatment, using activities such as card games where the hands are particularly visible. Discussion in a small group can include the subject of appearance, and the therapist can introduce and steer this in a constructive way. Again, if any deeper problem is suspected (such as prolonged denial or avoidance) the clinical psychologist should be involved.

Other therapeutic interventions

Many types of intervention are within the scope of the hand therapist. Some may need specific liaison with the psychologist, whereas others are obvious treatments for the psychological or social need that is apparent. Under the pressures of a busy hand trauma department it is easy for such factors to be overlooked, so the following list may serve as a check. The interventions judged to be important should be incorporated in the patient's programme and are best undertaken by therapists with the relevant skills and experience or by staff other than hand therapists (e.g. art therapists or occupational therapy technicians). Many of the following factors are particularly relevant to occupational therapists, especially those with postgraduate experience in psychosocial specialties.

- stress management
- anxiety management
- relaxation
- dietary advice – especially following extensive injury
- sleep – restoration of sleep pattern; reduction of pain; lack of tiredness caused by reduction of normal activity
- achievement and creativity – particularly for building confidence and self-esteem
- physical fitness – hand-injured patients may quickly lose their fitness due to pain, inactivity and loss of employment, with debilitating effects on their physical health and particularly on their ability to cope with stress
- leisure – restoration of patterns, interests, participation and social roles
- fun, laughter and humour – perhaps even 'laughter therapy', as developed by Madan Katari in Bombay
- desensitization to the workplace/scene of accident
- work hardening.

Group therapy
Patients often form their own groups or pairs during treatment or, commonly, in the waiting room. It is natural to seek mutual support, information and 'fellow-sufferer' links, as these are all coping mechanisms. Conversely, some patients find it difficult to do this as they are lacking in confidence or self-esteem; this may be a sign of social isolation due to depression.

Group treatment, education and support are powerful tools for the therapist. They can be exceptionally efficient and cost-effective, but need to be monitored to prevent misinformation and scaremongering. Patients can derive immense support and motivation from their peers, and many lifelong friendships start with such contact.

Groups can be structured, informal, patient-organized etc. They are particularly useful for patients whose treatment cannot be furthered but who still need some ongoing support, or as an acceptable way to wean patients who have necessarily become dependent on the treatment environment.

MANAGEMENT CONSIDERATIONS

Teamwork
A well co-ordinated professional team is the essential framework for providing the physical and psychological needs of the patient (Hunter, 1986). Teamwork underpins education, compliance, trust, professional learning, stability, confidence, and the psychological support of both the patients and the staff. Secure teams engender confidence and success, while disorganized teams misspend their skills and energy and have poor treatment outcomes.

Involvement of the patient's family and friends
Involvement of the patient's family and friends is always highly desirable; the patient will need their understanding, encouragement and support throughout the treatment. This will be particularly true once the initial drama and stimulus of the accident, however negative, has faded. The subsequent troughs and highs of treatment, recovery, setbacks, further surgery and financial difficulty, and simply the sheer effort of being a patient make exceptional demands on close relationships. Those who are involved, whether willingly or otherwise, will also need education regarding the injury, surgery, pain control, home care and exercises, and the understanding and support of the hand therapist.

Many close relatives find it helpful to attend at least some treatment sessions (with the permission of the patient), and in long-term therapy to participate in patient/relative support groups.

Client-centred practice
The concept of working as a partnership of patient and professional is gaining in both emphasis and research. Essentially, treatment decisions are made with rather than for the patient. This involves consent, agreement, and a level of responsibility and control of the treatment process. It may also include 'contracts' for compliance, which are agreed between the patient and the therapist. Haese (1985) found that hand-injury patients lacked responsibility for their treatment, and that this was detrimental to progress and outcome. Perhaps a client-centred approach would have changed this?

Evaluation of patient satisfaction is another move towards understanding the needs of the service user (Macey and Burke, 1995).

Patient education
This is inherent in client-centred practice, as the patient can only be empowered in decision-making by the provision of information. This information is also the basis of compliance. Patients should be given a logical reason for every instruction that is delivered. If the patient is told to keep the hand elevated, he or she needs to understand why; what precisely is meant by this term; how high is 'high'; when; and for how long.

Effective education is delivered at the right time and in digestible portions, always repeated, repeated at suitable intervals, given in appropriate

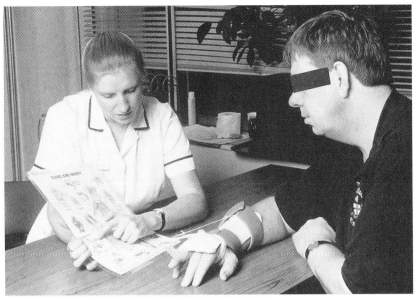

Figure 3.3 Education is the basis of motivation, compliance and patient empowerment.

language, accompanied by demonstration and visual aids, written down for the patient's future reference, and tested by questioning. The hand therapist is in a unique position to deliver this education, as the frequency and duration of treatment sessions fit the described criteria (Figure 3.3).

The author believes that education should occupy about 50 per cent of the patient's treatment. It can be comfortably combined with other treatment processes such as electrical procedures or splinting, when the patient's concentration is free enough to allow assimilation.

Honest, accurate information will inevitably include both welcome and unwelcome facts – for example, the length of time that nerve recovery will take following a nerve repair. This needs to be sensitively conveyed to the patient and adequate time and opportunity allowed for assimilation and questions – probably spanning the duration of several treatment sessions.

Compliance with treatment
Patients are often labelled as non-compliant, and therefore considered to be 'bad' patients (Finlay, 1997). Although it may take initial time and effort, it is worth attempting to discover the reasons for erratic attendance or failure to follow important instructions. Such problems may be the first indication that the patient is having more serious difficulties, such as depression, anxiety, sleeplessness due to night terrors, or marital disharmony. However, they may also be due to the therapist's failure to detect that the patient's appointments are at inconvenient times – for instance, when the children need collecting from school, or during employment

hours. Inconvenience has been shown to be a significant factor in non-attendance. Patients may hesitate to assert themselves when making appointments as they feel their therapist is so busy, and if they are suffering from psychological problems, lack of confidence or self-esteem, they may be afraid to be a nuisance. It must be remembered that such patients need more rather than less consideration and support from the hand therapist.

The principles described in this chapter under teamwork, client-centred practice, patient education and trust all have significant effects on compliance. Compliance can be improved by a number of additional strategies (Groth and Wolf, 1995), including speedy appointment setting for the first intervention, immediate follow-up of broken appointments, appointment reminders, establishing positive encouragement and reinforcement, and realistic and achievable home splinting and exercise regimens.

Trust
Compliance is also dependent on trust. Patients need to be sure that their treatment is correct and is being given by professionals who are competent. They will soon be wary if they are given conflicting information about their hand or prognosis. Sound teamwork and professional loyalty are therefore fundamental to rapport with the patient, as well as to the effective co-ordination of hand rehabilitation.

Listening, empathy and regard for the patient's difficulties and interests are all signals that engender trust. The simple acknowledgement that they might need a cup of tea or time for a sandwich after a long wait for hospital tests shows the patient that the therapist is concerned and humane.

Setting time aside to hear the patient's views and to answer questions is essential to this process, as is the assurance of confidentiality and privacy, particularly during assessments and note-taking.

Trust is also dependent on the approach to the patient's discomfort and pain. Handling the patient must always be preceded by questioning and verbal assessment of the degree and sites of pain.

Consideration and control of pain

Pain control by medication should be integral to treatment, except in the rare circumstances when it is contraindicated during evaluation or for reasons of patient safety.

Fear greatly exacerbates pain, and measures such as preparation, education (fear is often the product of ignorance), relaxation and increase of patient control are therefore effective.

In circumstances where pain is a safeguard during hand therapy – e.g. in joint mobilization – the patient must be told when discomfort is expected and be given a method to control the therapist's actions. There should be no psychological pressure to exceed personal pain tolerance, and treatment should also proceed at a speed that is in the patient's control. Patients' jokes about 'PT standing for pain and torture' and 'OT for only torture' can be a humorous way of coping, but may also be a sad reflection of their care and indicate the underlying reality of their hospital visits.

Rheumatoid arthritis

Patients with rheumatoid arthritis may experience many of the psychosocial difficulties that occur in hand trauma, except that there is no sudden accident with the attendant sequelae of trauma, and their disability has a slower onset and longer duration. The shock or series of shocks to their body-image, self-esteem and confidence may be no less disturbing (MacKinnon *et al.*, 1994); they merely have longer in which to adapt and mourn, and to develop their coping strategies. They too suffer pain, loss of function, loss of independence, and unwelcome changes in the appearance of their hands (Wiskin, 1998). They may have to accept that there will be slow deterioration rather than gradual improvement. Added to this, they frequently feel very unwell and are unable to anticipate when a flare-up of disease may occur. This makes it difficult to plan such things as going on holiday, getting washed and dressed in the morning, and going to work (see p. 272).

A notable cognitive-behavioural approach to develop coping skills for the worker with rheumatoid arthritis is described by Wiskin (1998).

Amputations

The psychological effects of traumatic amputations have all the elements of other types of hand trauma and, as can be expected, there is usually a significantly increased level of loss. As described previously, the perceived severity of trauma is subjective and can only be quantified by the patient. The medical calculation of physical loss may therefore be disproportionate to the psychosocial effect on the individual.

All patients with amputation, however major or apparently insignificant, should also have professional psychologist services available throughout their treatment. Early in their treatment they should be made aware that cosmetic prostheses can be supplied and given information on accessing the prosthetic services. This information should include details of private, international prosthetics suppliers of high repute, whether or not the patient is thought to be able to afford such expense.

Self-inflicted injury and factitious conditions

Wounds that do not heal and unexpected or illogical patterns of sensory deficit must all raise questions for the hand therapist. Early detection and investigation are of course preferable, but in reality most cases are complex and prolonged. Whenever possible the true diagnosis must be sought (using hospitalization and observation, if necessary) to prevent the reinforcement of inappropriate treatment and to allow the correct approach and psychological help for the patient (Grunert *et al.*, 1991b; Friedman *et al.*, 1998).

Hand injuries due to attempted suicide usually present as lacerations at the wrist, and all treatment should be co-ordinated with that of the psychiatrist. Guidance will be needed on the approach to the patient and the timing of assessments in relation to the patient's readiness for realization of problems and deficits, particularly those that will have an effect on personal relationships and functional capacity.

Psychosocial considerations are discussed further in Chapters 8, 9, 11 and 13.

Psychological assessments

Psychological assessments that are commonly used and referred to in the treatment of physical trauma include:

- Health Assessment Questionnaire (HAQ)
- Symptom Checklist 90 Revised (SCL-90-R)
- McGill Pain Questionnaire (MPQ)
- Revised Impact of Events Scale (RIES)
- Hospital Anxiety and Depression Scale (HAD Scale)
- Hassles and Uplifts Scale
- Coping Responses Inventory
- Significant Other Scale
- Minnesota Multiphasic Personality Inventory (MMPI).

REFERENCES

Bear-Lehman, J. (1983). Factors affecting return to work after hand injury. *Am. J. Occ. Ther.*, **37(3)**, 189–94.

Bronowski, J. (1973). *The Ascent of Man*, p. 116. British Broadcasting Corporation.

Cone, J. C. P. and Hueston, J. T. (1981). Psychological aspects of hand injury. In: *The Hand* (R. Tubiana, ed.), Vol. 1, pp.704–14. W. B. Saunders.

Finlay, L. (1997). Good patients and bad patients: how occupational therapists view their patients/clients. *Br. J. Occ. Ther.*, **60(10)**, 440–46.

Friedman, B., Yaffe, B., Blankstein, A. *et al.* (1988). Self-inflicted hand injuries: diagnostic challenge and treatment. *Ann. Plast. Surg.*, **20(4)**, 345–50.

Groth, G. N. and Wulf, M. B. (1995). Compliance with hand rehabilitation: health beliefs and strategies. *J. Hand Ther.*, **8(1)**, 18–22.

Grunert, B. K., Devine, C. A., Matloub, H. S. *et al.* (1988a). Sexual dysfunction following traumatic hand injury. *Ann. Plast. Surg.*, **21(1)**, 46–8.

Grunert, B. K., Smith, C. J., Devine, C. A. *et al.* (1988b). Early psychological aspects of severe hand injury. *J. Hand. Surg.*, **13B(2)**, 177–80.

Grunert, B. K., Devine, C. A., McCallum-Burke, S. *et al.* (1989). On-site work evaluations: desensitisation for avoidance reactions following severe hand injuries. *J. Hand Surg.*, **14B(2)**, 239–41.

Grunert, B. K., Matloub, H. S., Sanger, J. R. and Yousif, N. J. (1990). Treatment of post-traumatic stress disorder after work-related hand trauma. *J. Hand Surg.*, **15A(3)**, 511–15.

Grunert, B. K., Matloub, H. S., Sanger, J. R. *et al.* (1991a). Effects of litigation on maintenance of psychological symptoms after severe hand injury. *J. Hand Surg.*, **16A(6)**, 1031–4.

Grunert, B. K., Sanger, J. R., Matloub, H. S. and Yousif, N. J. (1991b). Classification system for factitious syndromes in the hand with implications for treatment. *J. Hand Surg.*, **16A(6)**, 1027–103.

Grunert, B. K., Devine, C. A., Smith, C. J. *et al.* (1992a). Graded work exposure to promote return to work after severe hand trauma: a replicated study. *Ann. Plast. Surg.*, **29(6)**, 532–6.

Grunert, B. K., Devine, C. A., Matloub, H. S. *et al.* (1992b). Psychological adjustment following work-related hand injury: 18-month follow-up. *Ann. Plast. Surg.*, **29(6)**, 537–42.

Grunert, B. K., Hargarten, S. W., Matloub, H. S. *et al.* (1992c). Predictive value of psychological screening in acute hand injuries. *J. Hand Surg.*, **17A(2)**, 196–9.

Haese, J. B. (1985). Psychological aspects of hand injuries. Their treatment and rehabilitation. *J. Hand Surg.*, **10B(3)**, 283–7.

Hunter, J. M. (1986). Philosophy of hand rehabilitation. *Hand Clin.*, **2(1)**, 5–24.

Johnson, R. K. (1986). Psychological evaluation of patients with industrial hand injuries. *Hand Clin.*, **2(3)**, 567–75.

Johnson, R. K. (1989). The role of psychological evaluations in occupational hand injuries. *Occ. Med.*, **4(3)**, 405–18.

Johnson, R. K. (1993). Psychologic assessment of patients with industrial hand injuries. *Hand Clin.*, **9(2)**, 221–9.

Lee, P. W., Ho, E. S., Tsang, A. K. *et al.* (1985). Psychosocial adjustment of victims of occupational hand injuries. *Soc. Sci. Med.*, **20(5)**, 493–7.

Macey, A. C. and Burke, F. D. (1995). Outcomes of hand surgery. *J. Hand Surg.*, **20B(6)**, 841–55.

MacKinnon, J. R., Avison, W. R. and McCain, G. A. (1994). Rheumatoid arthritis, occupational profiles and psychological adjustment. *J. Occ. Sci.*, **1(4)**, 3–10.

Murray Parkes, C. (1972). Components of the reaction to loss of limb, spouse or home. *J. Psychosom. Res.*, **16**, 343–9.

Napier, J. R. (1966). Functional aspects of the anatomy of the hand. In: *Clinical Surgery: The Hand* (ed. Pulverstaft, R. G..), p. 1. Butterworths.

Pratt, J., McFadyen, A., Hall, G. *et al.* (1997). A review of the initial outcomes of a return-to-work programme for police officers following injury or illness. *Br. J. Occ. Ther.*, **60(6)**, 253–8.

Rusch, M. D. (1998). Psychological response to trauma. *Plast. Surg. Nurs.*, **18(3)**, 159–62.

Sims, A. C. P. (1985). Psychogenic causes of physical symptoms, accidents and death. *J. Hand Surg.*, **10B**, 281–2.

Tubiana, R.(1984). Architecture and functions of the hand. In: *Examination of the Hand and Upper Limb* (R. Tubiana, E. Mackin and J.-M. Thomine, eds), p. 90. W. B. Saunders.

Wiskin, L. F. (1998). Cognitive-behavioural therapy: a psychoeducational treatment approach for the American worker with rheumatoid arthritis. *Work*, **10**, 41–8.

FURTHER READING

Bradley, E. (1996). *Counselling People with Disfigurement*. British Psychological Society.

Brand, P.(1988). The mind and spirit in hand therapy. *J. Hand Ther.*, **Jul–Sep**, 145–7.

Grunert, B. K., Devine, C. A., Matloub, H. S. *et al.* (1988c) Flashbacks after traumatic hand injuries: prognostic indicators. *J. Hand Surg.*, **13A(1)**, 125–7.

Malick, H. M. and Carr, A. C. (1982). *Manual on Management of the Burns Patient*. Harmarville Rehabilitation Center, Pittsburgh, pp. 104–28.

Mendelson, R. L., Burech, J. G., Polack, E. P. *et al.* (1986). The psychological impact of traumatic amputations. *Hand Clin.* **2(3)**, 577–83.

Thieffry, S. (1981). Genesis and development of manual aptitudes. In: *The Hand* (R. Tubiana, ed.), Vol. 1, pp. 493–8. W. B. Saunders.

Winspur, I. and Wynn-Parry, C. B. (1998). *The Musician's Hand. A Clinical Guide*. Martin Dunitz.

OTHER RESOURCES

Occupational Therapists in Mental Health, Specialist Section of the College of Occupational Therapists, 106–114, Borough High Street, London SE1 1LB.

British Psychological Society, 48 Princes Road East, Leicester LE1 7DR.

British Association of Hand Therapists, Woodlands, 25 Mountview, Billericay, Essex, CM11 1HB.

4 Pain

Victoria Frampton

INTRODUCTION

The relationship of injury to pain and the changes of sensation and behaviour after injury have been well described (Wall, 1984). The immediate response to injury is frequently no pain at all; the second response is one of agitation, aggression and guarding; and the tertiary response is one of quiet, solitary, antisocial behaviour. This description of an animal's response to pain can be quickly identified with the behaviour demonstrated by many patients suffering from pain. In many conditions, pain can be a serious limiting factor to rehabilitation of hand and upper limb injuries. Pain may be described as 'an unpleasant sensory and emotional experience associated with actual or potential tissue damage, or described in terms of such damage' (International Association for the Study of Pain, 1994; Merskey, 1979). Pain is a 'complex, perceptual experience. There is a uniform sensation threshold in all people. However, the pain perception threshold may vary'. The perception threshold may be influenced by previous experience, upbringing, cultural influences, situation and suggestion. Inhibition of pain is commonly experienced in extreme situations. For example, in the height of a battle the pain experienced from the loss of a limb or digit may not be experienced; only when the battle is over and the immediate threat to life has passed will the full force of the pain be experienced.

A clear understanding of some of the mechanisms involved in the perception of pain, and when it is an indication of actual damage or just an emotional experience, will help to focus and direct treatment methods in the rehabilitation of hand injuries. The modulation of the central nervous system (CNS) by drug therapy reflects the most recent advances in pain management and the practice in pain clinics. However, modulation of pain by physical means still provides the most accessible treatment methods, and few advances or changes have been made over the past 5–10 years.

PAIN MECHANISMS

Bowsher (1994a) discusses the existence of two pains. The first pain is sharp, well-localized and carried quickly to consciousness, but ceases as soon as the stimulus is removed (for example, a pinprick). The second pain, or true pain, is dull, throbbing or aching, not localized, but may spread well beyond the original site of the injury. The existence of two pains can be illustrated by the example of hammering a nail into the wall. If the hammer slips and strikes the thumb, a sharp, intense, well-localized pain on the thumb is felt ('fast first pain'). This is immediately followed by a dull, throbbing ache, which no longer is localized to the site of the initial blow but has spread well beyond the thumb and possibly up the forearm ('slow second pain').

Pain is transmitted from the periphery to consciousness via different pathways. Nociceptors (pain receptors) connect with small, unmyelinated, slow-conducting afferent-C fibres. They also connect with small, myelinated, faster-conducting afferent Aβ fibres. These two nociceptive pathways lead to the convenient hypothesis that first pain (or acute pain) is carried by the fast-conducting Aβ fibres, and second (or chronic pain) is carried by the slower-conducting C fibres. Clearly the actual process of pain transmission and perception is more complex. First pain results in a reflex response; the hammer is dropped and the hand withdrawn. Second pain results in spasm and guarding. The detection of injury and painful stimuli via the activation of nociceptors and associated nerve fibres provides an understanding and basis from which normal afferent pathways may be modulated to provide pain relief (Figure 4.1).

The concept of the gate control of pain relief (Melzack and Wall, 1967) established the basis for understanding pain-relieving mechanisms. Although this has been revised since, it still may provide an explanation for the therapeutic value of

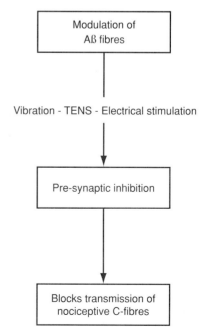

Figure 4.1 Summary of modulation of normal afferent pathways to relieve pain.

many modalities used for the relief of pain – for example, transcutaneous electrical nerve stimulation (Wall and Melzack, 1987). The theory suggests that painful stimuli transmitted by the smaller slow-conducting afferent fibres may be blocked by stimulating the large fast-conducting afferent Aβ-sensory fibres effecting presynaptic inhibition. Presynaptic inhibition prevents the continuing transmission of a painful stimulus to consciousness.

A well-known example of the mechanism is the instinctive response to rub a pain better. The large low-threshold cutaneous mechanoreceptors and Aβ fibres are susceptible to stimulation such as vibration, rubbing and electrical currents. These fibres provide the vehicle for pain modulation.

NERVE INJURY

When a peripheral nerve is damaged there are a number of profound physiological changes that take place, both peripherally and centrally (Wall and Gutnik, 1974):

1. Abnormal spontaneous electrical discharges occur at nerve endings. Electrical firing may spread from the neuroma site (the cut proximal end of nerve, where sprouting nerves have formed a knot of nerve fibres) and proximally along the length of the nerve. Nerve sprouts arising from the proximal stump are very sensitive to the slightest mechanical stimuli. They are spontaneously active. In a regenerating nerve, tapping over the neural sprouts will reproduce a referred sensation in the part of the skin that used to be supplied by that nerve (Tinel, 1915; Moldaver, 1978).
2. Increased sensitivity of C-fibre activity following nerve damage produces symptoms of sympathetic disturbances (Loh and Nathan, 1978). The sympathetic system is itself normal. It is the abnormal response of the C-fibre sprouts that produces an increase in sympathetic disturbances (Wallin *et al.*, 1976), and this may give the basis for the symptoms seen in complex regional pain syndrome. In such cases apparent minor injury can produce significant symptoms that are not consistent with the extent of the original injury.
3. There is increased firing of dorsal horn cells (Loeser and Ward, 1967).
4. Abnormal central patterns of pain are established (Wynn Parry, 1981).

The changes that have occurred and the constant barrage of abnormal peripheral discharges may well lead to the consequent changes and effects that occur at spinal level and higher centres. These central changes may in themselves produce further abnormal peripheral nerve discharges. It is not surprising that a small but significant proportion of patients experience pain following nerve injury

(Withrington and Wynn Parry, 1984). The autonomous circle of peripheral and central effects of nerve damage must be interrupted in order to modify chronic pain (Frampton, 1994, Wynn Parry and Withrington, 1984).

Pain from nerve injury may result from only minor trauma. For example, a relatively straightforward carpal tunnel decompression can lead to severe hyperaesthesia and hyperpathia (abnormal painful response to light touch), resulting in the patient being totally unable to tolerate light touches to the hand. The abnormal sensation often associated with symptoms of sympathetic dysfunction may result in the total loss of function of that part, and the danger of a chronic state of disuse and the subsequent development of contracture and disuse atrophy are high. The more the abnormal patterns of sensation are allowed to develop and establish themselves, the more abnormal patterns are set up centrally, and the patient is caught in a downward spiral of loss of function and consequent major disruption to everyday life. Phantom pain, which is the result of deafferentation to the spinal cord, is more commonly experienced in amputations of the upper limb. This might be due to the unusually large representation the hand has in the cerebral cortex. Interestingly, slow destruction of the limb, such as occurs in Hanson's disease, does not result in phantom pain or sensation. The 'central' pain phenomenon, or deafferentation pain, is also a feature of avulsion lesions of the brachial plexus.

CHARACTERISTICS OF PAIN

The characteristics of acute and chronic pain differ, and although they have some similar traits it is important to differentiate between the two types (Tables 4.1, 4.2).

The term 'central pain' is often used to describe a very specific type of pain that is completely different from the types of pain already described. Conditions that cause this type of pain are avulsion lesions of the brachial plexus (Wynn Parry, 1980), phantom limb pain following amputation, and spinal cord injuries. The hypothesis to explain the central pain phenomenon may be that it results from a barrage of abnormal firing of dorsal horn

TABLE 4.1
ACUTE PAIN CHARACTERISTICS

- Immediate onset
- Spontaneous
- Sharp
- Localized
- Hyperpathia*
- Intermittent

*Associated with nerve injury.

TABLE 4.2
CENTRAL PAIN CHARACTERISTICS

- Burning
- Crushing
- Electric shock
- Constant
- Paroxysms of pain
- Insidious onset

cells that have lost their normal afferent input (Loeser and Ward, 1967), and this unsuppressed firing of cells results in a loss of normal central inhibition. This type of pain is not always spontaneous and may develop over a 10-day–3-week period (Wynn Parry, 1981), and this clinical observation is certainly compatible with experimental findings (Loeser and Ward, 1967).

In essence, the therapist is faced with acute pain, chronic pain and intractable pain. It is the recognition of the different types of pain and the mechanisms that produce them that is essential for the understanding and the consequent successful treatment of pain. This brief overview of some aspects of pain mechanisms just touches the surface of a very extensive subject, the full range and detail of which is beyond the scope of this book (see also Bowsher, 1994b; Wall and Melzack, 1987).

PAIN ASSESSMENT

The initial clinical evaluation of pain provides a baseline of information. Careful analysis of the subjective and objective examinations will indicate the pain pathology and help to identify whether it is central or peripheral in nature. This enables treatment programmes to be established that will appropriately target specific areas for intervention. More importantly, the initial assessment of pain provides the basis for an ongoing comparative record by which the success of treatment can be monitored.

Pain behaviour

Questions relating to the behaviour of pain will build up a profile of the pain. Evaluation should include:

1. Description of the type of pain
   - burning
   - sharp
   - shooting
   - cramping
   - aching
   - stabbing
   - tingling.
2. Location of the pain
   - map out the painful area on a body chart
3. Assessment of the irritability of pain
   - which factors aggravate pain?
   - which factors relieve pain?
4. The pain state
   - is pain increasing, decreasing or static?
5. The frequency and pattern of pain
   - is pain present at night?
   - does it disrupt sleep?
   - is it present in bursts?
   - if so, how long did these last and how frequently did they occur – every 5 minutes twice a day, half-hourly, continuously etc.?
6. Pain onset
   - when did the pain start and how?
7. Pain medication
   - what and how much analgesia is being taken?

If part of the subjective assessment includes an objective measurement – for example, pain present only within a certain range of movement – then this should be recorded and will provide a baseline for comparative data. More than one type of pain may be described, and each individual pain may behave differently; for example, pain 1 may be a constant burning and pain 2 a stabbing pain that occurs once an hour and lasts 5 minutes. All these specific details should be recorded. It is important to demonstrate to patients that even if pain cannot be eliminated it can be altered and reduced, thus enabling them to carry out an activity for longer or perform a task they could not do before. This concept of small gains in pain behaviour must be recognized by chronic pain sufferers; it is an essential tool to motivate them in their own rehabilitation.

Quantitative assessment of pain

The intensity of pain can be recorded using a visual analogue scale ranging from no pain to maximum pain. This can be recorded verbally or on a chart using 10-cm lines; the latter has the added advantage of visual feedback (Figure 4.2). Pain ratings can also be taken before and after treatment, which can provide constructive feedback to patients who report no change in pain subjectively but can recognize a small gain on the pain visual analogue chart (Frampton, 1996).

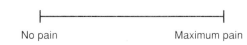

No pain   Maximum pain

Figure 4.2 Visual analogue scale.

Pain questionnaires

This method of assessment provides patients with an opportunity to identify their pain using descriptive questionnaires; an example of one of these is the McGill pain questionnaire.

PAIN MANAGEMENT

Pain may accompany injury and disease. The dilemma facing the therapist is that the natural response to injury may be guarding, enforced rest and immobilization of the damaged part. In many cases this may be appropriate – for example, following nerve repair or an unstable fracture. However, in many cases rehabilitation may be a balance between rest to promote healing and mobilization to maintain function.

Certainly pain is not necessarily a contraindication to mobilization. It is not always a symptom of potential tissue damage. A good example of the balance between pain and mobilization is that following tendon repair and, particularly, tenolysis. Active movement of the fingers or wrist results in pain around the incision line; however, if movement is not established the potential function of the tendon is jeopardized by adhesion.

Oedema is a limiting factor to movement, and often causes severe pain. Unless movement (and thus improved venous return) is re-established, the oedema will organize and may lead to permanent contracture and loss of function. Similarly, the burnt hand poses an enormous problem because contracture can occur so quickly. It is essential to establish early movement despite often intense pain.

If fractures of the fingers are treated by immobilization, this may lead to loss of movement and dysfunction. Early mobilization, despite pain, must be encouraged once the fracture is stable.

Pain arising from arthritis, whether degenerative or inflammatory, can be managed by a closely supervised drug regime and therapeutic techniques. Identification of the cause of pain is vital, and it may be that the major cause is instability within a joint. Splinting to provide joint protection may be an essential component of pain control.

Clearly in many cases it is essential to establish good pain control prior to and during mobilization in order to restore normal function. A wide battery of pain-relieving modalities can be exploited and, when critically selected, can aid relief of pain and resolve function.

CHRONIC PAIN-RELIEVING MODALITIES

Relief of pain/oedema can be achieved by elevation, compression/flow pulsation, Coban wrapping, compression garments, Diapulse, contrast baths and interferential treatment. Relief of pain/ arthritis can be achieved by Diapulse, laser or ultrasound treatment, splinting or interferential treatment.

Transcutaneous electrical nerve stimulation

Pain resulting from nerve damage can be modified or reversed by the application of electric currents, and it has been shown experimentally that the application of vibration or an electrical stimulus proximal to the cut end of a nerve damps down and reduces the abnormal electrical discharges that occur at the nerve stump (Wall and Gutnik, 1974). Transcutaneous electrical nerve stimulation (TENS) has established itself as a valuable and economic tool in the management of these difficult cases (Frampton, 1994). As the name implies, an electrical stimulus is applied via the skin. TENS is thought to provide pain relief by the following mechanisms:

- the presynaptic inhibitory mechanism (stimulation of the large Aβ afferents, which gate off or block transmission of nociceptive C-fibre afferents)
- direct mechanical inhibition to subdue an abnormally electrically active firing nerve
- restoring an artificial input in cases of deafferentation, for example phantom limb pain, brachial plexus avulsion injury (Wynn Parry, 1980) and spinal cord injury
- the role played by endogenous opiate peptides (morphine-like substances naturally produced within the body, which may be released through stimulation by many techniques including TENS).

TENS can only form part of a whole treatment programme for patients suffering from chronic pain (Frampton, 1994). Central changes that have occurred as a result of chronic pain mechanisms must be reversed or modified (Withrington and Wynn Parry, 1984). A full programme of normal functional activities must be employed in conjunction with TENS so that normal use can be restored to the affected part once pain has been reduced or relieved.

TENS – machine parameters

TENS may be described as producing an asymmetrical biphasic modified square waveform output. There is a zero net DC component, the area of the positive wave portion equal to the area within the negative portion (Figure 4.3). The amplitude of the current can be adjusted from 0–50 ma, with an electrode impedance of 1 kΩ. This range is standard for almost all TENS machines, and does not vary from one manufacturer to another. Pulse width is usually fixed at 200 ms, although some machines provide variable pulse widths ranging from 50–300 ms. A wide pulse width has an application in denervated brachial plexus injuries or in any

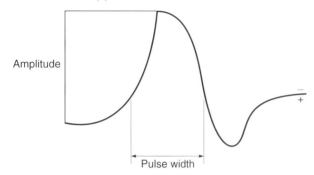

Figure 4.3 Biphasic asymmetrical square wave with a zero net DC component.

condition where deafferantation and denervation exists (normally innervated muscles would be stimulated and lead to contraction of muscle fibres, an unwanted response).

Pulse frequency is variable on almost all machines, varying from 1–150 Hz, and burst and frequency modulated output wave forms are also available. One of the criticisms of TENS in the management of chronic pain is that the benefits tend to fall with time (Loeser *et al.*, 1975). It has been suggested that this may be due to the adaptation of the nervous system to regular repetitive stimuli (Thompson, 1986; Pomeranz and Niznick, 1987), and it is for this reason that variable frequencies and burst-type stimulation are advocated. Patients should be encouraged to try a variety of different frequencies and modes of stimulation to find their optimum parameters for pain relief (Frampton, 1994). The stimulus from the machine is delivered to the patient transcutaneously via lead wires or cables and conductive electrodes. The principles of electrode placement are based on an understanding of the pain mechanisms involved. If deafferentation is the predominant feature, then one large pad should be placed over the appropriately damaged dermatome (provided there is some residual afferent input) and the other pad may be placed over the

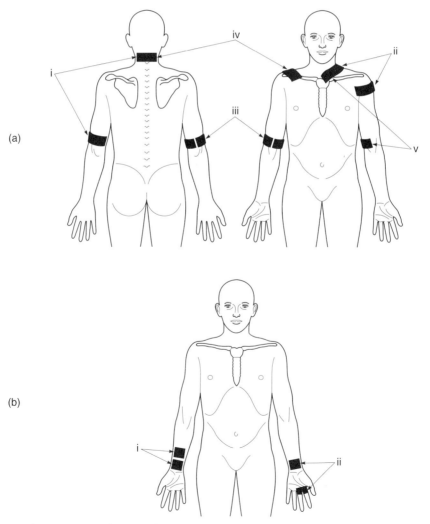

Figure 4.4 Suggested placement for TENS electrodes in brachial plexus lesions (a) and carpal tunnel syndrome (b).

nerve trunk at the appropriate root level of damage (Figure 4.4a, position i).

Other positions of placement can be seen in Figure 4.4a, positions ii, iii, iv and v.

With peripheral nerve damage, such as carpal tunnel syndrome, pads may be placed directly over the affected nerve with one electrode proximal to the site of damage where the affected nerve is nearest the surface (Figure 4.4b). Small pads may be adequate in these cases.

Fundamental guidelines with regard to placement are to place the pads:

- over the peripheral nerve where it is most superficial, proximal to the site of pain
- over the affected dermatome, or the adjacent dermatome
- over the nerve root
- above and below the painful area;
- not over anaesthetic areas
- over areas which still allow for functional use of the limb or part
- over trigger points (Melzack *et al.*, 1987).

One or more of the above principles of placement may be employed in one treatment. Systematic application of electrodes over successive sessions will lead to a more successful outcome (Woolf *et al.*, 1981). Prolonged stimulation (for example, 8 hours per day) is indicated to provide sufficient relief to allow normal use of the hand and limb, as active use is essential to allow restoration of normal sensory patterns and movement. When applying TENS it is important to advise patients that they might feel a mild, tingling sensation, and to emphasize that a mild sensation is all that is required – it should not be strong or painful. Careful monitoring is essential for successful results with TENS.

Possible reasons for poor results can be attributed to different factors, ranging from patient treatment techniques to basic technical faults or inappropriate patient selection. Successful treatment will depend on an accurate assessment of the patient – whether an individual is a suitable candidate for TENS. Objectives must be clearly set out prior to treatment. It must be explained that TENS may only reduce the pain at first and not obliterate it – patients' expectations must be rationalized without dampening their hope of pain relief. The need to encourage and motivate chronic pain patients is an extremely important facet of treatment, and the need to gain patients' confidence is vital.

Hazards
Few hazards exist with TENS, and these are avoidable using common sense. Many of the contraindications quoted by manufacturers are given as a precaution, and act to protect the supplier:

1. TENS is not to be used in the area of the carotid sinus nerves or elsewhere in the region of the front of the neck or in the mouth
2. TENS is not to be used near the eyes
3. The safety of TENS in pregnancy or childbirth has not been fully established
4. TENS should not be used when operating vehicles or hazardous equipment
5. Patients with known heart disease or defects should only use TENS following full examination by the referring physician and careful patient instruction
6. TENS should be kept out of the reach of children
7. Skin irritation can occur under or around the electrode site
8. TENS should not be used for undiagnosed pain.

CASE HISTORIES
Carpal tunnel compression
A 58-year-old night sister had a 10-year history of paraesthesia in her right hand. She had pain at night, and difficulty in writing and manipulating small objects. EMG studies demonstrated that she had a moderately severe carpal tunnel syndrome. In July she had a carpal tunnel decompression. One week post-operatively, she was complaining of sharp, shooting pain at the wrist and hyperaesthesia in the palm. She continued to have tingling in her hand at night and in the median nerve distribution. Two months later she was referred for outpatient physiotherapy.

On examination, her hand was red and engorged. She complained of hyperaesthesia in the palm, a sharp pain at the wrist and paraesthesia at night and with manual activities, such as writing and opening bottles.

A single channel TENS unit was applied with standard 2×2-cm^2 pads in position 4.4.b.i. The patient was instructed in its use and requested to leave it on for a minimum of 8 hours and return the following day with the TENS in place so that correct positioning and application could be monitored. She wore the TENS for 11–13 hours per day for 3 weeks, and was able to continue working with the TENS in place. At the 3-week follow-up, her symptoms were much improved and the hyperaesthesic area was reduced by 50 per cent. At 5 weeks post-TENS, the hyperaesthesic area was reduced by a further 25 per cent, leaving only a small area of hyperaesthesia around the scar. She reduced the hours of stimulation to 6 hours a day.

Eight weeks after the first application the patient discontinued TENS, and on discharge she had no pain or hyperaesthesia. However, she did have some residual clumsiness owing to a degree of loss of sensory proprioception.

A painful scar

A 60-year-old lady sustained a dislocation of her proximal interphalangeal joint and laceration of the palmar surface of her right middle finger. Five weeks later she was referred for physiotherapy. On examination, she had a swollen proximal interphalangeal joint with a range of motion from +20° to 90°. Although the finger was tender, her main symptoms contributing to loss of function of the hand were due to the painful scar of the laceration. She complained of hyperaesthesia over and around the scar, with a sharp, stabbing pain when pressure was applied to a nodule that was in the scar. She was unable to use the hand for washing and carrying due to these symptoms.

Single channel TENS was applied in position 4.4.b.i using standard 2×2-cm^2 electrodes. She wore the TENS for 6–8 hours a day. She was reviewed after one day for correct positioning and application of the TENS. At the 1-week follow-up she had minimal relief, so position 4.4.b.ii was applied using a small finger electrode for the distal pad and she continued with the same number of hours of stimulation. Three weeks post-application of TENS, the pain in the scar had completely resolved. TENS was discontinued and her range of movement had improved to +15° to 115° with function fully restored, except for some residual joint tenderness that limited her ability to carry heavy bags.

In this case it was necessary to remove the distal pad closer to the laceration to achieve pain relief. A successful outcome of the dislocation may have been compromised if the hyperaesthesia had not been treated.

Brachial plexus lesion

An 18-year-old man was involved in a motorcycle accident while travelling at 66 km/h (40 mph). The front wheel of the motorcycle hit a hole in the road and he came off the machine and hit a telegraph pole. The patient sustained a right brachial plexus lesion (BPL) involving the roots of C5–T1. C5 and C6 were diagnosed as postganglionic lesions, and C7, C8 and T1 as preganglionic lesions. Two weeks later he developed a constant severe burning pain in all his fingers and the ulnar border of his forearm, with sharp shooting pain in his middle, ring and little fingers occurring every 5–10 minutes. Although the pain varied little, he found that distraction was the only means of providing some degree of relief, as drugs had no effect.

His life was affected dramatically by the pain, as he had to stop to grip the arm with every stab of pain. He had been fitted with a flail arm splint (Robinson, 1986; Frampton, 1990) to restore some function to his paralysed arm, but was unable to use it because of the pain.

Following sensory assessment he was found to have sensation to light touch proximal to the elbow, but no sensation below that level, and his VAS score was 10 (the maximum). It was decided to apply TENS, and the position seen in Figure 4.4.a.v was used. A high intensity, moderate frequency and wide pulse width were used. After only a few hours' stimulation, he had obtained good relief of pain. He was then encouraged to use his flail arm splint to restore some afferent input from the deafferented side. He was discharged 3 weeks later, using TENS for 8 hours a day. Although he still had the constant burning pain, the frequency of the stab of pain was reduced to once daily and his VAS score dropped to two. After 2 months he was using TENS one morning per week, and had ceased using it altogether at the 7-month follow-up. When seen 2 years after his accident, he was still not using TENS and was working full-time as a television engineer.

COMPLEX REGIONAL PAIN SYNDROME

The onset of the controversial condition known as complex regional pain syndrome (CRPS) or reflex sympathetic dystrophy (RSD) frequently occurs following minor trauma, sprains or Colles' fractures, or after minor surgery such as carpal tunnel decompression. It is important to distinguish true CRPS and disuse atrophy. There are still many who speculate that CRPS is purely a response to lack of motivation from a patient following minor trauma, and that it is, in effect, self-induced. Undoubtedly, the effect of disuse or lack of mobilization following minor surgery or minor injury where bruising has been present will lead to a stiff and painful hand. However, true CRPS can spontaneously occur and have significant symptoms. The hand can become painful, red, hot and swollen, and this is associated with severe pain and disability. If allowed to progress without intervention, patients may develop complete alienation of the hand from the body – they may cease to recognize the hand as part of the complete body image and are often seen to carry the hand like a parcel. The debate on diagnosis of complex regional pain syndrome led to further classification by some workers (Lee-Lankford, 1990). This particular author felt that classification of the different clinical types was helpful in identification of the condition.

- Minor causalgia is subsequent to damage to a minor peripheral nerve, resulting in symptoms affecting a small part of the hand – for example, the superficial branch of the radial nerve, palmar branch of the medial nerve, neuroma and dorsal superficial branch of the ulnar nerve.
- Minor trauma is related to no specific nerve but produces symptoms following minor injury such as a crushed finger, fracture dislocation or sprain, or a penetrating wound.

- Shoulder hand syndrome is a characteristic pain in that it originates in the shoulder and spreads to the whole upper extremity. The cause may be an initial shoulder injury such as irritated cuff injury or some other factor such as capsulitis, and it may also develop secondary to heart disease or stroke.
- Major traumatic dystrophy is the symptom that is produced following a major trauma such as a crushed hand or Colles' fracture of the wrist.
- Major causalgia is when a major nerve sustains a partial nerve injury. The symptoms of major causalgia are well recognized and, although extreme, can be related to those of minor causalgia.

Abnormal sympathetic reflex

The normal sympathetic reflex of the body to injury is to promote vasoconstriction of the small vessels to stop bleeding, and this is then followed by vasodilatation to continue the healing process. Sympathetic reflex is stimulated by the C fibre afferent in response to injury. If for some reason the sympathetic arc does not shut down at an appropriate time, sympathetic activity is increased and the consequent sustained vasoconstriction produces ischaemia in the tissues, leading to more pain and consequently more C fibre activity, reactivating the sympathetic arc and leading to increased sympathetic nerve activity (Lee-Lankford, 1990).

In 1994, the International Association for the Study of Pain (IASP) renamed and reclassified RSD into complex regional pain syndrome types I and II:

- Type 1 is sympathetically maintained pain from no initial injury
- Type 2 is nerve-related pain following actual damage or injury.

Consequently, recommendations have been advocated for management of the two types of CRPS.

Reclassification has not significantly changed the therapist's management of this difficult condition. People still present with the same characteristic problems, and management must still be based on recognizing and appropriately applying treatment modalities after a problem-orientated assessment.

Clinical experience confirms that some people predispose to CRPS. Poor or disturbed circulation, such as in Raynaud's disease, is often found to be a common condition in patients who have CRPS. Equally, slightly hot and clammy hands may predispose to CRPS and should be identified for review post-operatively if undergoing even minor hand surgery.

Current management of this condition is most successful if the condition is recognized early and there is early intervention, mobilization and control of pain, and also treatment for the sympathetic symptoms if they predominate. In the author's opinion there is no recipe book remedy for the successful treatment of CRPS. Certainly if there is not early mobilization of the hand and re-education of its functional use, this will quickly lead to a more severe and permanent disability.

Reclassification has not changed the ultimate management, and for this reason it will be approached in three stages. The priorities of choice of treatment may vary depending on the stage of the syndrome.

Stage 1 (early stage)

A stage 1 patient presents with burning pain, which may be of 3 months' duration. The hand is soft, swollen and hot, and frequently sweaty. The pain is intense and increasing. Frequently, hyperpathia (abnormal painful response to light touch) is present. Osteoporosis is not present before 3 weeks, but may be evident after the fifth week.

Clearly management of CRPS is likely to be more successful if treatment is aimed at reducing or modifying some of the abnormal neurophysiological effects associated with nerve damage – for example, modulation of the abnormal C fibre activity sustaining the abnormal sympathetic symptoms seen in CRPS. Any medical management must be accompanied by active therapy. Guanethidine blocks are certainly the first choice of treatment when abnormal sympathetic symptoms predominate (Withrington and Wynn Parry, 1984), but the blocks must be given in conjunction with therapy and may have to be repeated.

Medical management – guanethidine blocks

There are varying ways of administering these blocks. However, in the author's experience the following regime has proved to be most successful (Withrington and Wynn Parry, 1984).

The patient must be conscious and able to participate in the whole procedure. The patient lies flat and an automatic pneumatic cuff is applied above the elbow and inflated to just above systolic pressure. Using an intravenous cannula, 10 ml 0.25% marcaine, 20 ml normal saline and 20 ml of guanethidine are introduced, and the cuff remains inflated for 20 minutes. It is essential that once pain is relieved normal sensory stimulation is encouraged, and the hand or part concerned should be stimulated by gentle manual stimulation, stroking the skin and attempting to get the patient to move the hand in normal patterns of movement. The sooner more normal patterns of movement can be restored, the more likely it is that the relief of pain will be maintained. The blocks may be repeated and given every 2 days if necessary. The need for careful monitoring is essential to evaluate the response and encourage active movement. The patient remains on bed rest for 2 hours prior to commencing intensive rehabilitation in the therapy department.

If repeated blocks are unsuccessful, it may be necessary to consider other more permanent procedures, such as sympathectomy. If symptoms of shooting pain are present, then the use of antispasmodic drugs such as carbamazepine may be helpful.

Therapy management

Therapy management of CRPS differs according to the stage of the syndrome. However, therapy modalities should be introduced appropriately in direct response to the current symptoms and to the patient's tolerance. The 'staged management' is therefore only a guide.

The initial instinct of any therapist when faced with a stiff and painful hand is to mobilize it aggressively. Therapy management of CRPS must be co-ordinated with pain relief. Precautions must be taken to avoid any increased vascularity with active movement, which may add to an already highly vascularized hand.

Successful treatment relies on:

- realistic and attainable goals
- a clear understanding of the pathology
- accurate and appropriate application of treatment
- management of pain in the context of the complete rehabilitation.

Active movement must be accompanied with aggressive, effective and consistent elevation.

Ice and contrast baths are popular modalities for pain relief, but their use in CRPS is questionable.

Other modalities, such as Diapulse and interferential, all have their value. However, treatment of CRPS is time-consuming, and often only limited progress is made even with long treatment sessions. The use of equipment that requires immobilization and inactivity for periods of 20 minutes may not be the first choice of treatment, despite the alleged therapeutic value, especially as this may alienate the hand even further.

TENS is very valuable in management, as it affords pain relief whilst simultaneously allowing active movement. Placement of electrodes must be close to the painful area but not touching it if hyperaesthesia is a major symptom (see Figure 4.5). If pain is predominantly on one aspect of the hand only, for example anterior, pads can be placed on the same anterior aspect in parallel (Figure 4.4.b.i).

As already discussed, continuous stimulation for prolonged periods is essential for good results. Active and passive mobilization can commence once a degree of pain relief is achieved. As osteoporosis may be present after 5 weeks, it is vital that no undue force is employed because this may result in permanent tissue damage. Conversely, movement must be effective, otherwise 'placebo wiggling' will result.

More recently, the use of continuous passive motion as part of the management of CRPS has proved to be very promising (Woods and Withrington, 1992), and the period of rehabilitation and the need for intensive therapy have been shown to be significantly reduced by this. In their study, Woods and Withrington used continuous passive motion (occasionally in conjunction with guanethidine blocks) for 24 hours and removed patients from the machine twice daily for active movement. The time on the continuous passive motion machine was reduced over a 2–3-week period, and stopped at between 4 and 8 weeks. The most significant improvement was demonstrated in the first 2 weeks. Contrary to what might have been

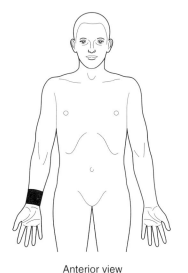
Anterior view

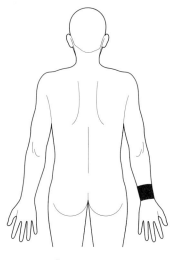
Posterior view

Figure 4.5 Placement of TENS electrodes for CRPS. Pain on both aspects of hand.

expected, pain was significantly less while patients were on the machine. In this study, 90 per cent of function was restored in the cases discussed.

Splinting may be used. Loss of movement may be total, involving flexion and extension of the fingers and wrist, and mobilization is a balance between gaining one movement and not compromising the opposite movement. Flexion gloves can be a useful adjunct to treatment, but application should be for very short periods and closely supervised. These gloves are modular splints whereby the patient slips the hand into the glove and the fingers are held down with Velcro™. The application of flexion gloves may not be tolerated in the early stages, but can be introduced as pain reduces. Bilateral activities must be encouraged at an early stage. Ideally rigid splinting should be avoided, but there may be certain circumstances where splinting may be necessary – for example, if a rapidly advancing flexion contracture is developing.

To establish an effective and reproducible hand exercise regime is quite difficult. Few but effective exercises should be taught, and the Wehbe–Hunter exercise regime used following tendon repair is a useful method (Wehbe and Hunter, 1985). The aim of active exercise is not only to maintain a full range of movement of the joint, but also to maintain the elasticity and full excursion of all soft tissues (Figure 4.6; Van Strien, 1990).

Stage 2 (middle stage)

In stage 2, the pain increases, there is a change in the swelling from soft to hard, the redness and heat are reduced and there is less sweating. Demineralization may increase and continue for the next 9 months.

There are a wide variety of dynamic splints that can restore function and prevent contracture. Again, if splinting can be avoided this may be preferable. The fabrication of splints and the frequently severe difficulty in applying them to CRPS hands may prevent their use. Treatment can also

focus on the splint so that this becomes the most important feature and distracts from the hand itself, and this reduces useful active treatment time. Frequently, if the splints are effective and producing the correction that you wish to achieve, they are not tolerated. They may also serve to further isolate the hand as part of the body, as the splint acts as a reminder of the loss of function of the hand.

Time is a scarce and valuable resource, and must be directed at the most efficacious use leading to the best outcome. This may mean making choices of treatment modalities. Flexion gloves and Coban wrapping for contracture and oedema respectively are both useful tools in the therapist's repertoire.

Stress loading programmes remain a practical solution to providing sensory inhibition and evoking the gating mechanism to painful stimuli, and can work well as part of a full rehabilitation programme (Carlson and Kirk Watson, 1988). In this activity the patient is encouraged to put pressure through an extended arm for 3 minutes and alternate with holding a carrier bag weighted with between 500 g and 3 kg for 3 minutes.

Stage 3 (late stage)

In stage 3 the symptom of constant pain may be reduced although it is still present, particularly on movement. Pencil pointing of the fingers presents with shiny, wasted fingers, and this may last for 2 years. The shiny, atrophic appearance and osteoporosis may be the main features at this stage, together with complete dysfunction and alienation of the hand.

This is possibly the most difficult stage, as contracture may be present and osteoporosis profound. It may be that only surgical intervention will replace movement. However, it would take a brave surgeon to operate on any CRPS hand. Certainly, early intervention for treatment of CRPS may prevent progression to the final stage. Successful treatment will depend on early intervention, a co-operative patient and perseverance of the therapist.

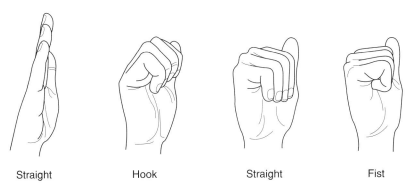

Straight   Hook   Straight   Fist

Figure 4.6 Tendon gliding exercises. (Reproduced with permission from *Rehabilitation of the Hand*, 3rd edn (Hunter, J. M., Schneider, L. H., Mackin, E. J. and Callahan, A. D., eds), p. 401. C. V. Mosby.)

CONCLUSION

No exact recipe exists for pain management, and each case must be taken individually. A wide variety of modalities and treatment techniques exist, but not all are available or accessible to all therapists. It is vital that therapists have a comprehensive understanding of pain mechanisms, and that through innovative and imaginative practice they can exploit resources that are available in their own environment.

Pain is the most frequent symptom that limits or hinders rehabilitation of the hand. Unless there is an understanding of the cause of pain, then effective treatment will not be possible. Successful treatment relies upon accurate diagnosis, realistic and attainable goals, and full co-operation in partnership with the patient.

REFERENCES

Bowsher, D. (1994a). Acute and chronic pain and assessment. In: *Pain Management in Physiotherapy*, 2nd edn (P. Wells, V. Frampton and D. Bowsher, eds), pp. 11–17. Butterworth Heinemann.

Bowsher, D. (1994b). Anatomy, neurophysiology and pharmacology. In: *Pain Management in Physiotherapy*, 2nd edn (P. Wells, V. Frampton and D. Bowsher, eds), Section 1. Butterworth Heinemann.

Carlson, L. K. and Kirk Watson, H. (1988). Treatment of reflex sympathetic dystrophy using the stress loading program. *J. Hand. Ther.*. **1(4)**, 149–54.

Frampton, V. M. (1990). Therapist's management of brachial plexus injuries. In: *Rehabilitation of the Hand* (J. M. Hunter, L. H. Schneider, E. J. Mackin and A. D. Callahan, eds), pp. 630–39. C. V. Mosby.

Frampton, V. (1994). Transcutaneous electrical nerve stimulation and chronic pain. In: *Pain Management in Physiotherapy*, 2nd edn (P. Wells, V. Frampton and D. Bowsher, eds), pp. 89–91. Butterworth Heinemann.

Frampton, V. (1996). Transcutaneous electrical nerve stimulations. In: *Claytons Electrotherapy*, 10th edn (S. Kitchen and S. Bazin, eds), pp. 287–305. W. B. Saunders.

International Association for the Study of Pain (IASP) (1994). *Classification of Chronic Pain: Description of Chronic Pain Syndromes and Definitions of Pain Terms*, 2nd edn. IASP Press.

Lee-Lankford L. (1990). Reflex sympathetic dystrophy. In: Rehabilitation of the Hand (J. M. Hunter, L. H. Schneider, E. J. Mackin and A. D. Callahan, eds), pp. 763–86. C. V. Mosby.

Loeser, J. D. and Ward, A. A. (1967). Some effects of deafferentation on neurones of the cat spinal cord. *Arch. Neurol.*, **17**, 629–30.

Loeser, J. D., Black, R. G. and Chirstman, A. (1975). Relief of pain by transcutaneous stimulation. *J. Neurosurg.*, **42**, 308–34.

Loh, L. and Nathan, P. W. (1978). Painful peripheral states and sympathetic blocks. *J. Neurol. Neurosurg. Psychiatr.*, **41**, 664–71.

Melzack, R. and Wall, P. D. (1967). Pain mechanism: a new theory. *Science*, **150**, 971–8.

Melzack, R., Stillwell, D. M. and Fox, E. J. (1987). Trigger points and acupuncture points for pain. Correlations and implications. *Pain*, **3**, 3–23.

Merskey, H. (1979). Pain terms: a list with definitions and notes on usage. (recommended by the IASP subcommittee on Taxonomy. *Pain*, **6**, 249–52.

Moldaver J. (1978). Tinel's sign. Its characteristics and significance. *J. Bone Joint Surg.*, **60A**, 412.

Pomeranz, B. and Niznick, G. (1987). Codetron, a new electrotherapy device overcomes the habituation problems of conventional TENS devices. *Am. J. Electromed.*, **First Quarter,** 22–6.

Robinson, C. (1986). Brachial plexus lesion. Functional splintage, Part 2. *Br. J. Occup. Ther.*, **49(10)**, 331.

Thompson, J. W. (1986). The role of transcutaneous electrical nerve stimulation (TENS) for the control of pain. In: *International Symposium on Pain Control 1986* (D. Doyle, ed.), pp. 27–47. Royal Society of Medical Services.

Tinel, J. (1915). Le signe due 'fourmillement' dans les lesion des nerfs peripherique. *Press. Med.*, **47**, 388.

Van Strien, G. (1990). Post-operative management of flexor tendon injuries. In: *Rehabilitation of the Hand*, 3rd edn (J. M. Hunter, L. H. Schneider, E. J. Mackin and A. D. Callahan, eds), p. 401. C. V. Mosby.

Wall, P. D. (1984). Changes of sensation and behaviour after injury. In: *Textbook of Pain*, 1st edn (P. D. Wall and R. Melzack, eds), pp. 13–14. Churchill Livingstone.

Wall, P. D. and Gutnik, M. (1974). Properties of afferent nerve impulses originating from a neuroma. *Nature*, **248**, 740.

Wall, P. D. and Melzack, R. (eds) (1987). *Textbook of Pain*, 2nd edn. Churchill Livingstone.

Wallin, G., Torebork, E. and Hallin, R. (1976). Preliminary observations on the pathophysiology of hyperalgesia in the causalgic pain syndrome. In: *Sensory Function of the Skin in Primates* (Y. Zotterman, ed.), pp. 489–502. Pergamon Press.

Wehbe, M. A. and Hunter, J. M. (1985). Flexor tendon gliding in the hand. Part I. Differential gliding. *J. Hand*, **S10–A**, 575.

Withrington, R. H. and Wynn Parry, C. B. (1984). The management of painful peripheral nerve disorders. *J. Hand Surg.*, **9B(1)**, 24–8.

Woods, Z. and Withrington, R. H. (1992). Continuous passive motion as a treatment modality in reflex sympathetic dystrophy. *Proceedings from the British Society for Surgery of the Hand*, Autumn meeting.

Woolf, S. L., Gersh, H. R. and Rao, V. R. (1981). Examination of electrode placements and stimulating parameters in treating chronic pain with conventional transcutaneous electrical nerve stimulation (TENS). *Pain*, **11**, 37–47.

Wynn Parry, C. B. (1980). Pain in avulsion lesions of the brachial plexus. *Pain*, **9**, 41–53.

Wynn Parry, C. B. (1981). Pain. In: *Rehabilitation of the Hand*, pp. 126–46. Butterworths.

Wynn Parry, C. B. and Withrington R. H. (1984). The management of painful peripheral nerve disorders. In: *Textbook of Pain*, 1st edn (P. D. Wall and R. Melzack, eds), pp 395–441. Churchill Livingstone.

5 Treatment

Maureen Salter and Carole Bexon with contributions from Dominique Thomas

In order to achieve good results following hand trauma and other disorders, it is preferable that therapists are involved in both the pre- and post-operative management of the hand. It is erroneous to consider that hand patients can regain sufficient function by themselves. Skilled therapy is essential for acceptable outcomes, and many hand surgeons hold the view that 50 per cent of the treatment is by the surgeon and 50 per cent by the hand therapist.

The essential elements for successful hand therapy are:

1. Skilled assessment
2. Knowledge peculiar to the hand
3. Education
4. Patient motivation
5. Support for the patient.

Without guidance and direction it is likely that patients may not even know the extent to which they should exercise or rest their injured hand, may find the principles of hand therapy difficult to comprehend and, even though well motivated, be unlikely to have the suitable means with which to work at home.

Some patients will only need advice and minimal supervision, whereas others may need extensive treatment. It is not always obvious from the initial assessment into which category the patient will fall, as the extent of injury does not necessarily correlate with the amount of therapy input required. All patients will benefit from skilled management, and problems may well arise without it.

PATIENT REVIEW

Hand patients are reviewed within the therapy process as follows:

- initial assessment
- treatment planning
- treatment implementation
- evaluation
- review to ensure that progress is maintained.

This process is most successful when the patient and the entire team work towards common goals. The value of this team approach cannot be over-emphasized, since it benefits everyone, especially the patient. As discussed in Chapter 2, the team comprises a surgeon, hand therapists, nurse, social worker, clinical psychologist and, most importantly, the patient. A disability employment advisor (DEA) is involved if the patient is likely to experience difficulty in returning to work.

Regular multidisciplinary clinics

These supply the framework for the team approach, providing the opportunity to discuss progress and any problems that may have arisen in various departments. The clinics:

- give everyone the opportunity to discuss any difficulties that may have arisen during treatment
- allow each team member to become aware of the patient's progress in the various departments
- ensure that all aspects of the patient's needs are covered.

Roles of therapists

The roles of the occupational therapist and physiotherapist vary from one hand unit to another, but in the UK hand therapy is generally given by both the occupational therapist and the physiotherapist. To avoid confusing the patient it is essential that the occupational therapist/physiotherapist team has common goals and clear methods of communication. The workload can then be suitably divided:

- the physiotherapist taking a prominent role in regaining a specific range of movement combined with re-education of muscles and use of electrical treatments such as pulsed diathermy and ultrasound
- the occupational therapist focusing on the use of activity as a treatment modality for restoration of function, splinting, activities of daily living and return to employment.

The patient thus receives highly specialized treatments, with the therapists working as a sub-team and giving each other academic and managerial support.

Hand therapy conforms easily to a problem-solving approach, and problem-orientated medical recording (POMR) provides a useful framework to detail the progress in treatment as well as for assessment (see Chapter 2). A plan of treatment, with aims for each problem, can be based on the initial problem list. Treatment plans must be written in clear behavioural descriptions, with no ambiguity.

Reassessment

Reassessment of the patient's hand on a weekly basis enables specific progress to be measured. However, a longer interval between assessments may be indicated to prevent a patient who is making only slow progress and seeing little improvement from becoming discouraged. The results of the reassessment will identify those problems:

- that have been resolved
- that will continue
- that are new and have have recently arisen.

The aims and plans of treatment can then be modified accordingly.

Provision of rehabilitation

The provision of adequate rehabilitation for hand injuries should have high priority in all therapy departments.

1. Intensive early treatment, which means at least two or three times a day, should commence within a few hours of the patient leaving theatre. Over a short period this can be more effective, especially for severe injuries, than limited treatment over an extended period.
2. Problems such as pain and residual joint stiffness should be attended to urgently.
3. A large proportion of severe hand injuries affect people of working age. Their needs, both in getting them back to work and in looking after their leisure interests, must take priority over some of the more chronic work of the department. The cost of this treatment will be justified when a patient returns to work instead of becoming a burden to the state by becoming permanently disabled.
4. Full-time treatment might make all the difference between a poor result and an efficiently functioning hand.
5. If large numbers of hand patients require treatment, for example if there are a lot of fractures and sprains caused by icy road conditions, it may be necessary to treat them within a group (see Group treatment, below).
6. As a general principle, patients with hand injuries must not be placed on a waiting list, otherwise poor outcomes are likely. Even though patient numbers may be extremely high, all injuries must be treated adequately.

A severe hand injury can have a devastating effect on the life of the patient. For successful overall care, the emotional, psychological and social needs of the patient should be handled sympathetically and with urgency. The therapist plays an important role in listening to the history of the injury and the patient's feelings and worries, providing reassurance, and being alert to any covert cues that might herald depression. The social worker and clinical psychologist should be advised of problematical developments.

STAGES OF REHABILITATION

The management of hand injuries progresses continually and steadily through the various stages of healing and rehabilitation. This gradual progression from initial to final stages is described in the following pages. The timings given for the commencement of treatments (such as adding resistance and applying stretch) are a rough guide only,

and definite timings must be agreed between surgeon and therapist so that damage is not caused by starting treatment too soon or too late. The stage at which intensive treatment may commence depends on:

- the degree of injury
- the surgery performed
- the stage of healing
- the patient's progress.

This process of recovery following major hand trauma can take many months or even years, and some patients may possibly be left with permanent disabilities or problems, depending upon the extent of their injury. The maximum gain from therapy is likely to be achieved during the early rehabilitation and the later intensive phases of treatment. When the rate of progress begins to slow or plateau, it is important to re-establish the patient in a normal environment and not to prolong therapy. On discharge, it is possible that not all problems will have been resolved. However, most will have improved significantly, with adequate function restored.

Early stage following injury and operation (1–5 days)

Surgical procedures are performed within the first few hours in the majority of severe injuries, and therapy should be commenced immediately postoperatively – that is, as soon as the patient regains consciousness. Sessions lasting 15–30 minutes and repeated two or three times a day are desirable. Surgery for some specific tissues may need a further few days rest, but positioning with elevation must be catered for immediately.

At this early stage, only a few of the assessments described in Chapter 2 can be made, so careful questioning of the patient and observation of the hand is recorded in the POMR regarding:

- pain
- resting position
- swelling
- colour
- any active movement of the affected part, if allowed
- range of movement of non-immobilized joints
- sensory changes.

A check must be made that bandages and plasters are not too tight, as this could lead to the development of a neurapraxia, and ischaemia of the soft tissues. Patients must be taught to check themselves for any warning signs in the fingers and hand distal to the lesion, such as:

- pain and throbbing
- change of colour
- change of temperature

- oedema
- sensory changes such as 'pins and needles' or numbness.

Injury of the soft tissues inevitably results in cellular damage. At first an inflammatory process occurs, which is followed within 5 days by the onset of healing and repair. A number of factors can accelerate or retard this healing process (Evans, 1980), and the formation of collagen resulting from tissue damage can be influenced by early treatment (Kesson and Atkins, 1998).

The state of the healing process must be carefully observed. If early treatment is too aggressive it can exacerbate a greater inflammatory reaction, which in turn results in the production of more extensive fibrosis. Some rest of the injured structures may be necessary following surgery before exercise can commence; however, therapy undertaken during the first 24 hours will have the greatest impact on the long-term outcome.

The main aims of treatment at this stage are:

- reduction of pain
- positioning of the joints of hand and arm for safe immobilization
- prevention or reduction of oedema
- gentle active movement of the injured part, if permitted
- movement of joints proximal to the injury, especially the shoulder, which is liable to stiffen (particularly in the elderly)
- attention to the patient's chest function following surgery
- attention to activities of daily living (ADL)
- attention to social, domestic and employment problems.

General fitness of the patient should be considered throughout all stages of rehabilitation, including this early stage after injury and operation.

Intermediate stage (6 days–6 weeks)

Stitches are removed between 10 and 14 days post-operatively, depending on the degree of healing. The assessments described in Chapter 2 should be carried out now. They enable:

- the problems to be identified
- a plan to be drawn up with specific aims and objectives
- a baseline to be formed from which treatment can be evaluated.

Continuing measurements are important, as they provide the objective means by which patient and therapists can identify improvements. For example, it is usually not possible to see changes of only a few degrees range of movement without regular and accurate measurement. Patients may not be able to identify their own progress without an objective hand assessment.

An increase in the treatment regime is usually suitable at 3–4 weeks after surgery or injury. Time must not be lost in recovering movement as stiffness of the joints occurs extremely quickly, especially in the presence of gross oedema. Joints that are immobilized for 6 weeks or more are liable to become permanently stiff, and soft tissues will lose their elasticity.

Treatments are concentrated on:

- reduction of any pain
- reduction of any residual oedema
- softening of the skin and indurated areas
- achievement of a full range of those joints not immobilized
- free active movements – usually resistance may be gradually added at 3 weeks
- functional activities
- attention to any remaining social, domestic or employment difficulties.

Later stages (6 weeks onwards)

The main aim of hand therapy during the later stages is for the patient to resume as normal function as possible and return to employment. This will be dependent on a number of factors such as:

- range of movement
- sensation
- normality of movement patterns
- grip strength
- dexterity
- manipulative skills.

Therapy must be aimed at restoring these skills, and the intensity of any treatment programme should match the patient's needs realistically:

1. A daily session may be all that is necessary for routine conditions.
2. Full- or part-time rehabilitation should be available for the patient with severe injuries. This can achieve a better result than from only one treatment session daily, when any gain in one day may well be lost by the next.
3. Early recovery and return to work makes sound economic sense. The patient will be earning a living and will not need disability or unemployment benefits, and this is of significant psychological benefit.

Case conferences should continue to be held weekly to discuss progress. It may be decided that a more strenuous form of treatment is appropriate, with:

- increased activity and greater resistance to active movement
- passive stretching
- serial splinting

- strenous workshop activities
- attention to employment requirements
- the solving or improvement of any social, domestic or psychological problems.

The availability of a rehabilitation unit that offers full- or part-time treatment with workshop facilities can prove invaluable at this time for maximizing hand function.

PLANNING TREATMENT

It is vital for patients:

- to become experts in their own hand and the injury
- to be involved in setting the treatment goals
- to understand the purpose of therapeutic activities.

Patient education is essential from the onset of treatment, with the therapist taking a major role as educator. The patient should understand some anatomy of the hand and how it relates to the damaged structures, together with the process of recovery and prognosis for the injury. For example, a detailed description of the progression and time-scale for the recovery of nerve lesions enables the patient to make sense of the delay before activity occurs in the muscles, and the sensations that are likely to be experienced. This understanding of injury and approach to treatment helps to improve motivation and co-operation, and allows the patient to feel more in control, with some responsibility for the outcome.

Teaching, advice and counselling will need to be an ongoing process throughout rehabilitation.

Therapists should design the treatment using the problem-orientated approach, based on the problem list drawn up following the assessment (see Chapter 2). At times during treatment only one or two problems may be seen as the priority, but usually the therapist will be addressing several problems simultaneously.

A typical treatment session may progress through the following sequence, but priorities must be determined for each individual patient and not all these treatments will necessarily be needed:

1. Reduction of oedema and improvement of circulation
2. Reduction of pain
3. Care of scars and soft tissues
4. Mobilization of joints – active and passive range of movement
5. Re-education of muscle activity and the establishment of normal patterns of movement
6. Improvement of dexterity and manipulation
7. Muscle strengthening
8. Sensory re-education
9. Attention to specific problems, such as cold intolerance and machine phobia.

Following major hand trauma where there are multiple problems, the physiotherapist and occupational therapist should designate which problems each will treat so that time is not wasted by duplication. Problems can often be treated simultaneously – for example, oedema, joint stiffness and loss of dexterity will all be improved by a carefully selected functional activity in elevation. Therapy resources must be utilized as efficiently and effectively as possible.

PREPARATION AND WARM-UP

A short preparatory warm-up session improving the circulation and carefully stretching the muscles should be given prior to any specific treatment, as is undertaken by normally fit sportsmen and women prior to strenuous activity. A warm-up can take the form of simple exercises, possibly performed to music, at the start of morning and afternoon sessions. Alternatively, the patient may exercise the hand for a few minutes in an arm bath of warm soapy water or saline.

GROUP TREATMENT

Group treatment has various patient benefits besides ensuring that large numbers can be treated at once when departments are busy. However, in the first instance every patient must be assessed and treated on a one-to-one basis, including a thorough explanation of the injury, the proposed treatment programme, and the progress expected.

Some of the advantages of group treatment are that:

- the patient meets and works with others who have similar problems
- activities are easily adapted to the individual patient requirements – e.g. padding of racquet handles, and selection of size and weight of apparatus and equipment
- general fitness will be improved
- activities are fun, which is very important
- the competitive spirit between patients often achieves greater gains than those from formal, individual treatments.

Patients should be seen individually for at least a few minutes at each attendance of class therapy:

- each should be able to demonstrate that he or she remembers the home exercises and is practising them sufficiently, and a list of activities should be taken home by each individual as a reminder
- measurements taken should confirm that satisfactory progress is being maintained
- problems such as pain and joint stiffness must be addressed urgently and treated individually.

(See also later stages of group treatment, p. 110.)

SPECIFIC TREATMENTS

Hand-to-hand contact is the most natural occurrence in our lives from infancy onwards, and the therapist's use of his or her own hands to make contact with the patient's injured one is extremely important. The patient will be aware that the difficulties can be detected and therefore much better understood by the palpation of the damaged hand. The willingness of the therapist to touch and handle a possibly unsightly hand also has the added benefit of providing reassurance and helping the patient to regain lost confidence. Therapists must wear masks and gloves when handling the patient if dressings are to be removed before skin healing has occurred, to retain aseptic conditions.

Oedema

Increased swelling, or oedema, is a serious complication that frequently occurs following both hand injury and surgery. Good circulation in the hand is essential for healing and recovery, and insufficient arterial supply to the soft tissues may contribute to permanent disability. Oedema caused by the escaping exudate creates an increase of pressure within the tissues of the hand, and this pressure in turn damages structures such as the small arteries, veins, capillaries, nerves and lymphatic system. If the blood supply to the hand is jeopardized, ischaemia of the skin and muscles can occur. This damage may be irreversible if it is not identified and treated quickly. The median nerve within the carpal tunnel is particularly vulnerable to compression in the oedematous hand.

Oedema is easily observed when the hand is uncovered. The therapist should enquire for diagnostic symptoms such as tingling in the index and middle fingers and the thumb, especially in the absence of a traumatic lesion of the median nerve. Median nerve damage, either through trauma or compression, can predispose to the additional secondary problem of complex regional pain syndrome.

Oedema tends to collect where the skin is loose and elastic, e.g. over the volar aspect of the wrist and the dorsum of the metacarpals, and on both aspects of the fingers. The swollen hand and wrist therefore adopts a typical posture of wrist flexion, metacarpophalangeal joint extension and proximal interphalangeal joint flexion. In this posture the joints are in the loose-packed position, and if not treated rapidly a permanent deformity will result, which is difficult to reverse. The metacarpophalangeal joints quickly become fixed in extension, and it can be extremely difficult and time-consuming to regain full flexion. The proximal interphalangeal joints are also particularly vulnerable to soft tissue flexion contracture with loss of joint extension, which is difficult to regain. The oedema

that remains in the hand will consolidate with the formation of fibrous tissue.

The oedematous hand:

- feels stiff to the patient
- is awkward and often painful to move
- is displeasing to look at
- is dysfunctional.

For all these reasons, and particularly because of the risk of consolidation, it is vital that swelling is reduced quickly and effectively, with the majority eliminated within the first 6 weeks following trauma. Any oedema remaining after this time is likely to disperse very slowly, and residual swelling may remain for many months.

Oedema of the hand requires fast and active intervention, and the patient must understand clearly the importance of reducing the swelling. The patient's education, understanding and co-operation in its treatment is the first line of attack in solving the problem.

Elevation

The fundamental approach to oedema treatment is elevation, combined wherever possible with active movement. The patient must elevate the hand at every practical opportunity, enabling the excess fluid to drain away from the hand with the assistance of gravity. This can range from elevation of the whole arm, with almost full shoulder flexion and elbow extension, to resting with the hand held at least at shoulder height. Instruction must be given on positioning at home during the day, with the hand elevated on pillows on a table set alongside the armchair. At the same time, extension of the wrist is encouraged because a flexed wrist will hinder efficient drainage.

Elevation of the hand helps to lower the pressure in the blood vessels and assists the lymphatic drainage of exudate caused by the soft tissue damage. The decrease in tissue pressure greatly helps to reduce the intense pain of a severely oedematous hand.

The upper limb is supported with the hand in an elevated position both when the patient is in bed and when ambulant. In bed, the whole arm is elevated, using either a Bradford sling (Figure 5.1) or a roller towel suspended from a drip stand. The edges of the towel are pinned together to hold the hand in place, and pillows used to support the upper arm. A broom handle can be used at home as a substitute for the drip stand if the patient is discharged early and elevation at night is still necessary. It can be fixed head upwards to the bed, and the Bradford sling or a towel suspended from the broom head as described above. Alternatively, the arm can be rested on a large pile of pillows.

When ambulant, the hand should be supported initially in a high triangular sling, remembering always that the hand should be held higher than

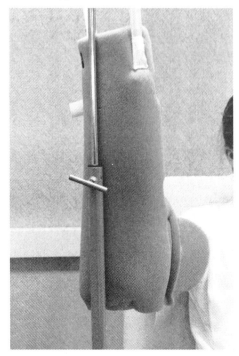

Figure 5.1 Elevation in a Bradford sling.

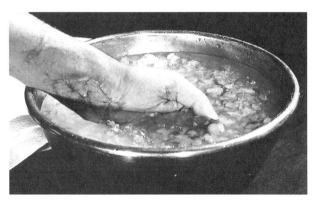

Figure 5.3 A mulch of ice and water.

the elbow. The angle of the latter must not be too acute, as this may restrict drainage. *Hand above heart* is a useful *aide memoire* to ensure that the principle of elevation is applied correctly.

Slings The patient should use a sling whilst moving around during the day, and several varieties are available. The triangular sling can be replaced by a continuous strap or Boscombe sling as the swelling decreases (Figure 5.2), with the weight of the injured hand and arm taken by the shoulder of the uninjured side rather than round the neck.

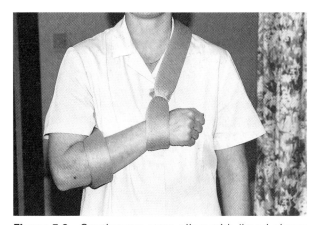

Figure 5.2 Continuous strap sling with 'hand above heart'.

Cooling and the use of cold as a treatment

Vasoconstriction of capillaries helps to prevent excess exudate, and this can be achieved most simply by cooling. Cooling in the hand and arm can be produced by use of a fan, or by application of cold towels to the skin.

Ice packs should not be used during the first few days as they can produce an undesirable local vasodilation that could exacerbate the inflammatory reaction and possibly also induce cold intolerance.

Wet towels, wrung out in iced water, can be applied to available skin as a cold treatment when the hand is kept elevated. They are renewed in the cold water when they warm, and are applied for 4–5 minutes.

Ice baths consisting of a mulch of ice and water help to reduce oedema when the hand is free of dressings, by causing vasoconstriction of the capillaries (Figure 5.3).

The patient can exercise the hand in the ice slush by flexing and extending the fingers for 2–3 minutes at a time, or less if the hand becomes very uncomfortable. During the brief rest period the hand should be dried. Tolerance to this treatment will increase quickly and improved mobility usually results, mainly because of the reduction of oedema.

A small area of oedema can be treated locally using an ice cube or compressed crushed ice, rubbing it over the affected area for 1–2 minutes.

Caution: Ice packs must be used with great care in order to avoid an undesirable vasodilatation or ice burn of the skin. Ice is contraindicated for patients with a peripheral nerve lesion, because the autonomic disturbance results in the hand becoming very cold and the time taken to warm again is increased considerably. (See Cold intolerance, p. 118.)

Movement

Movement provides a pumping action of muscles, which assists venous return and helps to both improve lymphatic drainage and prevent the return of swelling. The patient must be encouraged to exercise the arm, hand and wrist regularly whilst in elevation, particularly using the small intrinsic muscles of the hand when possible.

Active movements of adjacent unaffected joints should be performed immediately post-operatively, and gentle muscle contractions of the affected area encouraged as soon as possible. This activity provides the best means of assisting both lymphatic and venous drainage, and will not aggravate the inflammatory process when undertaken correctly.

The interval between surgery on the injured hand and the commencement of active or passive movement of the repaired structures will depend on the nature of the injury and the treatment regime prescribed by the surgeon. In most cases movement commences as soon as the patient is conscious, i.e. within a few hours of surgery:

- each patient's needs must be considered separately and carefully
- gentle active movements give a natural stretch to the damaged tissues but must be introduced with extreme care in order to improve and not damage the quality of healing
- isotonic contractions are made, initially through a small range of movement only
- isometric contractions can also be included, and are possible even though the hand may be totally covered in dressings and splints
- range is gradually increased as the condition improves.

This movement is necessary to ensure that the collagen forming in the scar tissue is laid down in an effective linear structure. Premature passive movement and energetic exercises are contraindicated, as they are likely to increase the inflammatory process and thus exacerbate the degree of fibrosis. Fibrous tissue continues to contract for at least 6 months after healing, and will need regular stretching throughout this period.

Caution: Early exercises must not involve contraction of muscles and tendons that have been recently repaired, unless the early active motion regime has been chosen.

Elevated tables

Hand tables enable physiotherapy treatments and occupational therapy activities to be performed in elevation in the therapy department. The tables:

- are adjustable in height (Figure 5.4)
- are relatively simple to make from a wooden board fixed to a metal pole
- must be of sufficient size both to support the hand and forearm, and to use for large activities
- can be either free-standing or slot into brackets on the side of a chair leg (it is worth dedicating a chair for this purpose and adapting it for both left- and right-sided use)
- are made comfortable and hygienic by draping the table top with a towel, which is easily changed
- are hinged to the wall from the upper edge (Figure 5.5)
- are supported at the bottom at varying distances from the wall, thereby creating different angles of slope – the most useful slope is about 30–40° to the vertical

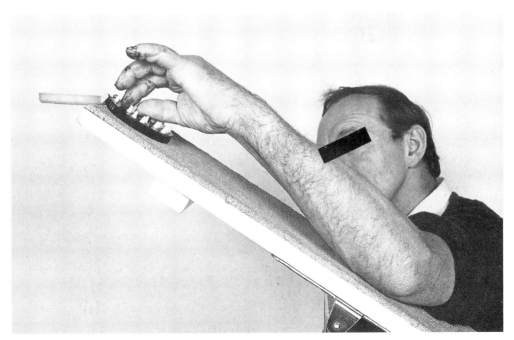

Figure 5.4 An adjustable elevated table.

- have a ledge at the lower edge of the table, which safely supports the weight of each activity (e.g. a large draughts board).

Simple exercises such as making a fist, extending, abducting and adducting the fingers and thumb, and intrinsic movements can be performed while the patient waits for the therapist's attention. Remedial games may be played with other patients, resting in elevation when the others take their turn. A wide variety of board games can be adapted for use on this sloping surface, with the patient moving pieces into the holes cut away in the game board. If non-resisted movement is necessary, for instance following tendon repair, it is essential to provide pieces that can be moved freely. Pieces attached by Velcro or magnets should not be used too soon, since the resistance might be sufficient to rupture repairing tendons.

Large board games and activities can be positioned on a high shelf (Figure 5.22) if neither a hand-table nor a wall-table is available.

Alternatively the patient can sit on a low stool in front of a normal height table, with the hand elevated whilst undertaking the exercises and activities. Wrist extension is maintained by supporting the activity on a bookstand. Another option is for the patient to rest the arm on the raised backrest of a plinth (Figure 5.6).

For safety reasons great care must be taken to ensure that all activities are adequately supported,

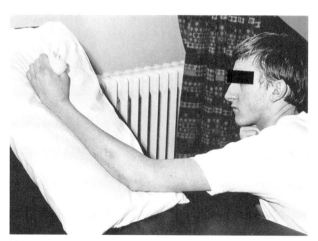

Figure 5.6 Patient's arm elevated on the raised backrest of a plinth.

and the game board should be clamped to the sloping table to ensure that it cannot fall.

Functional activities such as painting or varnishing can be performed in elevation, and small basketry projects tackled from a sloping elevated wall-table. Macramé can be undertaken from an overhead gantry when damaged tendons are able to take some resistance. Workshop tasks can encourage elevation, e.g. by the use of pillar drills with elevated handles.

Electrical therapy

Pulsed electro-magnetic fields (PEMF) Early treatment with high frequency pulsed diathermy is advocated to reduce oedema and limit the degree of fibrous tissue formation (Barclay *et al.*, 1983). The quality of healing, particularly the regeneration of nerves, is accelerated and improved (Wilson and Jagerdeesh, 1976; Raji and Bowden, 1983). A higher dosage can be given than for continuous diathermy, since the heating effect of the pulsed current is minimal. This allows the technique to be used safely even in the presence of metals.

Ultrasound Early use of ultrasonics has been recommended for improving the quality of fibrous tissue repair, probably through the effect of streamlining the collagen fibres (Dyson and Suckling, 1978) and the heating of the collagen (Low and Reed, 1994). A pulsed, low-dose treatment should be used.

The area immediately surrounding sutured tendons should not be treated with ultrasound for at least 5 weeks post-operatively, as this has been shown to delay and even prevent healing (Roberts *et al.*, 1982). It is advisable to allow a similar delay before treating sutured nerves.

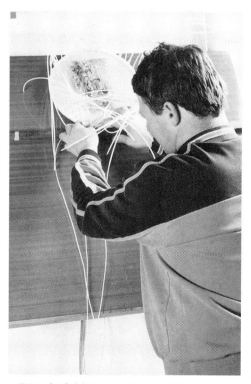

Figure 5.5 Activities can be positioned on a wall mounted elevated table.

Interferential Interferential treatment has been found to assist in the dispersal of persistent oedema. Its effect must be monitored carefully, especially if the patient has autonomic disturbance in the hand.

Heat treatment

Warm water arm baths are a useful means of warming and exercising a hand, improving the circulation (especially in cold weather), and for a preliminary warm-up. Hot water should not be used.

Wax baths and other forms of heat are contra-indicated for the acutely oedematous hand. Heat can cause the hand to swell, especially after recent trauma, and wax treatment immobilizes the hand and is therefore not desirable. Poor circulation and loss of sensation make the hand susceptible to burns at a lower temperature than normal, so care must be taken.

Intermittent pressure therapy

Intermittent pressure therapy (IPT) can be useful both in preventing and reducing oedema. The specially designed sleeves or bags apply pressure to the patient's hand and arm while elevated, helping to press and pump the oedema out of the limb. The bag goes through a regular and repeated cycle of inflation and deflation by the use of an electric pump.

Closed environmental therapy (CET) may have been selected post-operatively for the patient by the surgeon. CET involves elevating the whole hand and arm inside a single-layer sealed plastic bag into which sterile air is blown at above normal atmospheric pressure. The patient is able to exercise the hand, if this is suitable, while it is in the bag. The timing and pressure can be adjusted as required.

A double-walled sleeve may also be used. This is specially designed for the hand and forearm or the full arm (sleeves are also available for the leg), and the hand and arm are placed inside it. This is a particularly suitable treatment in a therapy department and for use at home for reducing oedema. Great care must be taken to prevent any creasing of the double-thickness wall of the bag, as this could traumatize the skin when the pressure is applied. The bag should be rested on an elevated hand table, raised plinth or piled pillows (Figure 5.7), and the amount of pressure applied is adjusted by the therapist and should not be too high since this can be unnecessarily painful. Care must be taken to avoid unwanted passive movement of the fingers after flexor tendon injury or surgery, when tendons are at risk of rupture. A loose boxing glove-style of bandaging will protect the hand. Similar principles should be applied for extensor tendon injuries.

Massage

Massage can be used effectively to disperse oedema, particularly in small areas such as the web spaces. Effleurage and gentle kneading should be given, combined with elevation, and the therapist must be careful not to traumatize delicate skin and scar tissue by using too deep a pressure with the fingertips. Transverse scars across the dorsum of the hand frequently cause problems by trapping the oedema distally in the hand, and creaming and massaging the scar helps to break down scar tissue to allow lymphatic drainage. Straps used to hold splints can similarly exacerbate oedema, especially over the dorsum of the hand. Gentle effleurage will assist in its dispersal, together with care taken to avoid any future problem.

Massage can be time consuming, and may not be the most time- or cost-effective treatment for large

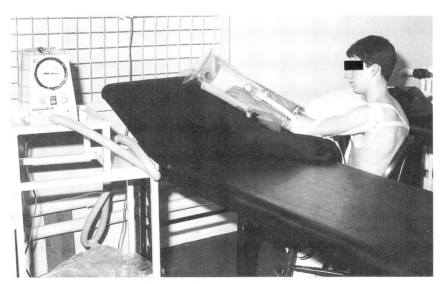

Figure 5.7 Intermittent pressure therapy in elevation.

areas of oedema. It may be appropriate for the massage to be performed by a trained therapy helper, and it can be combined with the use of aromatherapy oils, making it a relaxed, pleasant session for the patient. Both patient and family can be taught hand massage so that it can be undertaken at home.

Wrapping (or roping)

The technique of wrapping, or roping, can be used to squeeze oedema out of the fingers.

A narrow Coban bandage (2.5-cm wide) provides a gentle stretch in the acute stages, and is wound around the finger, commencing at the tip and working proximally. On reaching the base of the finger the bandage is unwound, and the procedure is repeated several times each hour for each finger. A check must be made that there is no compromise to the patient's blood supply, so the very tip of the finger should be left uncovered.

As the oedema reduces pressure can be increased by using a rubber strip (approximately 40 cm × 3 cm), which is wound similarly around the finger (Figure 5.8). Initially the therapist should complete the wrapping, particularly if healing tendons are at risk, but later the patient can perform his or her own wrapping.

The technique can also be used for gross oedema over the dorsum of the hand, but here it is less effective. The hollow of the palm must be padded, and a wider bandage or strip used.

Rubber or plastic tubing may be used as an alternative to a rubber strip. Orthopaedic cord, if used, must be applied with special care in order not to traumatize stretched and delicate skin and newly healed tissues.

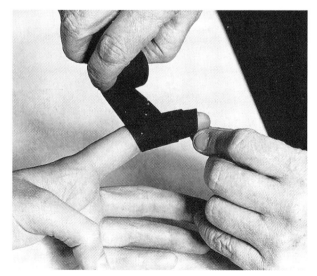

Figure 5.8 Wrapping using rubber strip.

Pressure garments

Pressure garments help to reduce persistent oedema, which is liable to occur where the volume of damaged soft tissue is high (for example in a crush injury). Garments that fit both the fingers and the whole hand are available commercially in a range of sizes, although some elasticated gloves must be specially measured, made and fitted to be effective.

The use of a whole-hand pressure glove should be a rare event, but a glove with just the fingertips cut away can improve the functional use of the hand. It may prove to be an impractical proposition in the work situation, and the patient must discover the best regime for wearing the glove.

Oedema frequently persists in one or two digits even when the bulk of the hand oedema has subsided. In these cases it is possible to use small elasticated sleeves that are fitted over the fingers or thumb (see Chapter 12, p. 242).

1. Sleeves are available commercially in long rolls, and come in a variety of width fittings (Edema Sleeves™). The appropriate width and length of sleeve can be quickly cut off for the patient (Figure 5.9a).
2. Lycra™ finger-stalls are easily custom-made with the use of a sewing machine (Kennedy *et al.*, 1998).
3. Double-thickness Tubigrip™ may be used if neither sleeves nor Lycra are available. A double finger-stall, if required, can be made by stitching down the middle (Figure 5.9b and c), and two double stalls can be used if all four fingers are swollen.
4. Gloves can be made of Lycra or Tubigrip if commercial ones are not available, but may not be as efficient.

Caution: Tendon healing should be complete before these garments are used because of the risk to unhealed tendons when pulling them on and off.

Circulatory disturbance

Circulation in the hand will be considerably reduced following damage to blood vessels or extensive soft tissue injury. Normal response to temperature changes will be slower, especially when there is nerve damage, so care must be taken not to burn the patient, by either heat or cold.

The collateral blood supply can be improved by the use of contrast baths. The patient soaks the hand alternately for 2 or 3 minutes first in a bowl of warm and then in cool water. The effect of this alternate vasodilatation and vasoconstriction of the capillaries will help to improve the response of blood flow in the affected area.

An adequate circulation must be maintained to encourage healing and regeneration. A warm glove

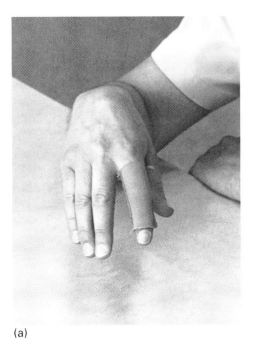

(a)

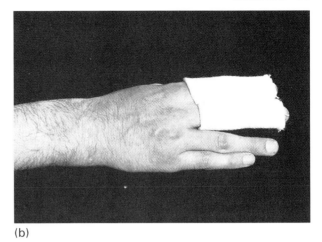

(b)

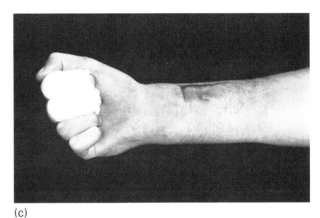

(c)

Figure 5.9 Finger sleeves to control oedema: (a) Lycra, (b) and (c) Tubigrip.

or mitt must be worn in cold weather to keep the hand warm, particularly for those patients with nerve damage. The patient must also be encouraged to perform general whole arm and aerobic exercises, if suitable, which will increase the cardiac output and overall level of circulation. (Whole arm exercise is contraindicated if there is any infection of the limb.)

Pain

Pain relief will be provided initially following trauma or surgery, and for the majority of hand patients pain is not usually a priority problem. However, patterns of pain can be set up very rapidly and unexpectedly, so a regime for prevention is essential.

Patients suffering from severe pain need their problem recognized and treated quickly, as chronic pain can be extremely difficult to resolve (see Chapter 4).

Scars and soft tissues

Skin

Following both injury and surgery the skin becomes dry and scaly (Figure 5.10), but this can be improved quickly by treatment.

An arm bath of warm soapy water and a few minutes soak will help to soften dry skin (if there are still open wounds, warm saline should be used). The hand can be exercised in the water for 3–4 minutes, as described in the general preparation. Hot water and wax should be avoided, as these are likely to increase oedema.

Softened dead skin can be removed with the towel while the hand is being dried, and the application of a hydrous ointment will assist in improving the skin condition. When the hand is

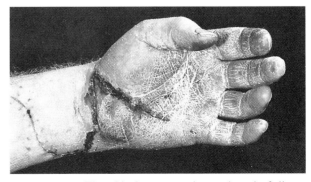

Figure 5.10 The skin becomes dry and scaly following injury and surgery.

first taken out of the post-operative splint, this warm water treatment may need to be undertaken by the therapist or a nurse. As confidence is gained patients can do this for themselves, and should be encouraged to cream the skin at least four or five times a day.

The care of anaesthetic skin and the danger of burns must be taught to patients urgently. Burns (with resulting blisters) can be caused by a variety of means, and patients must be reminded frequently to watch the hand if near to or using anything hot. The authors have encountered patients who have burnt themselves:

- on radiators, kettles and teapots
- by letting a little finger slip down onto an iron
- picking up and peeling a hot potato
- with a lighted cigarette burning across anaesthetic fingers.

Cold burns and friction can also blister anaesthetic skin. Patients must be warned that anaesthetic or partially anaesthetic skin is more fragile than normal skin and is liable to burn at a substantially lower temperature than the unaffected hand.

Blisters, if they do occur, should not be pricked and should be left uncovered unless they are likely to be damaged. If they burst, they must be dressed to avoid the risk of infection. A lesion of this type will usually take much longer to heal than normal, owing to the poor nutrition resulting from the nerve lesion.

As hand function improves, patients must gradually toughen up the skin. Many patients will have delicate new skin, and manual workers' hands in particular will have become much softer than before injury. The skin must be toughened in the later stages of treatment prior to returning to the original job, and it is most important to avoid causing any blisters during this toughening process. In the early stages the therapist should monitor the skin condition frequently and change activities regularly. At first the tools used should offer little friction – e.g. be made of smooth metal, or have handles covered with foam or Rubazote. Gradually, rougher handles such as planed timber may be used, and when the skin begins to toughen, equipment and materials that have raw finishes may be introduced.

Nails

When necessary, the nails should be cut very carefully or filed using an emery board and the cuticles manicured by the nurse or therapist to ensure that patients do not damage themselves with scissors. The nails of the uninjured hand will also need attention.

Soft tissues

The soft tissues of the hand are at risk of losing their suppleness and are prone to contracture following injury, especially during immobilization. Contractures must be prevented wherever possible, and the natural suppleness of the hand maintained through daily stretching. The volume of soft tissue damaged by direct trauma should be considered as well as the actual structures divided and lacerated. There is a high potential for disability following a crush injury due to the extent of soft tissue damage.

Injury in the forearm can also cause loss of movement in the hand. Both vascular damage (which causes a Volkmann's ischaemic contracture) and direct trauma to the muscle bellies can result in loss of full contractile and extensile properties of the forearm muscles. Contracture of the flexor muscles may cause loss of extension in the distal joints of the hand. In severe cases of ischaemic contracture both the extensors and the flexors, together with the small muscles of the hand, can be affected. Contracture of the intrinsic muscles may also develop as the result of an injury distal to the wrist. Frequently this is due to vascular damage.

Soft tissue mobility can be maintained by movement, preferably active but if necessary passive. Passive movements must be performed carefully and without jeopardizing the healing of other structures. Daily stretching of the web spaces and mobilization of the hand into its functional postures will help to preserve the tissue elasticity.

The intrinsic muscles are particularly prone to contracture, and if they become contracted they are extremely difficult to stretch because they are so small. Maximum extensibility may be achieved by metacarpophalangeal joint extension combined with interphalangeal joint flexion (Figure 5.11). Any splinting to stretch an intrinsic muscle contracture must attempt to achieve this position.

Massage, combined with the use of a hydrous ointment in the early stages, is effective for maintaining soft tissue mobility. When the structures are sufficiently healed the therapist should apply effleurage and kneading, paying special attention to the thenar and hypothenar eminences. At the same time, some traction should be applied at the tips of the fingers and thumb.

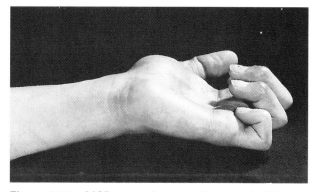

Figure 5.11 MCP extension combined with PIP and DIP extension.

Soft tissues and webs that are already contracted should be given a deep kneading massage, followed by active movements and gentle but firm passive stretching. The therapist should aim to give a long, slow stretch in order to allow the tissues to adapt and lengthen. The same degree of stretch can be maintained for an hour or longer by the use of splints (see Chapter 12). At the appropriate time the patient and family must be taught how to complete the soft tissue massage and stretches at home.

Caution: Further tissue damage caused by too strenuous a passive stretch, either manually or by the use of splints, must be avoided.

Scars

Scar tissue needs treatment, especially when adherent and surrounded by indurated subcutaneous tissue. Severe scarring can cause considerable disability, as tendons frequently become tethered in the scar tissue and occasionally a painful neuroma may form if a nerve becomes trapped in dense tissue. It is not always possible to predict the amount of scar tissue formation; some patients heal with considerable collagen and fibrous tissue production while others form very little. The choice of siting and type of incision by the surgeon is crucial for minimizing scar formation. Release of adhesions can improve tendon gliding, and the softening of scars will improve both the range of movement and the comfort of the patient's hand.

Scars, especially those that are grossly adherent to skin or underlying tendons, respond to intensive treatment by:

- massage
- suction
- vibration
- exercise combined with massage and pressure over the scar
- exercise combined with active and passive stretching
- electrical stimulation
- percussion and desensitization to painful neuromata.

Massage Before full healing has occurred, scars should be massaged gently with a soft hydrous ointment. Deep massage directly over the scar should be avoided initially, as it may cause blistering of delicate new skin and lead to further fibrous tissue formation.

The massage, applied with some Lanolin ointment, should gradually deepen as the scar tissue strengthens. Lanolin makes a comfortable, tacky contact with the skin, and prevents both the sliding that can occur with use of hydrous ointment and the painful frictioning of the skin if no medium at all is used. The surrounding area of induration is also massaged deeply, as this has an efficient softening effect and improves the local circulation.

Suction Suction therapy proves effective in the freeing of adherent scars, commencing at the stage when massage can be safely introduced (Otthiers, 1998). Utilizing a plastic tube connected to the hospital central suction system, with a valve for control, small areas of adherent scar may be treated by moving the end of the tube continually over the skin and scar. About 10 minutes per session daily is adequate.

Vibration Vibration is of value in helping to soften and break down scar tissue. Using a small hand-held battery-operated massager, available commercially, careful vibration can be used over scars at about 5 weeks post-tendon repair.

It may also be applied through sanding machines in the workshop when passive stretching of flexor tendons is allowed. Many air-compressed sanders have a flat on/off lever that is operated by the extended hand. The sander creates vibrations through the extended fingers as the patient works. Additionally, the therapist can passively stretch the patient's fingers into extension and encourage combined wrist extension.

This vibration has produced dramatic improvement in scar tissue by breaking down adhesions around the flexor tendons and thereby improving tendon pull-through. The patient can safely work on an air sander for about an hour a day.

Massage combined with exercise and stretching When it is safe to perform resisted movement and passive stretching, massage can be combined with exercise as below. The following techniques should *not* be used during the first few weeks following tendon and nerve repair.

1. Tension should be applied to the scar site, first in a caudad and then in a cephalad direction. The patient flexes the fingers until further movement is prevented by the adherence of the scar, and the therapist frictions the scar over the taut tendons (Figure 5.12a).
2. This is then repeated in the opposite direction, with the therapist extending the fingers passively whilst applying deep frictional massage over the adherent scar (Figure 5.12b).
3. Strong active movement may be combined with a passive stretch. The patient tensions his or her tendons by strong muscle contraction, whilst the therapist applies a quick passive stretch at the moment that further range is prevented by the scar and tendon adhesion. This exercise should be repeated several times.
4. In another combined active and passive technique, the therapist places a hand firmly on the skin immediately proximal to the scar and asks the patient to flex his or her wrist and fingers. The scar is stretched when the adherence moves

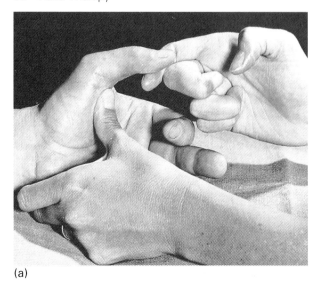

(a)

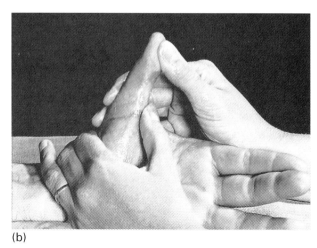

(b)

Figure 5.12 Frictional-type massage given across and around the adherent tendon of the FPL. Tension is applied at the same time (a) by the patient's own active contraction against slight resistance, and (b) by the physiotherapist.

under the strong grasp of the therapist's fingers. In movements into extension, the hold should be distal to the adhesion.

These procedures can be rather uncomfortable for the patient, so the degree of movement and pressure should be both applied and increased gradually.

Electrical stimulation can also be effective for stretching or even totally freeing adhesions that are preventing full tendon gliding. (See Electroactive exercise, p. 121).

When all healing is complete, a commercial pressure garment may be used to soften and flatten scar tissue (Johnson, 1984). Because of the concave nature of some of the scars or the shape of the patient's hand, the pressure glove may not always apply uniform pressure over those areas of the hand where it is needed. Silicone elastomer putty, or silicone moulding compound is an inexpensive compound when obtained from the manufacturer or the direct agents (for suppliers, see Appendix A). It can be used to bridge any gap and ensure that even pressure is applied. The putty is made from two components, one of which is a catalyst, which harden after mixing. There is time whilst it is still pliable to apply it to the patient's hand and achieve an exact impression of the scar.

Use of highly conforming thermoplastic material, applied with pressure, is also an effective method for softening scar and indurated tissue, especially for small areas. It can simultaneously provide a stretch to the part.

Gross adherence of tendons in scar tissue can cause considerable reduction in function. When conservative treatment fails, surgery may be neces-

sary to free the adherent tendons (tenolysis). Therapy should be commenced immediately following the operation in order to retain the movement gained at surgery.

Joint range of movement: active and passive

A priority aim is to establish a full range of pain-free movement for all joints of the hand. This involves maintenance of the mobile joints and mobilization of those that have become stiff. Hand functions most essential to the patient should be ascertained so that priorities can be decided.

Before fully mobilizing a joint it should be considered whether or not active control is likely to be regained, as a permanently flail joint would be a handicap. Some function, however, can usually be returned to mobile joints because of the continual improvements in surgical techniques (i.e. tendon and nerve transfers). Hypermobility should always be avoided, and lively splints may be needed to avoid this occurring while waiting for recovery from a peripheral nerve lesion (see Chapter 12).

The most functional position of the wrist, thumb and fingers (especially important if there is residual stiffness) is when contact can be made between the tips of thumb, index and middle fingers. This occurs when the joints are in the close-packed range, and therefore has a bearing on both the position of immobilization and the direction in which the mobilization will later be necessary.

Position of immobilization

Following trauma, when immobilization is considered absolutely essential the hand should ideally be placed in the position of safe immobilization.

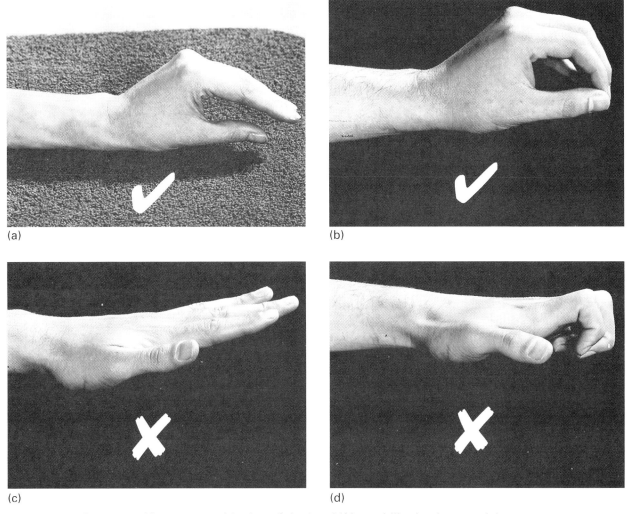

(a)

(b)

(c)

(d)

Figure 5.13 Correct and incorrect positioning of the hand if immobilization is essential.

The forearm should be in the mid-position, the wrist in some extension with slight ulnar deviation, the metacarpophalangeal joints in full flexion, and the interphalangeal joints in full extension. The thumb should be abducted and rotated medially. In this position the ligaments are on full stretch, the capsules spiralized and the joint surfaces maximally congruent. The hand should never be immobilized in either a fully flexed or fully extended position (Figure 5.13).

The duration of the immobilization must be specified, including whether it is to be continuous or interrupted by sessions of mobilization and exercise.

There is inherent danger of contractures quickly developing from immobilization, especially with burns and crush injuries, where there is considerable inflammation and oedema.

Post-operatively the position of immobilization is likely to be significantly different, and will be determined by the surgical procedure performed:

- following tendon repair, it will be necessary to take tension off the structures that have been repaired (see Chapter 7)
- following release (e.g. Dupuytren's contracture), extension may be necessary for a short period to maintain the stretch on the tissues
- where the injuries are complex and involve both the volar and dorsal aspects of the hand, the best compromise may be to immobilize the patient's hand in the position of function, with some flexion at both metacarpophalangeal (MCP) and proximal interphalangeal (PIP) joints.

Each case will need to be assessed on an individual basis, and the protocol of hand surgeons and hand units must be adhered to.

Direction of mobilization
If the hand has been in the position of 'safe' immobilization the subsequent mobilization is easier, since the direction of movement to be regained

is into the loose-packed range. Conversely, if immobilization has been in a loose-packed position, mobilization must be into the close-packed range and results may be disappointing.

Priorities of joint mobilization
The extended stiff hand that cannot flex is of little functional value, and is both extremely difficult and time-consuming to mobilize. It is important to improve the movements of grasp, pinch grip and finger flexion before extension. If the finger range of movement is likely to remain limited, MCP flexion is of the greatest benefit in improving function. Ideally the therapist aims to restore all the joints to full range, but in situations of compromise the following priorities should be considered:

- activities of daily living (ADL) needs of the patient
- employment
- leisure activities.

The radio-ulnar joint
Immobilization of the radio-ulnar joint is normally in the mid-position, and the first priority is to regain pronation because it generally has a greater functional value than supination.

The wrist joint
Included in the category of the wrist are the joints of the radius and ulna with the carpus, the intercarpal joints and the carpometacarpal joints. The order of priority for wrist movement is:

1. Wrist extension
2. Ulnar deviation
3. Wrist flexion
4. Radial deviation.

For most activities the hand will function more effectively with the wrist in some degree of extension, which enables the long flexors of the fingers to produce a stronger grip than with the wrist in flexion. However, flexion of the wrist is necessary for certain functions, such as placing food in the mouth with a spoon, playing the drums and percussion instruments, and bowling a cricket ball; eating may therefore be more difficult when wrist flexion is limited.

Ulnar deviation is necessary to achieve correct alignment of tools in activities such as using a knife, hammer or axe-handle.

Flexion combined with lateral rotation of the fifth carpometacarpal joint helps to deepen the distal palmar arch and allows pulp-to-pulp pinch of the little finger and thumb. This movement also needs to be maintained, because pinch grip is lost if the transverse distal arch becomes flattened or reversed. This flexion and rotation also applies in a special manner to the index finger. Normally, when flexing the fingers, the tip of the index converges with the tips of the other fingers towards the centre of the carpus. However the index finger is also capable of lateral rotation at the carpometacarpal (CMC) joint, to enable the pulp-to-pulp pinch of the index finger and thumb (see Chapter 1).

The joints of the fingers
The order of priority of finger movement is:

1. MCP joint flexion
2. IP joint extension
3. Full finger flexion
4. Full finger extension
5. Combined MCP joint extension and IP joint flexion.

It is not easy to increase MCP joint flexion and IP joint extension simultaneously when the joints are stiff, and it is simpler to mobilize the joints together, first into flexion and then into extension. Having achieved an increase in one direction the therapist should then switch to the opposite direction, ensuring that there is no decrease of the initial gain.

In the later stages, when the therapist can use passive stretch and serial splinting techniques, it is easier for mechanical reasons to regain extension than to regain full flexion. This is a strong additional reason for concentrating on improving flexion during the early stages of treatment.

The joints of the thumb
The order of priority of thumb movement is:

1. Palmar and radial abduction of the CMC joint
2. Opposition of the CMC joint
3. Adduction of the CMC joint
4. Flexion and extension of the MCP joint
5. Flexion and extension of the IP joint.

Co-ordination between the eye and the thumb is a highly developed function that allows the patient to grasp objects and pick up small items with accuracy. Restoring the thumb to a functional position and improving its range of movement will need urgent consideration, otherwise the patient may be severely handicapped.

Palmar abduction and opposition at the CMC joint must be adequate to enable the thumb to approximate to the tips of the fingers. A limited range of movement at either the IP or MCP joint of the thumb is of less functional significance, provided that there is some movement in one of these joints and CMC joint movement is good.

Techniques for joint mobilization
Joint mobilization should commence as early as possible, and the timing and choice of technique will depend upon the severity and nature of the injury. The therapist's decision must be based on information such as the diagnosis, details of the surgical

procedure and therapy assessment. Timing of activities, such as when resistance may be used and passive stretching commenced, should be agreed in principle with the surgeon. Complicating factors such as infection must be assessed for each patient.

The techniques for improving joint range of movement include:

1. Active mobilization
2. Passive mobilization including accessory movements
3. Passive stretching
4. Splinting.

The occupational therapist and physiotherapist must ensure that their aims are the same and that activities are complementary for each stage of treatment. The passive mobilization and stretching are usually performed by the physiotherapist, who should keep the rest of the team informed so that techniques in other treatment areas can be upgraded simultaneously. This upgrading should also be continued by the patient and family at home.

Active mobilization Active movement uses the available physiological range, and free or resisted exercise should be given whenever possible to maintain and increase joint range. Shoulder movement must be maintained because this joint is liable to stiffen following hand trauma, especially in the elderly.

A joint is particularly at risk from stiffness if the muscles are paralysed, and this risk is increased considerably if both agonists and antagonists are affected, as the accessory movements are totally absent. Range of movement in stiff joints, which could previously only be mobilized with passive movements and stretching, will improve more rapidly with the return of active movement.

Reciprocal relaxation of antagonists, and the relaxation that follows maximum contraction of the agonists (Sherrington, 1961), are techniques that can be used to improve the adaptive shortening of muscles. This shortening is likely to occur with lengthy immobilization of joints.

It is very important that all hand muscles are regularly put through their fullest movement, when this is permissible, from their most shortened to their most extended position. This will help to prevent adaptive shortening occurring, and includes:

- full and simultaneous flexion of MCP and IP joints
- full extension of MCP and PIP joints
- flexion of MCP joints together with extension of IP joints
- full flexion of IP joints with full extension of MCP joints.

Active mobilization may be given by both specific exercises and as functional activities (see Appendix B).

Contraindications to active mobilization include:

- recent surgery to nerves
- immediately following tendon surgery, except for the planned early mobilizing routine (see Chapter 7)
- the presence of adjacent fractures, unstable fractures and joint injury.

Passive mobilization Passive mobilization should be given to maintain the normal physiological range of movement of a joint, both when there is paralysis of muscles following nerve damage and when there is muscle weakness either following injury or during early nerve reinnervation.

A normal joint can be immobilized for 2–3 weeks before pathological changes occur. For any longer period of immobilization, one or two passive movements a day are necessary to retain the full mobility of a joint.

When muscles are paralysed but the joint is freely mobile, the movement can be maintained by taking the joint through its normal range of physiological movement. The proximal part is supported firmly and the distal component is moved through the full range of movement available. At the same time, the correct direction of accessory movement must be incorporated (Figure 5.14). Patients can be taught to do these for themselves or, if it is difficult to complete the movements one-handed, the relative or carer can be taught.

If the joint is stiff through part of its range, the free range must be maintained and the stiff extreme treated by small oscillations into that stiffness (see Chapter 6). Some distraction of the joint may help reduce any discomfort during passive movement.

For combined passive movements, all the joints should be passively mobilized together to mimic normal functional movement. For example:

1. First fully flatten and then deepen the distal palmar arch, combining this with full thumb flexion, abduction and rotation
2. Rotate all the fingers together, applying some traction
3. Hold the relaxed hand at the wrist, and shake or tap it loosely on to a pillow.

Continuous passive motion (CPM) may be beneficial in certain cases for maintaining joint mobility, for example following joint replacements and in some cases of complex regional pain disorder (or reflex sympathetic dystrophy; Woods and Withrington, 1992), and is especially useful for patients following tenolysis and burns. It is unable, however, to mimic the intricate movements of the hand.

A CPM machine may also be used to mobilize the patient's hand passively. The machine can be used for gross flexion and extension, and can be set to give different ranges of passive movement in each

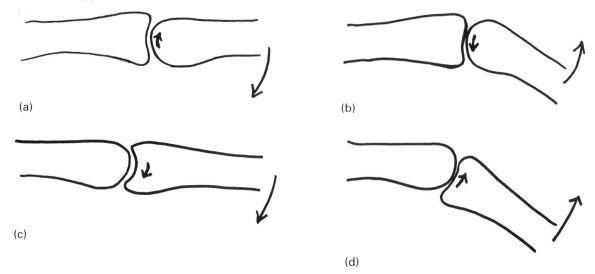

(a)

(b)

(c)

(d)

Figure 5.14 Direction of accessory movement is influenced by the shape of the joint surfaces: (a) and (b) concavo-convex; (c) and (d) convex-concave.

digit. In order to isolate the joints that need moving, it may sometimes be necessary to immobilize the mobile joints also. This enables the action of movement to be maximized on the stiffer joints. CPM should not be used if it might jeopardize any surgical procedures.

CPM is provided by means of a special battery-powered machine strapped to the patient's hand. This can be adjusted to alter the range of movement in the joints, and its frequency set by the therapist.

CPM is of value for those patients who find active exercise difficult or whose joints stiffen up at night. However, patients must understand that the machine cannot replace their own efforts and active input into the rehabilitation process.

Contraindications to passive mobilization include:

- swollen and inflamed joints
- intracapsular damage
- recent direct injury to the joint
- adjacent unstable fractures.

Passive stretching If progress with active and passive mobilization is slow, for example when joint stiffness is combined with soft tissue injury and adhesions, then passive stretching may be used. The technique is similar to passive mobilization, but involves the addition of controlled stretching. As with passive mobilization, the therapist should apply the same direction of accessory movement (Figure 5.14).

Passive stretching should not be used:

- before 6 weeks post-tendon and nerve repair. The time scale should be agreed with the surgeon
- if there is injury to the articular surfaces.

The therapist should firmly support the proximal part of the joint and move the distal component slowly whilst applying slight traction, stretching the joint gradually into the range of stiffness (Figure 5.15). The stretch should be slow and sustained, and never continued into a position that causes the patient undue pain. The therapist must watch the patient's face and stop the stretch immediately it appears to cause pain. The maximum comfortable stretch should be held for a few seconds. Sometimes the patient may feel that a few more degrees of movement may be attempted. Fast, jerky movements must be avoided as these may tear adhesions, with release of further fibrinogen, and cause an exacerbation of the scarring process.

At the end of the stretch the tension must be released gradually, since a fast release can be quite

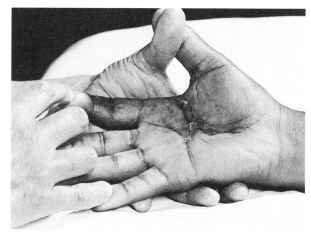

Figure 5.15 Support of the MCP joints must be given while passively stretching the interphalangeal joints.

painful; the discomfort should then disappear rapidly. Any pain that remains after a few seconds indicates that the stretch was too strong. If this occurs, only a minimal stretch should be given at the next treatment and the passive stretching increased very gradually thereafter.

The therapist must give a clear explanation of the purpose of the technique, as patients are likely to find this treatment uncomfortable and possibly painful. Most will cope with this discomfort once they appreciate that it will last for only a short time. Strong active exercise should always follow passive stretching to ensure that the range of movement gained is maintained by the patient. The active movement also appears to reduce any discomfort experienced from the stretch to the joints.

Passive stretching can also be incorporated by the occupational therapist into late-stage activities. The hand should be strapped or bandaged onto machine handles or tools that have been adapted to give the required amount of passive movement. However, the patient's safety is paramount and any machine handles to which the hand is strapped must be quickly and easily detachable from the machine. The hand may also be strapped to the handle of jigs that are used with specific machines; similarly the jig must be easily removable from the machine. In this situation the patient may be able to undertake a task for up to an hour whilst a gentle passive stretch is applied to the hand. The diversion achieved through activity helps the patient to tolerate the passive stretch.

Wrist extension may be improved by the choice of activity – for example, squashing pipes in a vice demands considerable effort and facilitates wrist extension because the body weight is taken through the hand. Other machines can be adapted so that wrist extension is achieved by using pressure.

Over-energetic passive stretching may cause a lasting painful reaction, in which case the patient must rest the hand until it is fully recovered. This wastes precious time, delays progress and makes the patient reluctant to have further stretching. It is therefore imperative that this treatment is given in a gradual and controlled manner.

Occasionally, the patient may experience an extreme reaction to a very mild stretch. This can usually be reduced by the application of TENS both before and during the stretch, and if necessary an analgesic may be taken half an hour beforehand. The degree of discomfort must never be so severe that it interferes with the rehabilitation that follows.

In the presence of dense, extensive scar tissue and adhesions, passive stretching may produce considerable discomfort actually in the joints. This is due to lack of tissue extensibility, especially in the joint capsule. On the application of stretch the joint surfaces are being compressed, and this can eventually become quite painful. If there is no improve-

ment over a 2–3-week period, further conservative treatment is unlikely to succeed. The patient should be referred to the surgeon, who may consider a surgical release of the contracted structures.

The therapist must constantly evaluate the effectiveness of passive stretching through accurate hand assessment.

Contraindications to passive stretching include:

- damage to joint articular surfaces
- recent repair of tendons and nerves (within 6–8 weeks)
- adjacent unstable fractures
- inflammatory disease of the joints.

Splinting Static splinting may be used to maintain and improve the range of movement in a joint, fundamentally using the same techniques of passive mobilization and passive stretching.

There is a wide range of splinting materials available commercially, offering different properties, and the therapist must design the splint for solving the patient's problem and select the most appropriate materials for that design (see Chapter 12). The purpose and use of the splint must be explained to the patient, and guidelines and precautions given for its use, together with a strong warning not to over-use the splint.

Serial splints maintain the stretch that the therapist has gained during the day. Splints should be worn regularly throughout the day – for example between treatment sessions, during meal breaks and, when possible, for up to an hour at a time whilst at work. As soon as the finger or hand can be lifted away from the splint, it should be adjusted to match the patient's current range of movement.

Caution: The splint must never stretch the finger or hand beyond the range gained by the therapist.

Initially the rate of progress is likely to be rapid, and the splint may need to be adjusted every couple of days. Modern thermoplastic materials make this a quick and simple procedure. The rate of change is likely to decrease as progress is made.

The patient will be able to wear the serial splint at night, but should be taught how to reduce the amount of passive stretch by slightly loosening the fastenings. This should ensure that the optimum position is maintained and the patient's sleep is not disturbed.

Boxing glove splints can be used at night to improve flexion of metacarpal and proximal interphalangeal joints. A rolled-up bandage is slotted in to the patient's hand, the roll size allowing the required amount of joint flexion, and a second bandage is used to pull the fingers down into flexion over the roll and is anchored round the wrist. The therapist should teach the nursing staff or patient's carer how to do this, as the patient will be unable to apply it. This method is more effective if the hand is fairly mobile. Joints that have a fixed extension deformity will need corrective static or lively splinting.

Strapping or taping may be used to stretch the IP joints of the fingers into flexion, at the same time stretching the intrinsic muscles. A non-stretchy strapping material, such as zinc oxide tape, is wrapped around the proximal and distal phalanges with the PIP and DIP joints flexed. The patient keeps the strapping on for a short period of time (e.g. 10 minutes). This procedure can be repeated at intervals during the day.

Dynamic (or lively) splints may be used as an alternative to static splinting (see Chapter 12). Patients often find it valuable to have a dynamic splint for daytime use and a static splint for night.

Plaster cylinders may succeed when very resistant stiff joints have not responded to any other mobilizing techniques. The day following application of the cylinder, a small piece of cork should be wedged into a slit made in the plaster, to increase the range in the desired direction. This is then worn for a further day or two, but no longer, as the immobilized joints must not be allowed to stiffen. This technique is particularly effective for increasing wrist extension and interphalangeal joint extension when other methods have not succeeded.

Contraindications for splinting may include:

- damage to the joint articular surfaces
- swollen and inflamed joints.

Some splints are designed specifically for joint articular damage and swollen joints (see Chapters 12 and 16).

Selection of mobilizing techniques

The choice of technique is determined by factors such as the extent of injury and disease, and the state of healing of bones, soft tissues and skin. The diagnosis of intracapsular or extracapsular joint injury is of particular importance.

Intracapsular injury Dislocations and fractures through the articular surfaces of the joint fall into this category. These joints need careful treatment, and the prognosis for recovery of a full range of movement is poor. Immobilization should be for as short a time as possible, and in either the 'safe' or the functional position. Therapy must be introduced gradually to avoid irritating the joint. The following techniques can be used:

1. Free active movements
2. Accessory movements when the joint is cool and pain-free
3. Gentle functional activities
4. Static splinting overnight to prevent loss of range regained actively.

The patient's response to treatment should be monitored carefully. Any increase of pain, warmth or swelling, or decrease of range of movement in the joint, will indicate over-treatment. Resistance and stronger functional activities may be gradually commenced if there is no adverse reaction to these techniques. Arthritic conditions of the joints must also be treated with special care (see Chapters 13, 14, 15 and 16).

Extracapsular injury These injuries involve damage to structures around the joint, whilst the joint itself may have no direct involvement. Tendons and nerves may be damaged, with the joint needing immobilization to allow these structures to heal, resulting in some temporary joint stiffness. Treatment should commence as soon as the surgeon will allow. Suitable techniques should be selected according to the diagnosis, the assessment and the time lapse since surgery. It is rare that all these methods will be required to regain maximum movement, but the following may be used:

1. Free and resisted active movement
2. Mobilizations including accessory movements
3. Passive movement including CPM
4. Passive stretching
5. Splinting.

Joints that have sustained ligamentous damage or are subjected to constant and repetitive stress (e.g. from sporting activities) may need extra protection during the rehabilitation period, and can be protected by taping or strapping (Macdonald, 1994). Inflamed joints are particularly at risk, and it is imperative that joint protection techniques relating to activities of daily living are taught.

See Chapter 12 for further management of joint injuries.

Muscle re-education and activity

Following injury and immobilization, active hand function must be restored as quickly as possible to facilitate normal patterns of movement with the correct sensory input. The concept of the plasticity of the nervous system is now widely accepted. The brain is able to recognize patterns of movement and individual joint movement, change the role of muscles and influence the properties of the fast and slow contracting muscle fibres (Kidd *et al.*, 1992). The hand has a high density of sensory nerve endings, and the therapist should use this to influence the motor response. Stimulation of the proprioceptors enhances the recognition of individual joint movement, and the low ratio motor units help in learning to contract muscles individually.

Hand-to-hand contact is a normal everyday experience, and the therapist should use the hands to facilitate exercise and improve motor function. Patients find that free active exercises are difficult to perform following injury or surgery, when they can achieve only a small amount of movement, as this allows very little sensory feedback. If muscles have been paralysed or immobilized for some time, the patient may have lost recollection of how to contract them. The maximal safe sensory input should be used to help patients to understand what they are trying to achieve and to facilitate the movement. In the early stages, this may need to be of the lightest touch.

Proprioceptive neuromuscular facilitation (PNF) concepts (Voss *et al.*, 1985) are of tremendous advantage both when working in total patterns of movement and in individual muscle re-education, especially when reinnervation of muscles is occurring after a nerve lesion. The therapist should exploit all physiological principles that will facili-

tate muscle activity. Maximum response can be facilitated by:

- irradiation of the anterior horn cells
- successive induction
- use of the stretch reflex by the application of a quick stretch to muscles both before and during contraction
- a suitable amount of resistance
- traction or approximation of joints
- application of the hands onto the patient's skin over contracting muscles
- encouraging the patient to observe the movement
- urging of a greater response.

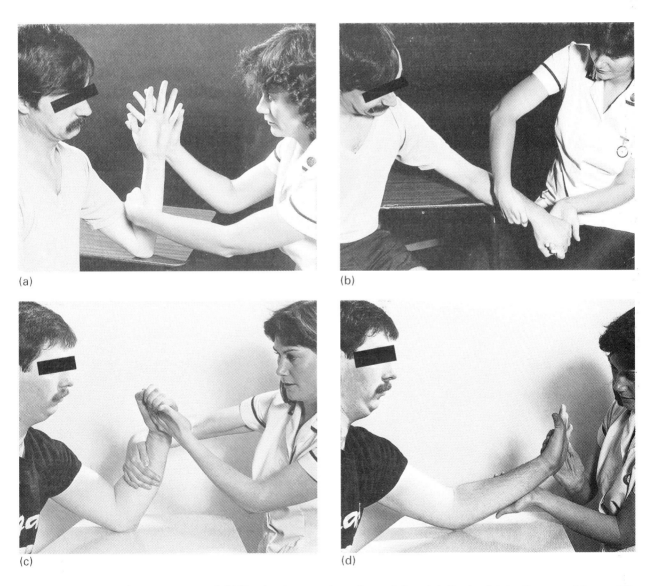

(a)

(b)

(c)

(d)

Figure 5.16 Modified patterns of PNF pivoting at the elbow joint: (a) flexion/abduction combines with supination and finger extension; (b) extension/adduction combines with pronation and finger flexion; (c) flexion/adduction combines with supination and finger flexion; (d) extension/abduction combines with pronation and finger extension.

Functional activities should also incorporate these physiological principles, as they are all part of normal movement and activity.

During most actions we can see what we are doing with our hands, and it is important that patients are able to watch their hands during re-education of movement. This is particularly so when there is a cutaneous and proprioceptive deficit as a result of a nerve lesion. Standard PNF techniques can be modified to be performed in a sitting position. The patient sits at a small table, preferably of adjustable height, with the elbow resting near the edge, either on a pillow or directly on the tabletop (Figure 5.16). Modified PNF patterns can be performed in this position with the elbow as the pivot. Only a small movement will take place at the shoulder, and full elbow extension is not possible, but the relationship of hand and eye facilitates improved function of the hand.

The main patterns to facilitate are:

1. Pattern 1 – the shoulder flexion, abduction and external rotation pattern combines with supination (elbow flexion when performed while sitting), wrist extension with radial deviation, finger extension and abduction (particularly index and middle fingers) and thumb extension.
2. Pattern 2 – the shoulder extension, adduction and internal rotation pattern combines with pronation, elbow extension, wrist flexion with ulnar deviation, finger flexion and adduction (particularly index and middle fingers) and thumb flexion.
3. Pattern 3 – the shoulder flexion, adduction and external rotation pattern combines with supination (elbow flexion when performed whilst sitting) wrist flexion with radial deviation, finger flexion and adduction (particularly ring and little fingers), and thumb flexion.
4. Pattern 4 – the shoulder extension, abduction and internal rotation pattern combines with pronation, elbow extension, wrist extension with ulnar deviation, finger extension and abduction (particularly ring and little fingers) and thumb extension.

Variations in thumb and finger movements can be made by slight alterations to the distal components of the movement pattern:

- thumb extension combines with pattern 1
- thumb adduction combines with pattern 3
- thumb opposition combines with pattern 2
- thumb palmar abduction combines with pattern 4
- index and middle finger MCP flexion and IP extension combine with pattern 2, replacing finger flexion
- ring and little finger MCP flexion and IP extension combine with pattern 3, replacing finger flexion

- finger abduction combines with patterns 1 and 4
- finger adduction combines with patterns 2 and 3.

Active movement is the crux of any therapy programme, and treatment time should be occupied largely by functional activities and specific exercises in order to regain normal use of the hand. Using only the unaffected hand may have become a habit, with the patient afraid to use the injured one, so frequent prompting may be necessary for automatic use to be re-established.

Therapeutic exercise needs to be planned, taking into account all the injuries the patient has sustained. It should proceed through stages of:

- individual muscle activity over one or more joints
- patterns of movement
- functional activities.

In the early stage, but depending on the treatment protocol, free active movements should be introduced within 24 hours of injury or surgery and progressed carefully. Reciprocal relaxation techniques (Kleinert *et al.*, 1973) may be utilized within 2 days after the suture of tendons, but under this protocol active exercise of these tendons is delayed for 3 weeks. An early motion protocol may allow controlled active movement within days of tendon suture (see Chapter 7).

In the later stages of rehabilitation, increasing muscle activity and strengthening is encouraged. The therapist must check that each muscle is performing its normal movement. Muscle activity may be weakened as a result of:

- injury
- immobilization
- inhibition due to pain
- lack of innervation due to a nerve lesion.

Following a peripheral nerve lesion, those muscles that are still working should be identified and those paralysed or in the early stages of recovery noted (see Chapter 2). If a muscle can produce only a flicker or a very weak contraction and becomes overpowered by stronger muscles when acting in a group situation, it should be re-educated and exercised individually or in as small a group as possible. This ensures that it will then function correctly in combined and intricate hand movements.

1. Some patients will find it easier to think in terms of moving a specific joint, rather then in attempting to contract a specific muscle.
2. Initially, weak muscles should be exercised with gravity eliminated. This may be necessary for the wrist flexors and extensors if they are unable to overcome the weight of the hand, and can be achieved with the forearm in the mid-position.
3. An extremely weak muscle, producing only a small amount of movement, will contract best in

its outer to middle range. As strength improves, the excursion will increase until the muscle is able to contract into its inner range also.

Exercises can follow methods similar to those given for muscle testing and charting (see Chapter 2).

The threshold of nerve activity is likely to be raised as a result of nerve damage and, when combined with long-term disuse, the patient may have lost all concept of movement. Electrical stimulation in conjunction with the patient's own efforts may be helpful in regaining movement (see Electroactive exercise, p. 121).

Muscle activity can be facilitated in the early recovery stages as follows:

1. Teach the patient the required muscle contraction and the movement on the normal uninjured side.
2. Ask the patient to attempt the same muscle contraction and movement on the injured side. Watch carefully, and tell the patient when the correct movement is achieved.
3. Apply a quick stretch to the muscle immediately before attempting another contraction.
4. Apply either a light touch or directional resistance to the moving part. This proprioception will enable the patient to *feel* what is being attempted.
5. Apply pressure over the muscle belly to facilitate muscle activity. This will be particularly necessary when educating the muscle into a new role, as for tendon transfers (see Chapter 7).

As strength improves, resistance may be increased gradually; however, following any tendon surgery this must be appropriate for the stage of healing to avoid the risk of tendon rupture. Since muscles respond best when working at their maximum capacity, progress must be monitored constantly and the activities upgraded accordingly.

Specific joint movements

All joints including and distal to the shoulder and shoulder girdle must be mobilized when necessary, with special attention paid to the radio-ulnar joints. This section, which is written in conjunction with Chapter 6, gives details of exercises and functional techniques for mobilizing the joints including and distal to the wrist.

The wrist joint The patient sits with the table parallel to the injured side, resting the forearm on the table with the injured wrist and hand extended over the edge. Single plane wrist movements (i.e. flexion and extension or radial and ulnar deviation) should be performed first. With the wrist in a neutral position, abduction of the fingers and thumb will produce a strong contraction of both the extensor carpi ulnaris (ECU) and abductor pollicis longus (APL).

A combination of diagonal and rotational movements are then introduced, providing a more functional approach to specific wrist exercise.

1. Combined wrist extension and ulnar deviation is important for strong grasp
2. Wrist flexion with some radial deviation is necessary for eating with a fork or spoon
3. Wrist extension while the fingers are flexed is also extremely important, as patients frequently attempt wrist extension by using the finger extensors; the co-ordination of this combined movement may be improved by the grasp of a light object such as a piece of plastazote
4. The ECRB helps to stabilize the wrist whilst the fingers are flexed during a gripping action; for a strong grip, both the extensor carpi radialis brevis (ECRB) and ECU will be needed
5. The forearm movements of pronation and supination may need increasing in range (see Chapter 6).

The finger metacarpophalangeal joints Flexion, extension, abduction and adduction of the MCP joints may be made in isolation, or combined with movement of the other finger joints.

1. *Flexion* of the MCP joints is produced strongly by the interossei, which simultaneously extend the interphalangeal joints. The patient should rest the supinated forearm on a table, palm uppermost. Flexion of the MCP joints whilst keeping the IP joints in extension should be practised (Figure 5.17). In the early stages of muscle recovery, if approximation is applied through the fingers to the MCP joints in this position, the muscle activity will be facilitated sufficiently for the patient to hold the position for a few seconds.

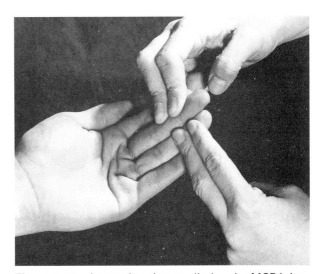

Figure 5.17 Approximation applied to the MCP joints in this position will facilitate a contraction of the interossei.

2. Contraction of both the flexor digitorum superficialis (FDS) and flexor digitorum profundis (FDP) will produce secondary flexion at the MCP joints, which can produce useful function when the intrinsic muscles are still denervated. The movement is called 'rolling flexion', as it starts at the interphalangeal joints and then 'rolls' into flexion at the MCP joints.

3. *Extension* of the MCP joints by the extensor digitorum (ED) should be taught, first with the IP joints flexed and then with the IP joints extended. The second movement depends on the presence of some intrinsic activity. Manual resistance should be added as early as possible.

MCP abduction and adduction by the interossei is performed most simply with the palm flat on a table or pillow and the fingers slightly abducted. The patient is asked to extend one finger whilst keeping the others in contact with the table, and then to move that finger from side to side. If this is difficult, the therapist may facilitate the muscle activity by moving the finger into abduction, giving the muscles a quick stretch and then asking the patient to adduct the finger and *vice versa* (Figure 5.18). A small amount of resistance is applied. The movement will be strongest in its outer range.

As strength improves, all the fingers are abducted then adducted together, and graduated resistance can be applied by the interlinking of the therapist's fingers with those of the patient.

Finger interphalangeal joints The patient should rest the hand on a table with palm uppermost.

It is usual and more functional to exercise the proximal (PIP) and distal (DIP) interphalangeal joints together. There are, however, occasions when it may be necessary to isolate the movement to each joint in order to re-educate the FDS and FDP

separately, e.g. following tendon repair. When the tendons are strong it is important to encourage this differential gliding between the FDS and FDP, as it will help to limit any adhesions that might form.

To isolate PIP joint movement:

1. The therapist should hold all the fingers in extension except for the finger to be exercised. This will eliminate any action of the FDP.
2. The patient is asked to bend the free finger, and any flexion that occurs at the PIP joint only is produced by the FDS. Resistance, if safe to be applied, may be given isometrically to FDS in this position.
3. If isolated FDS function is present, the DIP joint will feel floppy.
4. If the DIP joint flexes, it is likely to be the FDP that is also producing the movement at the PIP joint, and not the FDS.

To isolate DIP joint flexion:

1. The therapist should firmly support the middle phalanx of the finger and ask the patient to bend the tip of the finger so that the FDP flexes the terminal phalanx through its range.
2. Resistance can be added gradually.
3. A quick stretch will facilitate the muscle activity.
4. It should be possible for the therapist to palpate a contraction of the FDP tendon, by the finger or thumb supporting the middle phalanx.

If there is only minimal movement at this joint it is possible to be fooled by a trick movement – a quick active extension of the DIP joint followed by relaxation may appear as a small amount of DIP joint flexion. It is important to be sure that the patient is achieving an active contraction.

Combined flexion of the MCP and IP joints may be given using manual resistance and by the patient

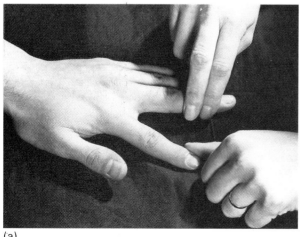
(a)

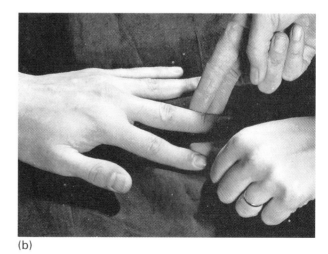
(b)

Figure 5.18 The therapist stabilizes the index finger and gives light resistance to the outer range movements of the middle finger.

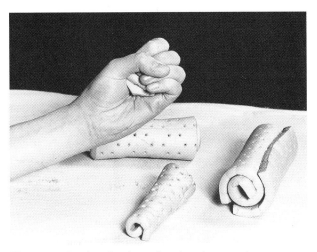

Figure 5.19 A selection of polystyrene grips.

grasping suitable objects – e.g. different sizes and shapes of foam and polystyrene blocks. Differing shapes and sizes will ensure that the patient can exercise through the whole and different ranges of movement (Figure 5.19).

Active finger extension is needed when the hand is preparing to grasp an object. IP joint extension is a complex movement, and should be re-educated with the metacarpophalangeal joints first in flexion and then in extension. Full finger extension requires the combined activity of the extensor digitorum communis (EDC) with the intrinsic muscles. Without the EDC there is no extension of the MCP joints; without the intrinsics the hand will claw into MCP extension and IP flexion.

Thumb carpometacarpal joint Effective hand function requires adequate thumb movement – i.e. the combination of flexion, extension, abduction, adduction and opposition. The carpometacarpal (CMC) joint is the most complex and mobile joint of the thumb. Its stability is provided by the short, bulky muscles of the thenar eminence.

Thumb flexion by the flexor pollicis brevis (FPB) at the CMC joint takes the metacarpal towards the little finger, close against the palm. Without the combined activity of abduction, this movement is not functional.

Thumb extension is achieved by the extensor pollicis longus (EPL) and extensor pollicis brevis (EPB), and is necessary for tasks involving span.

Thumb abduction enables the thumb and fingers to create a span in the thumb web sufficient to grasp an object. The abductor pollicis brevis (APB) abducts the thumb in a plane at right angles to the palm; the muscle contraction needs to be powerful enough to stabilize the thumb against the activity of the flexor pollicis longus (FPL). Its activity will help to stretch the thumb web, which frequently

becomes contracted during lengthy immobilization or when the APB is paralysed.

Thumb adduction by the adductor pollicis (Add. P) provides power for pinch grip and enhances the strength of power grasp.

Opposition by the opponens pollicis (Opp. P) rotates the thumb enabling the thumb pulp to make contact with the finger pulp, with the nails lying along the same axis. It is easier to re-educate this rotational movement in conjunction with the other movements of abduction, flexion and adduction of the thumb.

The activity of these small muscles of the thumb can be facilitated by the therapist by applying stretch, light touch or resistance with the fingers against the moving side of the thumb.

If movement is likely to remain limited, the thumb must be positioned in a functional position with abduction and opposition so that the fingers can be flexed to the thumb to achieve a pinch grip (see Chapter 12).

Thumb metacarpophalangeal joint The MCP joint movement of the thumb needs to be as stable as possible in order to perform both light precision movements and strong grasp.

Flexion is produced primarily by the FPB and secondarily by the FPL. The FPB is likely to be affected following a low level median nerve lesion. To isolate the FPB, the MCP joint is placed in flexion with the IP joint extended and the patient is asked to hold that position. Resistance may be added gradually. The FPB is most active when the thumb is opposed to the base of the little finger.

Extension is produced by the EPB assisted by the EPL. Support of the metacarpal enables the patient to localize extension of the MCP joint more easily. Resistance can be given over the proximal phalanx.

Thumb interphalangeal joint The thumb IP joint movement also needs to be stable. A flail joint, which has passive range but no active control, will lack both power and stability.

IP flexion is produced by the FPL, and *extension* by the EPL. The EPL is assisted by the APB, which has a slip insertion into the dorsal expansion mechanism of the thumb. The APB can extend the thumb following radial nerve lesions where there is paralysis of the EPL. Both the FPL and EPL may be exercised by supporting the proximal phalanx and resisting the movement of the distal phalanx, facilitating by successive induction.

A combination of CMC, MCP and IP joint movements can be produced by asking the patient to make an 'O' with the thumb and index finger. When there is only a little thenar muscle activity, a flat 'D' shape will be produced. As this activity improves, the 'D' will broaden and eventually become an 'O'. Activity of the first dorsal inter-

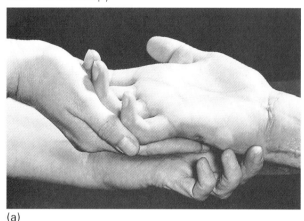

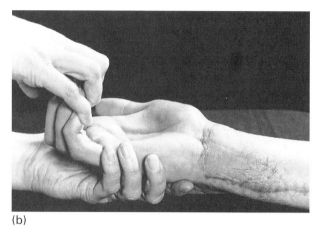

(a)   (b)

Figure 5.20   Manual resistance applied to finger flexors and extensors.

osseous is also necessary during strong pinch grip in order to stabilize the index finger.

Combined joint movements

The hand structure has the ability to conform to a wide variety of positions as a result of its number of joints and their mobility. Extension movements will flatten both transverse and longitudinal arches, and flexion in conjunction with opposition of the thumb towards the little finger will deepen these arches.

Movement is enhanced by sensory input, so resisted exercises (or purely light touch) should be given at the appropriate stage of healing. By using the hands the therapist can effectively apply resistance and sensory stimulation in the desired direction and at the suitable range, moving from one pattern of movement to its reverse (Figure 5.20).

Opposition of the thumb towards each finger is facilitated by touch or resistance. The therapist should apply a quick stretch to both the thumb and

finger away from each other at the start of the movement, and again when the full excursion has been reached (repeated contractions), in order to increase range and improve power (Figure 5.21). The tip of the index finger should rotate towards the thumb to give an efficient pinch grip. The normal index finger has the ability to rotate both towards the thumb and towards the other fingers.

When opposing the thumb to the little fingertip, facilitatation of the hypothenar muscles may be needed to achieve the flexion and rotation of the fifth metacarpal. This is necessary for deepening the distal transverse arch and, when strength improves, for providing a powerful grasp. In the absence of hypothenar muscle activity, for example following an ulnar nerve lesion, the grip will be extremely weak.

In the early stages following hand injury, the shoulder, shoulder girdle and elbow should be exercised, preferably in bilateral patterns since this

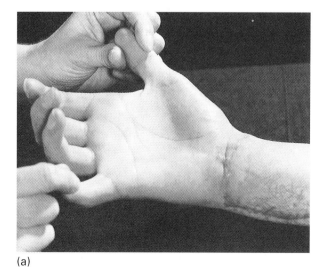

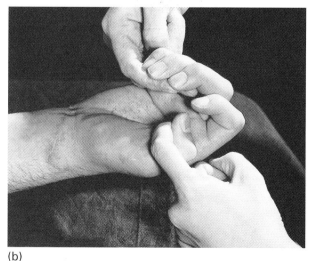

(a)   (b)

Figure 5.21   Attempted opposition of thumb to little finger, facilitated by quick stretch and repeated contractions.

is normal movement. The use of PNF is especially suitable.

Functional activities to improve joint movement and muscle power

The activity of picking up a soft ball, squeezing it and putting it down in a changed position requires more conscious effort than just sitting and squeezing it. If the patient is encouraged to incorporate exercises and use of the hand into purposeful patterns of movement and activity, disuse problems rarely occur. This approach needs to be encouraged from the earliest opportunity, as immediately following severe hand injury some patients may have difficulty in completing any activity at all.

For example, a patient with a median and ulnar nerve lesion and division of tendons was unable to flex the fingers except for a flicker of movement from full extension. By providing a piece of expanded polystyrene cut to slightly less than the distance between finger and thumb, the patient was able to pick up an object for the first time for several weeks. This success immediately raised morale, and the size of the polystyrene was reduced daily. Progress was increased considerably by the addition of this activity rather than by exercises alone.

The therapist should make use of remedial games and functional activities to restore active range of movement, clearly identifying the specific needs of the patient. How an activity can meet those needs must be evaluated, demanding the continuous process of activity analysis. The patient also must understand clearly the aim of the activity in order to achieve maximum benefit.

Activities can be used to meet the patient's needs by adapting the activity or adapting the patient.

Adapting the activity Games requiring a variety of different grips and ranges of movement are widely available commercially, and are easily adapted by the creative and lateral-thinking of the therapist. Many toy manufacturers already produce games in varying sizes, e.g. standard and travelling versions. The same game may also be adapted in a number of ways to achieve different ranges of movement. Patients playing together can use different types, shapes and sizes of counters which either meet their individual needs or to which they have to adjust. Flat, thin counters require the use of FDP in order to pick them off a tabletop.

Active range of movement should be regained (or at least improved) early after injury or surgery, but patients with tendon damage and/or fractures should not attempt to build muscle power until the structures are healed. This is generally about 6 weeks post-repair, but will depend on the surgeon's protocol. Most activities will consequently need to be adapted so that they offer light, non-resistive movements to the patient.

Adapting the patient The patient may also need to be adapted in relation to the activity, in a similarly creative way:

- range of movement can be facilitated by the relative positioning of patient and activity – e.g. the activity may be placed on a high shelf to improve elbow extension (Figure 5.22)
- a game such as three-dimensional noughts and crosses can be played holding the pieces with a pinch grip, either between thumb and index finger, or between the fingertips of a flat extended hand
- craft activities, although less specific, may also be used to improve range of movement.

A useful combination to employ is that of remedial games, which concentrate on specific movements, together with craft activities, which are more functionally biased.

The therapist must ensure that the patient is using a normal pattern of movement and not compensating for injured joints. This may need guiding and facilitating for the desired movement, or the use of equipment. As examples:

1. A patient may compensate for limited pronation and supination of the forearm by using shoulder abduction and trunk side flexion. A book held between the upper arm and body while working will prevent the shoulder abduction.

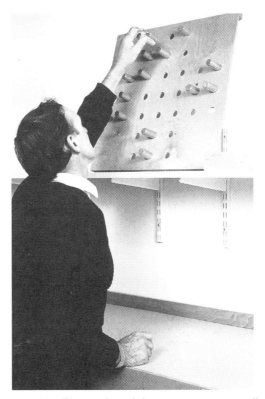

Figure 5.22 Elevated activity to encourage elbow extension.

2. If a patient is attempting to pick up something from beside him or her, it may be tempting to side flex the trunk to compensate for limitation of elbow extension. A crutch positioned under the shoulder will prevent this trunk side flexion.

3. Any trick movements, such as a rapid contraction then relaxation of finger extensors when the patient is attempting DIP joint flexion following tendon surgery (see Chapter 7), should be noted and re-educated.

4. The appropriate amount of effort for the movement may also need training. Some patients put so much effort into bending their fingers that both their flexors and extensors are working simultaneously in a co-contraction, with consequent lack of movement. This is frequently a problem for strong men who perform heavy work such as weight training. Range of movement needs to be regained initially as a light effortless task.

In the later stages, when some resistance can be tolerated, blocking splints can be used to prevent joints with full range of movement from compensating for those that do not. Frequently a MCP joint may have full range while a PIP joint is still limited. In such a case, a blocking splint could be used to prevent MCP joint flexion while facilitating improved PIP joint flexion. Blocking splints are also useful for encouraging thumb IP joint flexion. These splints:

- should be made individually for each patient
- are designed to be used during treatment sessions with remedial games.

As movement improves, the patient must be encouraged to maintain range without using the splint.

Biofeedback

Electromyographic biofeedback, using surface electrodes placed over the motor points, can assist the patient in the early stages of muscle reinnervation when little joint movement or muscle contraction is obvious. The apparatus can also be linked with a computer, which provides a variety of patterns with which the patient may work. The muscle contraction produces a small visual response, and the stronger the contraction the higher it appears on the screen. By increasing or slightly relaxing the contraction the patient is able to steer the light response through the patterns, which can be pre-set according to ability. Auditory signals are also available, but these may prove aggravating in a busy department. The patient's muscle strength can be recorded on a printout for future reference.

Manipulation and dexterity

As the range of movement improves, the patient needs to be encouraged to complete tasks involving more manipulation and greater dexterity.

Games can be adapted to include gathering and holding objects in the palm. They can be graded so that the objects in the palm have to be released in a controlled manner – e.g. by dropping them one at a time from the ulnar aspect of the hand, or moving them out from the palm with the thumb and index finger. The patient can hold a handful of mixed, coloured pegs and be required to select and sort out one colour using only the injured hand. This activity can then be applied to function by holding and counting out a handful of coins.

An improvement in speed should be aimed for by timing the completion of a circuit of exercises or tasks. Competition with others makes the activities more fun for the patients.

Functional activities such as macramé, basketry and type-setting are valuable in improving manipulation and dexterity, as long as compensatory movements are not allowed. For example, the patient should be encouraged to manipulate the piece of type into the correct orientation with the fingers, rather than by putting it down and then picking it up.

Muscle strength and power

In the later stages of treatment the patient should be:

- building up muscle power in the hand and arm
- increasing the strength of the pinch grips.

The timing of this stage must depend on the protocol of the surgeon and the quality of healing. Patients with an infection, large areas of unhealed or necrotic skin, or unstable fractures must not work on strenuous activities. Flexor tendon injuries may usually begin resisted work about 6 weeks post-repair (see Chapter 7).

Resisted exercise enables the therapist to influence the remodelling of scar tissue, for instance along the tendons, thereby promoting improved tendon gliding. For example, rubber bands attached to a bulldog clip can provide a resistance for finger flexion and extension (Figure 5.23). Power work should be carefully graded through a planned sequence from light to heavy activities. Work that is too strong and too early may cause further damage, in particular the possibility of tendon rupture.

Muscle groups of the upper limb, especially the shoulder muscles, may be strengthened by using the Westminster pulley, utilizing normal PNF patterns of movement either from a standing or a sitting position (Figure 5.24). The amount of weight lifted may be controlled easily, and:

- padding the handle with orthopaedic felt will enable patients who have poor finger flexion to hold the handle more firmly
- the amount of padding can be reduced as flexion improves

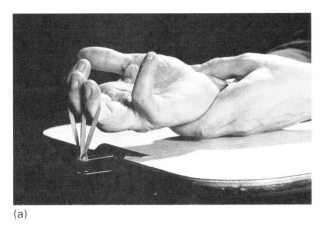
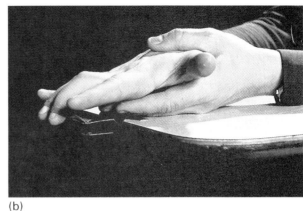

Figure 5.23   Elastic band resistance to finger flexors and extensors.

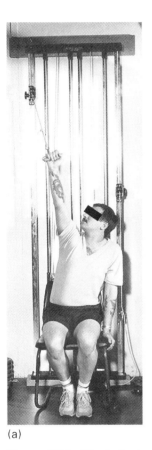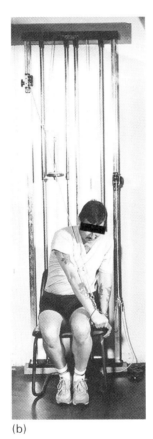

(a)   (b)

Figure 5.24   Westminster pulley for PNF patterns.

Flexion with radial deviation is a more difficult movement to perform into the inner range, but is necessary for eating with either fork or spoon, or when using the fingers.

The patient frequently finds that the combined action of finger flexion and wrist extension is extremely difficult to regain after a severe hand injury – when attempting to flex the fingers, the wrist automatically flexes also. Use of a handle and spring to practise wrist extension can be efficient in restoring this important pattern of movement.

Functional activities

Functional activities offer the best means for retraining the normal relationship between the brain and hand, and the emphasis of therapy should shift as soon as possible from specific exercises to a more functional treatment:

- differing activities demand a different amount of muscle strength
- machines may be adapted to increase the weight and resistance of the task – for example, the amount of muscle strength required increases by reducing leverage
- specific digits may be exercised by using on/off buttons on machines or tools that are operated by a single digit e.g. electric drill, staple gun.

There is no simple practical way, however, of measuring the force needed to complete the tasks or to operate the machinery. The occupational therapist must be familiar with the demands of the tasks being performed by the patient.

Remedial games can be adapted for pinch grip, for instance by using clothes pegs or tweezers to pick up counters. Pegs can be graded from a light to heavy pinch grip, first using a plastic one, then a wooden one, and finally a wooden peg with an elastic band wrapped around its bottom. Tweezers can be graded individually by their own resistance, then stiffened by placing a coin inside at the fulcrum.

- patients' fingers may be bandaged onto the handle if grasp is extremely weak.

Specific muscle groups of the hand and wrist can also be strengthened with a spring and handle (Figure 5.25). Diagonal movements may combine:

- flexion with ulnar deviation
- extension with ulnar deviation
- extension with radial deviation.

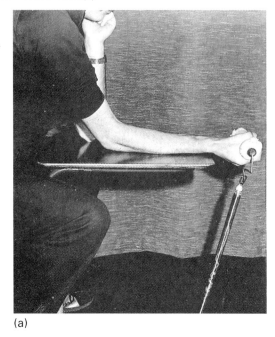
(a)

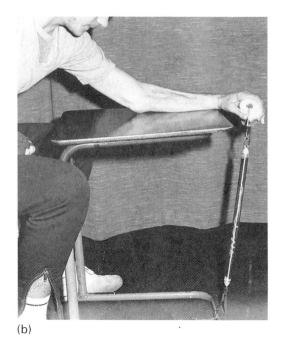
(b)

Figure 5.25 Spring-resisted work for wrist flexors and extensors.

Games can be adapted to strengthen finger extension and abduction by working against an elastic band or elastic material wrapped around the digits to strengthen abduction.

Functional tasks such as macramé, stool seating, printing and leatherwork are all appropriate as strengthening activities.

A heavy workshop is an extremely valuable facility for patients at this later stage of treatment. The weight of the task and the amount of time spent at work should be gradually increased. At approximately 8 weeks post-repair, the patient should be able to cope with activities such as:

- hand sawing
- belt sanding
- routing
- manually bending wrought iron
- moving timber
- hammering
- using hand tools
- lifting weights of 35–50 lb (16–23 kg) with two hands.

Patients can be safely programmed to undertake heavy workshop tasks for up to 6 hours a day if strength and endurance are necessary for their occupation or hobby.

Improving confidence

Lack of confidence and reluctance to use the injured hand may be caused by:

- the severity of the injury
- the number of operations
- pain
- fear or lack of therapy
- lack of information concerning the hand injury.

These factors may result in the patient becoming one-handed, and it is essential that normal posture, use and function is restored quickly. Altered posture and lack or abnormal use of the hand should be pointed out each time it is noticed, and it may help the patient to see the abnormal function recorded on a video. Bilateral movements and activities are particularly useful in correcting a one-sided habit.

The patient may need to regain confidence in the use of the hand as soon as the considerations of the immediate stage following injury and surgery no longer apply. Precautions and contraindications cease to be applicable in the later stages of treatment, and the patient must become confident that the hand can now be used without the risk of tendon rupture or the disruption of a fracture site.

Bilateral activities such as bouncing, catching and rolling of large but lightweight balls should be introduced. Beach balls are ideal for this purpose, ensuring that all the joints of both upper limbs are being used. Balance reactions, such as from sitting on a rocker board placed on a low plinth or on a gymnastic ball, also facilitate bilateral movements (Figure 5.26).

Class work in the gymnasium with other patients who have a variety of upper limb problems forms a most useful part of treatment, both physically and psychologically. A carefully matched and competitive atmosphere should help the patient forget

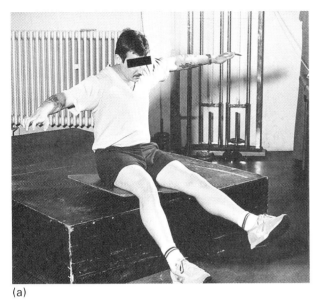 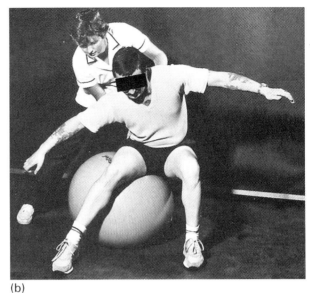

(a)   (b)

Figure 5.26   Bilateral balance reactions on (a) rocker board and (b) gymnastic ball.

worries and difficulties and once again have some fun (Figure 5.27). Specific treatment can be ensured by the careful selection of activities and by the use of adaptations, such as padding of handles for table tennis and badminton. Modifications should be made according to the degree of healing or the pain experienced.

Several benefits are to be gained from these activities:

- there is a 'fun' aspect in the competitiveness
- a degree of discipline is necessary while working with others
- many activities are bilateral
- there is plenty of verbal encouragement in the class

- a means is provided to stimulate both arm and hand with the maximum normal sensory input; this is especially beneficial for a patient with a mild complex regional pain syndrome or other associated painful condition.

Spontaneous use of the hand in everyday tasks, such as pushing open a door, may need encouragement. The patient should be incorporating the hand into normal body language, and games such as charades can help.

Contact with other people or objects should be introduced and increased gradually, and is especially important following a painful condition:

- use of the hand in tapping and striking movements should be encouraged (Figure 5.28), initially

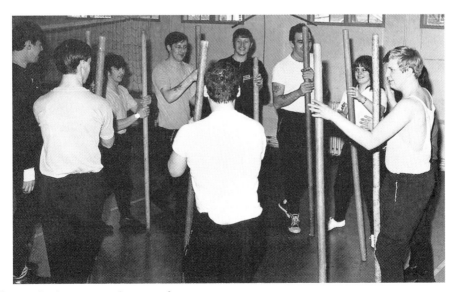

Figure 5.27   Games in the gymnasium are fun.

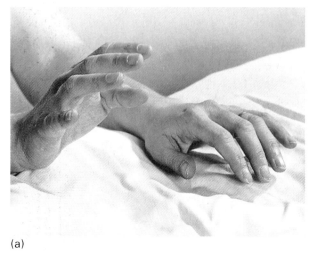

(a)

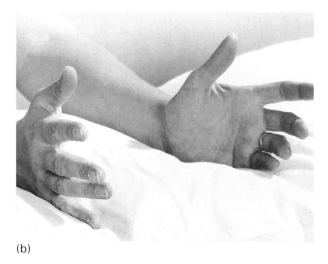

(b)

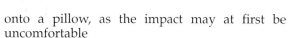

Figure 5.28 Contact activities.

onto a pillow, as the impact may at first be uncomfortable

- individual finger movements can be performed on a table, first with the fingers flat and then flexed, using the tips as in playing the piano
- hand clapping and the tapotement movements that physiotherapists learn are all suitable when the patient is less worried by the jarring effect
- games such as pat-a-cake and building up hands one on top of the other with the placing of the bottom hand on the top can be played by patients together
- card games such as 'snap', may involve sudden contact with other people's hands
- bouncing and catching a tennis ball and catching a leather 'mouse' in a flowerpot (Mousie Mousie) are appropriate games.

Leaning on the hand, either with the whole hand flat or on the fingertips, should be introduced (Figure 5.29). Pressing and weight bearing movements should be strengthened progressively (Figure 5.30). For the elderly it is essential that they can lean

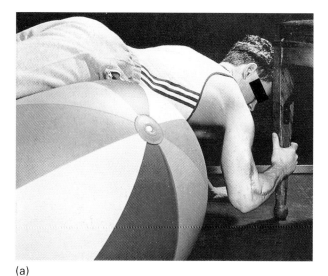

(a)

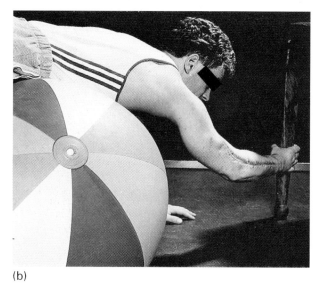

(b)

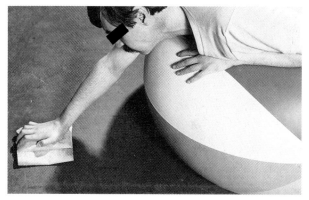

Figure 5.29 Taking weight on the outstretched hand.

Figure 5.30 Elbow flexion and extension movements with origins and insertions reversed.

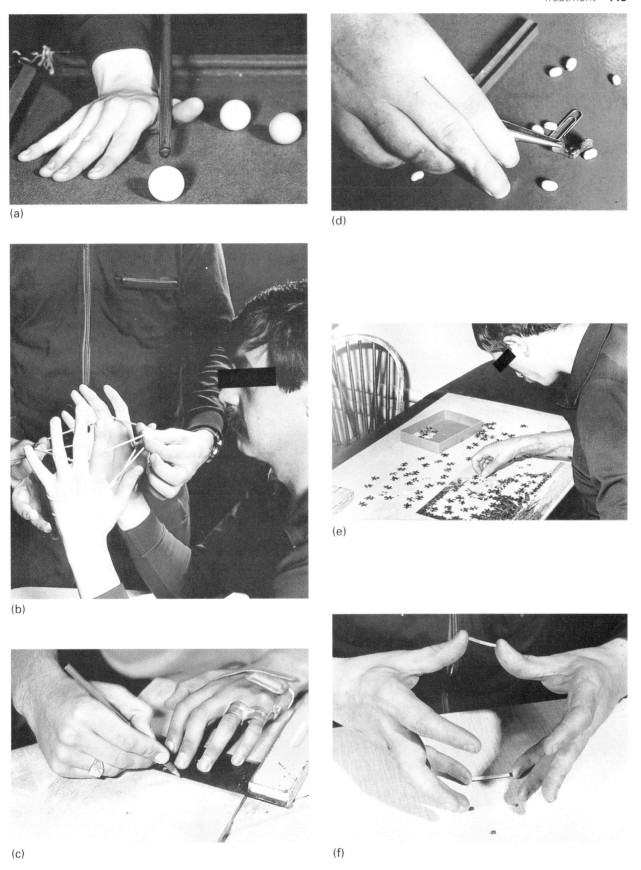

(a)

(d)

(b)

(e)

(c)

(f)

Figure 5.31   A selection of activities to encourage movement and dexterity.

on a hand for support. In young men, these movements may be practised in press-ups and applied to strenuous work.

As treatment progresses an increasing number of activities should be introduced, the selection depending on the patient's problems, future requirements, occupation and leisure interests (Figure 5.31). The heavy workshop also provides many valuable functional activities that help the patient to regain confidence.

Activities of daily living should also be checked at this stage of treatment. A patient who uses the hand correctly in therapy sessions might still be compensating badly in daily living skills. A wide range of tasks should be checked, such as:

● personal care
● dressing
● use of cutlery
● domestic tasks such as opening jars, tins and packets
● the method of carrying saucepans and kettles.

Usually all the patient needs is encouragement to perform these activities normally, and to be set 'homework' tasks. However, some patients may need more help and should be allocated a regular therapy session in the OT kitchen/daily living area to practice daily living skills. These patients may include:

● those who need more prompting and 'hands-on' guidance from the therapist
● those who will have to compensate and adapt their methods of working because of the type of injury (e.g. major amputation); these patients may need to use adapted equipment, e.g. jar openers etc., on a long-term basis.

Machine phobia

The therapist must be very alert to the possibility of the patient experiencing post-traumatic stress disorder or machine phobia (see also Chapter 3). The patient suffering from post-traumatic stress disorder may be very anxious, experiencing nightmares and flashbacks. The Hospital Anxiety and Depression Scale (HAD) and the Revised Impact of Event Scale (RIES) can be useful screening tools in helping to detect this problem. Some patients may have injured themselves on workshop machinery similar to that used as part of their treatment programme. The possibility of machine phobia must always be considered. If the patient has a persistent problem that does not seem to be resolving, help should be sought from a clinical psychologist.

Patients who have a machine phobia may need to undertake a desensitization programme under the guidance of a clinical psychologist. The occupational therapist should gradually introduce the patient into the workshop environment through a hierarchy of situations and machines, progressing from the least to the most threatening. This hierarchy should be planned and agreed with the patient. The patient uses relaxation techniques in the working environment, and when comfortable with one situation can move on to the next.

For example, if the patient has a machine phobia about a circular saw, a typical hierarchy might be as follows:

1. Work on a non-machine task in a room adjacent to a carpentry department that contains a circular saw (saw switched off)
2. Work on a machine task in a room adjacent to the circular saw (saw switched off)
3. Work on a machine task in a room adjacent to the circular saw (saw switched on)
4. Work on a non-machine task in the carpentry room containing the circular saw (saw switched off)
5. Work on a machine task in the carpentry room containing the circular saw (saw switched off)
6. Work on a machine task in the carpentry room (saw switched on)
7. Watch the circular saw being used
8. Stand next to the circular saw and touch the saw bed (saw switched off)
9. Stand next to the circular saw and touch the saw bed (saw switched on)
10. Operate the saw in a heavily jigged task
11. Operate the saw normally without jigs.

A few patients remain severely machine phobic, which may necessitate a change of career. The degree of machine phobia does not correlate to the extent of injury, and the occupational therapist should therefore not overlook the possibility that these problems might arise in patients with minor hand injuries.

Sensation

Without adequate sensation patients are unlikely to use their hand efficiently, except when they can watch what they are doing, as they will have neither sensory feedback to monitor movement nor stereognosis. The skill of the brain to interpret sensation correctly is the consequence of proprioception combined with tactile sensation, both of which function most effectively in a situation of movement.

Sensory recovery depends on a number of factors such as the site and type of nerve lesion, the type of surgical repair and the age of the patient. The patient should never be promised a full recovery and must be warned that the final stage of recovery may take many years. Three to four years is a good working figure for the time it will take for complete recovery from a lesion at the wrist level, but it does depend on the level and type of nerve damage. The patient should consider the return of all sensation as a bonus.

The process of sensory recovery and the stages of nerve regeneration that the patient may experience must be fully explained. Without forewarning and education, these normal processes may be alarming for the patient, especially as they are most likely to occur long after active therapy has finished.

Sensory recovery follows a gradual progression from anaesthesia, to hyperaesthesia, to hypoaesthesia and hopefully to normal sensation. Hyperpathia is an extremely painful response to light touch, but is a fairly uncommon phenomenon, and is more usually associated with brachial plexus lesions. Most patients will move through each stage of recovery, but this is not guaranteed and the process may halt at any stage.

Anaesthetic stage

In the early stage following division of a nerve, the patient will have a hand with total anaesthesia in the area supplied by that nerve. The patient must clearly recognize the areas of the hand that are numb and be taught about care of anaesthetic skin, learning to think for the hand and to check the skin regularly for damage. There is the risk of receiving burns from everyday objects such as kettles, saucepans, teapots, irons, radiators and hot food, and cold burns may occur from household freezers or carbon dioxide snow. Heat burns will be produced at lower temperatures than usual because of the absence of response to the heat. Blisters and resulting trophic lesions are slow to heal due to the poor nutrition of the area. Blisters can occur also as the result of friction.

The patient must be reminded frequently about the dangers of damaging the anaesthetic hand. The possibilities must be spelt out in great detail, as the consequences are unlikely to be fully understood. Regular reminders are therefore essential, and the patient must realize that every movement made must be watched, especially when near anything hot. Regrettably, no matter how often the therapist warns the patient, it often takes an injury before the seriousness of the situation is really appreciated.

The therapist must give advice about the length of time before some sensation is likely to return, to help the patient cope with what is usually a worrying but temporary situation. The rate of nerve growth can be explained to the patient as either 'an inch a month' or 'a millimetre a day', depending on which is the most understandable.

The majority of active rehabilitation will be undergone during the anaesthetic stage, and the patient must learn how to use the hand despite loss of feeling. A typing tutor package on a computer or word processor is a helpful activity in teaching patients how to use a hand that has little or no sensation, and is particularly valuable for patients who need keyboard skills in their job.

Sufficient range of movement and muscle power may have been regained for return to work whilst the hand remains anaesthetic. The patient must be encouraged to use the hand as normally as possible in a wide variety of workshop activities, whilst being aware of the risks and dangers to the hand. Strategies will probably be necessary to compensate for deficiency in sensation.

The patient with an anaesthetic hand will not be able to use the hand unless it can be seen. In many occupations (e.g. motor mechanic, plumber) the hands need to work blind, and this is impossible without sensation. The patient must learn to work normally in situations where the injured hand is in view, but to swap to the uninjured hand when it is necessary to work blind. As sensation improves, the patient must try using the injured hand in these blind situations.

For certain occupations the therapist can be inventive and enable the patient to return to work with the use of special tools. For example, a welder with an ulnar nerve lesion wished to return to work despite the risk of burns to the ulnar border of the hand. His glove was adapted with a small metal bar that passed from the anaesthetic ulnar aspect to the medial aspect of the hand where sensation was intact. The metal bar quickly transferred heat to areas of skin where it could be felt, warning the welder that the ulnar border was getting hot.

Hyperaesthetic stage

Hyperaesthesia, or pins and needles, is the first sign of some sensory regeneration. It is a sensation of acute sensitivity as a result of inadequate insulation from the myelin sheaths. As the myelin matures the hyperaesthesia will progressively lessen, but in older people it may remain a problem. Although fine sensory discrimination cannot be achieved at this stage, the hyperaesthesia should provide some sensory awareness and therefore protection from heat, cold and friction. The process of regeneration is from the proximal to distal direction.

The patient may also experience sudden unexpected pains, like electric shocks, shooting either up or down the arm. These sensations are often very alarming and are most likely to happen when the patient is unoccupied or tired, e.g. during the evening. Advice that these are quite likely, and are a normal feature of the regeneration process, should be given. The hyperaesthetic stage is likely to develop approximately 8 weeks after nerve repair.

An early preliminary exercise in sensory re-education is for the patient to run the hand slowly but frequently over different surfaces, coarse textures and the angles of large objects such as the edge of the table or chair. Test tubes containing hot and cold water can be used for temperature recognition. During this stage it is essential that the patient continues to use the hand despite the unpleasant sensations. The normal use of the hand will help to modulate painful afferent discharges and is an important ongoing process of sensory re-education

The use of TENS may be useful for reducing the unpleasant pins and needles sensation, allowing the patient to use the hand more comfortably. Very occasionally, however, TENS has been found to exacerbate the symptoms.

Hypoaesthetic stage and return to normal sensation

As the myelin sheaths continue to mature and provide better nerve insulation, the pins and needles sensation will disappear. It is replaced by sensation that is more normal but may be reduced, i.e. hypoaesthesia. Not all the sensory neurones will have been able to regenerate to their correct end organs, and some may well have gone astray and regenerated to muscle endplates. This reduced sensory recovery will produce a 'woolly' or distant feeling. When asked to compare the sensation of the injured with the uninjured hand, the patient may state that the uninjured hand has more acute sensation. Gradually a more normal sensation should occur.

Sensory re-education is commenced at the stage when the sensation of the palm has returned more or less to normal but the fingertips are still hyperaesthetic. There is no point in attempting sensory re-education in an anaesthetic hand. Dellon recommends that it is commenced when there is recognition of vibration at 256 Hz in the area of sensory disturbance. Many patients will reach this re-education stage long after they have finished active therapy. If the patient is functionally using the hand well, this will constantly provide situations that facilitate sensory re-education. However, it is necessary that the patient understands the principle and technique of sensory re-education so that this can be started at home at the appropriate time, with a reminder of the technique at a follow-up clinic.

Sensory re-education technique

Following the regeneration of nerves in the hand, the brain must re-map the new sensory information it is receiving. The therapist can help this remodelling process by use of sensory re-education. The technique involves the conscious process of linking three sensory inputs:

- normal input from the patient's uninjured hand
- abnormal sensory input from the injured hand
- vision.

Stereognosis provides a practical application for re-education of both sensory awareness and joint position sense. The technique involves the recognition of textures and objects without sight.

The sessions are performed with the patient's eyes closed or, if necessary, blindfolded. The patient can work with the hand through a screen, but this has the effect of psychologically separating the patient from the task and is best used for assessment purposes only. The therapist should explain the task in an introductory session, and ask the patient to describe a large but simple object, with prompts about its length, width, shape, material, texture, temperature and weight (Figure 5.32). This will help the patient to consciously consider and describe the object being held.

In the first instance the patient should be given objects that are easy to handle and made of a number of materials – e.g. the bristles and wood of a hairbrush. The objects used for training should not be the same as those used in assessment. The patient must not be allowed to become frustrated by being given objects so small that they cannot be felt, or by continuing a session for too long. Objects or textures that may be easily identified by sound should be avoided. A session of a few minutes several times a day will be sufficient.

If unable to recognize an object, the patient should be allowed to handle it in the uninjured hand, then open the eyes and look at the object. The patient should manipulate it once more in the injured hand, first whilst looking at it and then with

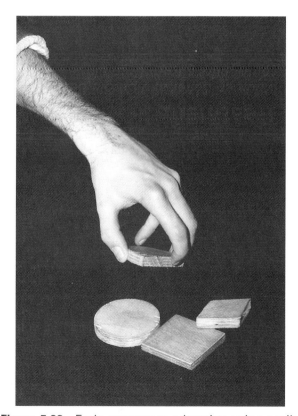

Figure 5.32 Early sensory re-education using easily described blocks.

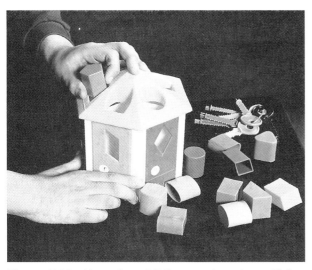

Figure 5.33   Use of a child's post box for utilizing proprioceptive abilities.

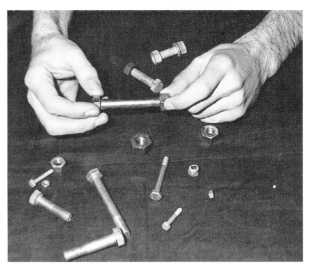

Figure 5.34   Nuts and bolts can reproduce a normal work environment and also be a competitive timed test.

the eyes closed. This activity should be repeated daily with the same and progressively smaller objects and different types of materials.

Patients can make their own individual sensory re-education kits by placing a large number of small, safe everyday objects and textures – e.g. a scouring pad, plug, eraser, screw, and material scraps – in a pillow case and feeling inside to attempt to identify the objects. If they cannot identify one, they bring it out of the pillow case into view. Alternatively, patients can carry a few objects or pieces of fabric in their pocket. They must be taught how to conduct their own retraining programme, as it may be impossible to take time off work to attend further therapy sessions, and therapy services may not have sufficient resources to provide this type of treatment. Well-trained patients can do much on their own with regard to sensory education.

As sensory awareness improves, the speed and ability of motor performance will increase. It is now useful to include tests of speed, with the blindfolded patient transferring objects from one place or container to another. Timed activities using children's toys, such as posting shapes into a post-box (Figure 5.33), a Tupperware™ ball with its numerous different-shaped pieces, a board with cut-out blocks, and nuts and bolts (Figure 5.34), provide both competition and interest for the patient. Most patients will rise to a challenge, particularly if there are several of them undergoing sensory re-education at the same time.

Specific training of proprioception is invaluable, as a considerable degree of gnostic ability is achieved by this means. Patients whose cutaneous supply from the median nerve remains limited can recover reasonable stereognosis and an adequate

sensory feedback if their proprioception is particularly efficient. The use of wooden letters (Figure 5.35) can provide an interesting medium in the re-education of this modality.

Localization training Localization is the ability to identify where the hand is being touched. After a complete or partial division of a nerve, localization may be altered, as it is probable that the axons will not regenerate to their original end organs. Training, along with the continual functional use of the hand, will help to correct this. If localization is inaccurate, patients will receive false and confusing information from their fingertips.

Areas with inaccurate localization must be determined (see Chapter 2). In each of these areas, the therapist applies a moving touch with the finger over one spot for a couple of seconds whilst the patient's eyes are closed. The patient is then asked to open the eyes and point to the spot where sensation was experienced. If correct, the therapist proceeds to the next area using the same method. If incorrect, the therapist strokes the same spot, but

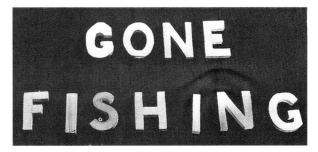

Figure 5.35   Wooden letters provide tactile and proprioceptive stimuli and the possibility of fun.

this time the patient watches. The touch is then repeated again, but with the eyes closed. As in sensory re-education, the patient is attempting to make a conscious link between where sensation is experienced, the stimulus, and vision. The patient is then able to recognize where he or she is being touched, even though the contact is felt somewhere else. This is the first step in localization training, and should be repeated at regular intervals during the day. The patient's family may be taught how to do the technique.

Eventually it should be possible to identify all areas correctly, and the patient's improving ability can be assessed by the speed of identification until hopefully an instantaneous and correct response is achieved. The technique can be upgraded by the patient to identify letters, numbers, shapes and words 'drawn' onto the palm and the palmar surface of the fingers.

Cold intolerance

Cold intolerance is a common and distressing problem of hand injury, occurring in a high proportion of severe cases. It can also follow relatively minor hand trauma, although is most likely to occur in conjunction with nerve damage. The problem is experienced most commonly when the patient moves to a cold environment or where there is a cooling effect (for example, when cycling the air currents over the hand create relative cooling). The patient's digit or hand turns blue and becomes stiff and painful as the circulation is disrupted. For some patients, the problem may occur quickly in even relatively warm environments. It can have a major impact on the patient's job and hobbies; for example, in the building trade, where most jobs are outside, the patient may be unsafe to climb ladders or unable to use hand tools.

There are four main symptoms of cold intolerance (Campbell and Kay, 1998):

- pain
- dysaesthesia (either numbness or tingling)
- stiffness
- change in colour.

One or more of these symptoms may occur, but pain is the most debilitating and change in colour the least.

Patients must be warned that these complications may occur. If they injure themselves in the summer, when cold intolerance is less evident, they must be forewarned that it may become a problem during the following winter. For some patients it can be a problem that persists for many years and is difficult to manage.

Suggestions for management include:

- keeping the hand as warm as possible, using waterproof ski gloves or mitts and heated hand pads (available from most camping shops and chemists)
- most importantly, keeping the body warm, with use of body warmers or thermal underwear.

USE OF ACTIVITY AS A TREATMENT METHOD

During the rehabilitation period following major hand trauma, patients will need to make the transition from being a patient to their previous roles – e.g. employee, parent, football coach. They will need to move from a passive role of dependence, illness and lack of control, to an active role of independence and self-sufficiency. The hand therapist will have an important part to play in this process. Although it is necessary to consider the specific problems that occur as a result of hand trauma, the patient as a whole person must not be overlooked.

Maslow (1970) describes a hierarchy of needs or motivational states for the individual, which fall into two distinct sets. First, there are those motivational forces that ensure survival by satisfying basic physiological and safety needs, and the need to be loved and to belong. Following major hand trauma, patients' primary motivation will be in satisfying these needs and being cared for in the early stages of trauma, surgery and rehabilitation. As they improve, these basic needs will be met, enabling them to explore the second set of the motivational states – self-actualization.

Self-actualization is the process by which a person realizes his or her full potential. This process will show great individual differences, and few people fully achieve it. Following major trauma, patients explore this process within the context of changed physical function. Activity is a critical part of the process of self-actualization, especially for people who have a strong practical orientation.

Early in treatment the therapist concentrates on achieving specific goals, e.g. reduction of oedema. As rehabilitation progresses, the emphasis changes to more functionally orientated treatment, helping patients to prepare physically and psychologically for return to their original lifestyle, or to adapt and re-evaluate in the light of their altered abilities.

Therapy goals must take into account other influences besides the hand trauma, including:

1. Psychological problems – underlying depression or mental illness, anxiety, fear, defence mechanisms such as denial or regression, alcohol or drug abuse
2. Social problems – domestic violence, family stress, care of elderly relatives and small children
3. Financial problems
4. Employment problems
   - the nature and demands of the work
   - if the injury occurred at work, the involvement of Health and Safety inspectors

- claims (possible litigation and compensation)
- the re-employment situation (whether the job will still be open to the patient)
- the amount of paid sick leave allowed.

5. Criminal proceedings – not uncommonly, hand trauma occurs as a result of criminal activity (e.g. actual bodily harm). The patient may therefore be involved in criminal investigations.

Factors such as these will give the therapist a broader view of some of the other influences that may affect the patient's behaviour. Detailed aspects of the patient's personality will also need to be considered and might influence the choice of activity, including:

- educational background and level of intelligence
- general practical ability and skills
- motivation
- hobbies and interests
- age
- overall level of health and physical fitness; secondary medical problems
- ability to concentrate
- awareness of safety, judgement and reasoning.
- reliability and amount of supervision needed.

Activities that are purposeful and meaningful can provide the patient with a sense of achievement as well as therapy for the specific goals. This can be a powerful motivating force for patients who have lost hope and direction.

Analysing the activity

The occupational therapist must analyse the activity if intending to use it as a remedial task. This is a core professional skill, and with regard to hand trauma the activities should be analysed under the following headings:

1. Physical skills needed to complete the task
2. Potential to adapt the task to meet specific therapy aims
3. The degree of complexity and the number of stages in the task
4. The social or cultural associations of the task
5. The potential for enjoyment or interest
6. Availability of equipment, materials and expertise.

Physical skills needed to complete the task
Consider:

- the range of movement needed at each joint
- patterns of prehension or pinch, e.g. pulp-to-pulp, tripod, cylinder grip
- the number of joints involved.
- the muscle strength needed
- patterns of movement and posture
- the degree of sensory input – is the task completed seen or unseen; can the patient sense

temperature; are there special safety considerations?
- contact with the skin (e.g. rough, wet)
- the other limbs or senses involved – e.g. bilateral activity, involvement of lower limbs in lifting and bending, need for good eyesight.

Potential to adapt the task to meet specific therapy aims
Examples of how activities can be adapted, and therefore graded, have been given within each section on specific therapy aims (e.g. changing the size of counters to change the range of joint movement required, elevating the activity to reduce oedema).

The degree of complexity and the number of stages in the task
Consider the degree of complexity and the number of stages in the task. For example, the task may consist of a single stage that is repeated, or of a number of stages which vary in the amount of physical demand and practical skill required. It may be appropriate that the patient only undertakes that stage or sub-task matched to his or her level of skill and present level of function. For another patient it may be appropriate to complete all the sub-stages of the task in sequence.

Examples Construction of a small wooden stool with a woven seat made from seating cord.
Patient A is in the early stages of treatment following tendon injury, and needs light non-resisted activity. He has an oedematous hand and no carpentry skills.
For this patient it would be appropriate to complete only one sub-task, varnishing or staining the stool frame, working from a high table with a low seat, with his hand in elevation.
Patient B is in the middle to late stages of treatment following tendon injury, and needs to begin to work for power grip and muscle strength. He has no major problems with oedema and no carpentry skills.
For this patient it would be appropriate to complete the woven seat on a pre-prepared stool frame. The stool seating cord will help to toughen up the skin condition, and the task becomes harder, demanding more grip strength and upper limb muscle power as it progresses. It would be appropriate for the patient to work standing at a normal working bench height.
Patient C is in the late stages of treatment, there are no contraindications and he needs to improve confidence in the use of his hand and its level of function. He is a carpenter by trade.
For this patient it would be appropriate to complete all stages of the task. This would involve him in the following:

1. Preparing the wood
   - selecting wood from a store and carrying the planks to the workshop (involving lifting)
   - cutting planks on a circular saw to create a straight edge
   - preparing wood through a surface planer
   - cutting planks into the required widths on a circular saw
   - pushing the strips through a thickness planing machine until the strips are of the required size
   - using a circular saw to cut the timber to the required length for the rails and legs.
2. Preparing the rails
   - preparing the dowels using a lathe
   - angling the dowels to 45° on a disc sander.
3. Preparing the legs
   - drilling holes in one end of the legs using a pillar drill
   - shaping a scallop along the length of the leg using a routing machine.
4. Assembling the stool frames
   - sanding the rails and legs with coarse, medium and then fine sandpaper, either by hand or with an electric sander
   - assembling the legs and rails to form the stools, using glue for the joints and supporting the frames with sash cramps
   - cleaning away any surplus glue and sanding off any dirty marks.

The stool frame would now be ready for staining and varnishing, and then weaving. It might be appropriate for this patient not to go on to seat the stool; this would also help to provide raw materials for patients A and B above.

The social or cultural associations of the task

The therapist must consider the social or cultural implications that the task might hold. Patients who never take any role in domestic chores may be very reluctant to attempt daily living skills such as cooking and ironing. There is little point in pushing such patients to do these tasks if they really do not want to. Do not make presuppositions about what tasks are appropriate for the patient to undertake. For example, a male patient went through a checklist of dressing skills to check his independence and was found to have no difficulties at all. However, when asked if he had any problems, he requested practice in unfastening bras one-handed!

Some tasks may have a very negative image. Some patients feel insulted by being asked to play games. Try to ensure that patients are matched against intellectually similar opponents to avoid frustration on both sides. Craft activities such as basketry can have a very negative image in the eyes of both the therapist and the general public. However, such activities do provide a very valuable

therapeutic medium – basketry provides a light non-resisted activity that can be adapted and done in elevation. Many patients appreciate tangible evidence of their efforts, and proudly take their tray home to show the rest of the family.

The therapist must always explain to patients what the purpose of the activity is, and the position in which it must be completed. Patients must take an active role in ensuring that the task they are doing is achieving the specified goals. The therapist must constantly monitor this.

The potential for enjoyment or interest

Occupational therapy activities should be interesting to patients so that they are positively engaged and participate. Consequently, the choice of activity will need to take into account the patients' practical and academic level of ability and interests.

Availability of equipment, materials and expertise

In considering the choice of activity, the therapist must ensure that the necessary tools and equipment are available, that they are well maintained and that the patient can be taught how to use them safely and correctly. For some patients it may be necessary to provide tools that have been specially adapted. Materials must be readily available, and the therapist must consider how to sell the finished product. The product must be of an acceptable standard without needing extra work from staff members, and the cost of the product must be reasonable. Do not assume that patients will want to buy what they have made – they should be under no obligation to do so. Hand trauma often imposes a considerable financial burden on patients, so there must be an outlet for the products that are made.

Choice of activity may also be determined by available expertise e.g. technical knowledge. The therapist will need a close productive relationship with the technical instructors and occupational therapy technicians within her team.

Conclusion

In summary, the choice of activity as a treatment method will depend upon many factors relating to the patients' problems and needs, their personality and the resources available to the therapist. The occupational therapist should be creative in using a wide variety of activities during treatment.

Details of activities the occupational therapist could consider are given in Appendix B (p. 310), and include:

1. Remedial games
2. Craft activities
   - Early stage – jewellery making, basketry, type setting, pyrography

- Middle stage – macramé
- Late stage – pottery, leatherwork, printing, stool seating
3. Woodwork
4. Engineering
5. Electronics
6. Gardening – indoor and outdoor
7. Cooking – making cakes, bread, chutney, soup and meals; handling hot pans and heavy dishes; cutting and chopping; lifting and pouring; opening packets and containers
8. Personal independence – in the early stages the patient may need help with certain aspects of care (e.g. dressing, washing, shaving), or need to compensate by using the uninjured hand; however, by the late stages the patient must be personally independent, if necessary with adapted equipment, and no longer using unnecessary compensatory movements
9. Domestic independence – cleaning, changing the bed, ironing, using keys (door and car), handling money, shopping etc.
10. Recreational tasks – playing cards, fishing (tying flies), electronic keyboard etc.
11. Communication and home administration – writing, keyboard typing, use of telephone etc.

The analysis of activity will enable the occupational therapist to use activities as a specific therapeutic method and to solve problems that the patient meets in relation to daily living – work, leisure, self-care, recreation and social.

Willard and Spackman (Hopkins and Smith, 1993) define occupation as follows:

Occupation is the dominant activity of human beings that includes serious, productive pursuits and playful, creative, and festive behaviours. It is the result of evolutionary processing culminating in a biological, psychological and social need for ludic and productive activity.

In conclusion, occupational therapists should be imaginative in their use of the fundamental skill of activity analysis so as to provide a successful and valuable form of treatment.

ELECTROACTIVE EXERCISE (BY DOMINIQUE THOMAS)

The application of neuromuscular electrical stimulation (NMES) both enhances and reinforces the rehabilitation of normally innervated hand muscles. The subject of denervated muscle stimulation will not be addressed.

History

The application of electrical stimulation for pain control was first documented by the early Greeks and Romans, who used live torpedo fish and organs of electric fish (Taub and Kane, 1975). Electrostimulation of normally innervated muscles arrived later in history (Watkins, 1972). In the twentieth century, up until the 1970s electrotherapy was mostly used for pain control, iontophoresis and denervated muscle stimulation. It was rarely applied to normal nerves or totally innervated muscles, because if muscles could be activated voluntarily there was no rationale behind applying electric current and no therapeutic effect could be expected. However, the locomotor system has been shown to gain from the long-term application of functional electrical stimulation (FES) to innervated muscles of upper motor neurone injured patients (Liberson, 1961; Rancho los Amigos, 1980; Gracanin, 1972; Merletti et al., 1978) and from the stimulation of healthy muscle to increase strength in athletes (Kots and Xvilon, 1977). In 1973, Braun implanted a modified cardiac pacemaker to maintain flexor tendon excursion after tenolysis.

Since then there has been application of NMES to normally innervated muscles in order to reinforce voluntary muscle contraction. This has been named electroactive exercise (Thomas and Frere 1979; Thomas, 1987). It is effective by overcoming:

- any inhibited motor control caused by nociceptive or defence reflexes
- motor image exclusion
- pain, which is common after injury or surgery.

Rationale for using electroactive exercise

Electrical stimulation is a modality that combines motor, analgesic and neuromuscular facilitation effects. The motor (efferent) effect is so powerful that motion induced in some muscle groups cannot be resisted at high intensities. Its use is justified in many clinical conditions (Cannon and Taylor Mullins, 1984; Moutet et al., 1988).

Creating an individual muscle contraction in combination with the analgesic and facilitation effects can be of clinical benefit. Mobilization produced by electrical stimulation is similar to active motion, producing physiological movement composed of both rotation and gliding. Passive mobilization induces joint rotation but little gliding, and as a rule should only be used when active motion is not able to maintain full range.

Clinical application of electroactive exercise

Before applying NMES to patients, therapists should be familiar with this modality and have experienced it personally at high intensity.

Stimulator selection

1. Portable battery-powered stimulators are user friendly and less intimidating to patients.
2. Ideally, two types of pulses (waves) should be available; rectangular monophasic and rectangular biphasic.
3. Most muscles respond to biphasic treatment, some muscles respond better to monophasic.
4. Stimulators should have manual triggering and automatic cycling for synchronizing electrostimulation with the patient's voluntary motion.
5. On-time should be adjustable up to 5–10 seconds to build an effective isometric contraction.
6. Off-time should be adjustable up to 40 seconds to allow muscle rest. Built-in synchronized visual and auditory feedback for reinforcement of electroactive exercise is an asset.
7. A timing device makes treatment easier to control for therapists.

Electrodes

These may be made of conductive rubber and applied with gel, or of metal, tin or stainless steel, which require felt, gauze or sponge squeezed out in tap water. Each has its own advantage; for example, to reach nerves such as the ulnar or median in the arm, electrodes need to be sufficiently rigid to be pushed into soft tissues. Metal has the advantage of easily being cut to size. Three electrode sizes cover all upper extremity and hand applications: 10×5 cm, 6×4 cm and 3×4 cm.

Application techniques

The classical methods of electrical stimulation suitable in the hand are monopolar and bipolar. The interferential technique is not suitable.

With *monophasic currents* (pulsed direct currents), one electrode is active and the other is called dispersive. Generally the negative electrode (cathode) is active. Pulsed direct currents:

- can be aggressive to the skin, resulting in burns
- quickly cause fatigue

- should not be used directly over metal, for instance over bone fixation material.

The larger dispersive electrode is placed proximal to the elbow, over the radial nerve for stimulating extensor muscles and over the ulnar and median nerves for the flexor muscles.

With *biphasic currents* both electrodes are alternatively positive and negative, which allows stimulation of two synergistic muscle groups at the same time. Biphasic currents:

- have no polar effect
- do not fatigue muscle as fast
- can be placed over metal.

With bipolar techniques the proximal electrode is placed below the common origin of the extensor muscles on the epicondyle, or of the flexor muscles below the epitrochlea (medial condyle). The distal electrode is placed on the muscle belly motor point.

Concentrating the muscle action on a given joint requires blocking proximally or distally. A pegboard is an indispensable accessory to electroactive exercise. With the wrist blocked on a pegboard it is easy to induce strong contraction of superficial flexor and extensor muscles (FDS, FPL, wrist flexors, thenar and hypothenar muscles, thumb, wrist and finger extensors). However, it is not possible to reach the deep finger flexors.

Proximal joint blocking allows the contraction of muscles in mid-range, at the point of greatest mechanical advantage. When metacarpophalangeal joints and the wrist are blocked, the finger flexors exert all their power into flexing proximal and distal interphalangeal joints. Conversely, when blocking finger flexion by holding a bulky object in the palm of hand, the finger flexors become wrist flexors.

Forearm blocking also maintains muscles in the same position throughout exercise, as pronation and supination modifies muscle position and muscle depth in relation to skeleton, skin and electrode placement. For instance, when applying a bipolar technique on finger flexors with the forearm in supination, stimulation reaches the FDS. The same electrode placement with the forearm in pronation will reach the ulnar part of the FDP.

Since it is impossible to target an individual muscle group without some irradiation to neighbouring muscles, proximal or distal joint blocking causes some muscles to contract isometrically while target muscles contract isotonically.

Joint blocking:

- helps to localize muscle action on target joints
- avoids the additional pain of full range of motion
- allows selective traction on tendon or muscle adhesions.

Recent application techniques

In order to reach the deep muscles, the therapists must think about the paths of least resistance that currents will follow, in spiral and diagonal directions through the hand and forearm, rather than purely the muscle planes of classical anatomy (Thomas, 1996).

The flexor digitorum profundus (FDP) to the fourth and fifth digits is posterior and medial, not anterior. Using a monopolar technique with the distal electrode placed medial to the ulna at mid-forearm level induces flexion of these two digits (Figure 5.36).

Simultaneous stimulation of extrinsic and intrinsic agonist muscles

Biphasic currents enable the stimulation of two synergistic muscles simultaneously. For example, stimulation of extrinsic and intrinsic flexors of the medial two digits produces full flexion of the MCP, PIP and DIP joints of those digits. One electrode is placed over the flexor profundus medially to the ulna and the other over the thenar eminence. This induces better MCP flexion than monopolar stimulation of the same muscles (Figure 5.37).

The irradiation phenomenon and use of diagonal electrode placement

The motor fibres of nerves and muscle tissue located closest to the electrode are progressively recruited as the stimulation intensity is increased, irradiating first through the intermuscular then through the interosseous membranes. Stimulating the thumb extensors and abductors causes progressive FPL recruitment with the IP joint pulled into flexion and the CMC and MCP joints remaining in extension. This phenomenon can therefore be used to produce combined movements and to reach deep muscles that are inaccessible from the anterior aspect of the forearm.

Combined movements of thumb opposition with wrist flexion, ulnar deviation and forearm pronation can be achieved with a proximal electrode on the ulnar and median nerves above the elbow and a distal electrode on the thenar eminence. This can be useful to treat stiffness of the wrist.

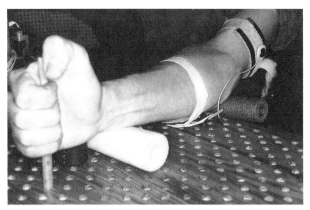

Figure 5.36 Stimulation of FDP, medial half, using the monopolar technique.

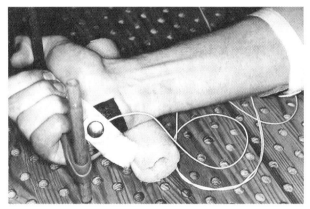

Figure 5.37 Simultaneous stimulation of extrinsic and intrinsic flexors of the last two digits.

Irradiation triggered from the anterior proximal electrode placed over the median and ulnar nerves proximal to the elbow and the distal electrode placed posteriorly like a wristwatch will reach the FDP and sometimes the index FDP, which is the most difficult muscle to stimulate (Figure 5.38).

Nerve trunk placement

Direct stimulation to the superficial sites of the median and ulnar nerves induces a powerful mass contraction of the extrinsic and intrinsic flexor muscles. It is the only technique to the median nerve that will consistently reach the FDP of the index finger. The proximal electrode is placed on the medial aspect of the arm at the mid-level of the trough between the biceps and triceps brachii, and the distal electrode is placed over the elbow flexion crease medial to the biceps tendon(Figure 5.39).

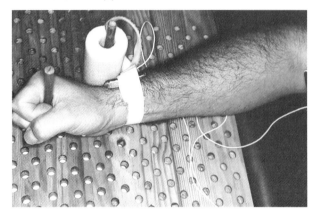

Figure 5.38 Diagonal electrode placement.

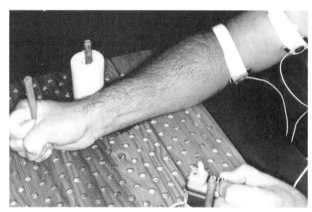

Figure 5.39 Median and ulnar nerve direct stimulation.

Direct radial nerve stimulation can be achieved with the proximal electrode placed over the triceps brachii and the distal electrode placed above the elbow and proximal to the epicondyle. This results in full elbow, wrist and finger extension.

Percutaneous implanted wire electrodes
Percutaneous implanted wire electrodes may be used in hand surgery in cases such as teno-arthrolysis. They are implanted in the same sites as surface electrodes except for the FDP in the index finger, the landmarks of which are the upper edge of the pronator teres and the medial aspect of the radius. Implanting a wire electrode enables checking of free tendon excursion during surgery, and makes post-operative rehabilitation easier (Thomas *et al*, 1993; De Soras *et al.*, 1994).

Practical pointers for stimulator adjustment

Finding the motor point (Table 5.1)

1. Use a manual switch.
2. Increase the intensity once the stimulation is on.
3. The proximal electrode need not be modified with monopolar stimulation. The motor point is found by sliding the distal electrode without lifting it from skin.
4. When using the bipolar technique, slight modification of either the proximal or distal electrode will alter the movement.
5. Stimulation may be unpleasant if the electrode is placed on a sensory nerve.

Adjusting the stimulator intensity
The stimulator intensity may differ according to:

1. Skin impedance (resistance). Ideally, the skin should be prepared by washing and warming it, otherwise the intensity increases when the skin becomes moist under the electrodes.
2. Adaptation and fatigue. Muscles adapt and contractions weaken as sessions progress. If sessions are too long or the off-time is too short, there is not enough time for the muscle metabolism to recover and therefore fatigue occurs.
3. Temporal summation and facilitation. At muscle contraction threshold intensity, the only muscles to contract are those that are closer to the electrode or types that respond better to stimulation pulse parameters. Temporal summation causes a facilitation effect, which produces an unexpected contraction that is unpleasant to some patients. This phenomenom occurs more with monophasic currents.
4. Variation in intensity. Never increase the intensity during the off-time, when the patient does not feel it, as the muscle contraction intensity increases several-fold once the contraction threshold has been reached. Do not turn the machine off during the off-time in case the potentiometer is turned the wrong way.
5. The patient's acceptance of electroactive exercise. Some patients may be unable to tolerate this form of treatment.

TABLE 5.1
ELECTRODE PLACEMENTS FOR PRINCIPAL HAND MUSCLE CONTRACTIONS

Muscle action	Technique	Proximal electrode placement	Distal electrode placement	Distal electrode polarity	Starting position	Range of motion	Contraction
		MONOPOLAR: For flexor muscles: over median/ulnar nerves, above elbow. For extensor muscles over radial nerve over elbow BIPOLAR: Unless otherwise specified For flexors: below common flexor origin on epitrochlea. For extensors: below common extensor origin on epicondyle					
STIMULATION OF EXTRINSIC MUSCLES							
Forearm supination	Monopolar		Below neck of radius on lateral side of common origin of extensors on the epicondyle	–	Pronation	Subtotal	Fair
Pronation	Mono or bipolar		Thenar eminence	– or +	Supination	Near total	Good
Wrist & finger flexion	Mono or bipolar		Junction of lower-middle thirds of anterior aspect of forearm	+	Midline supination of 'ref' position	Total	Excellent
Flexor sublimis digitorum	Mono or bipolar		For III, IV et V: center of anterior aspect of forearm. For II: Junction of lower middle-thirds of forearm on lateral side of forearm midline.	–	Supination or intermediate position, wrist blocked in slight extension	Total	Excellent
Flexor profundus digitorum, medial half	Mono or bipolar		Center of posterior forearm surface on medial side of ulna	– or +	–	Total for IV & V, sometime for III	Excellent
Flexor profundus digitorum, lateral half. D.I.P. flexion of the index	Diagonal	As for monopolar placement	Posterior forearm lower mid-third between ulna and radius ('wristwatch point')	+	Supination, wrist blocked	Subtotal	Fair
Mass flexion of all digits	Diagonal	Anterior lateral aspect of forearm upper mid-third	Posterior forearm lower mid-third between ulna and radius 'wristwatch point'	+	Midline or pronation wrist block in slight extension	Total	Good fair for index
Mass flexion of all digits	Bipolar	Nerve trunk, mid-arm, medial aspect, along groove between biceps and triceps	Nerve trunk along groove between biceps and triceps 2 inches below the proximal, above elbow		Midline; block wrist	Total	Excellent
Mass flexion of all digits and specifically index finger	Bipolar	Nerve trunk, proximal electrode same as above	Distal electrode over cubital fossa insertion of biceps tendon	–	Midline, block wrist	Total	Excellent
Flexor longus pollicis	Mono or bipolar		Junction of lower and middle third anterior lateral aspect of forearm	–	Supination, wrist blocked	Total	Good
M.C.P. flexion	Monopolar		Base of the hypothenar eminence	–	Supination, wrist blocked	Total	Good
Wrist and finger extension	Mono or bipolar		Middle posterior aspect of forearm	–	Pronation	Total	Excellent
Index extension	Mono or bipolar		Posterior-lateral aspect of forearm upper mid-third	–	Pronation	Total	Good
Little finger extension	Mono or bipolar		Posterior-medial aspect of forearm middle third	–	Pronation	Total	Good
STIMULATION OF INTRINSIC HAND MUSCLES							
Interossel	Monopolar		• Hypothenar eminence • Thenar eminence • Dorsal aspect of hand over metacarpal region	–	Supination or pronation	Total	Good
SIMULTANEOUS STIMULATION OF EXTRINSIC AND INTRINSIC HAND MUSCLES							
M.C.P.–P.I.P.– D.I.P. flexion of III, IV and V			Two electrodes, same size • One on base of hypothenar eminence • One on posterior aspect of forearm junction of upper and middle thirds medially to ulna	– or +	Supination, wrist blocked	Total	Excellent
D.I.P. and P.I.P. extension			• One on dorsal aspect of hand over metacarpal of concerned digit • One on extensor digitorum and extensor indicis or extensor digiti minimi	– or +	Pronation or intermediate position	Total	Good
SIMULTANEOUS STIMULATION OF TWO EXTRINSIC HAND MUSCLES							
Thumb, III, IV and V flexion			• One small electrode on flexor longus policis • One larger electrode on flexor profundus	–	Supination, wrist blocked	Total	Excellent

Clinical indications for electroactive exercise

Indications for electroactive exercise application are similar to those for voluntary active exercise:

- it can be used immediately post-injury or post-operatively, or when rehabilitation begins after immobilization
- it is used mainly to maintain or to improve joint range of motion and soft tissue excursion
- it is an efficient tool in preventing or loosening soft tissue adhesions by the powerful muscle contraction it induces
- it should be used as soon as the therapist realizes that patient's active mobilization is insufficient to maintain range of motion
- the timing of application to individual muscle groups is dictated by the fragility of the soft tissues and skeleton, and by related muscle group power. Application should also take into account human error – e.g. the possibility of mistakenly setting the intensity too high.

Examples
1. On a crush injury to the hand without a fracture, stimulation of the extrinsic flexor and extensor muscles can be applied immediately. However, application to the intrinsic muscles must be delayed a few days so as not to damage the new vascular network.
2. On a fracture stabilized by osteosynthesis, in order to maintain joint range of motion and soft tissue excursion, application is immediate on extensor muscles since their power is not sufficient to displace bone reduction and fixation. However, application on the flexor muscles must be delayed because flexor muscles are so powerful that an error in intensity setting can displace an internal fixation.
3. Electroactive exercise is one of the most efficient tools to loosen adhesions. It can be applied while adhesions are maintained in a maximally stretched position. When adhesions are located between the skin and underlying tissues, the scar can be blocked by hand or by a large rubber band while the muscle contracts in the opposite direction. Thus, adhesions are either pulled between the static skin and contracting muscle, or between adherent skin and tendon excursion.

Contraindications to electroactive exercise

Contraindications are the classical ones of neuromuscular electrical stimulation (Low and Reed, 1990):

- a demand-type pace-maker
- emotional hypersensitivity
- soft tissue and/or skeletal fragility
- skin conditions.

Surface electrodes cannot be placed on open wounds, surgical sutures or certain dermatological conditions

Possible side effects
These may result from too high an intensity, too early or too long an application, or inadequate skin care, and include:

- dryness of skin leading to mycosis
- electrical burns (rare with modern stimulators)
- rupture of the repaired tendon by using the incorrect intensity or too early an application
- fracture displacement
- tendonitis, particularly 'tennis elbow' after extensive extensor muscle stimulation to loosen adhesions.

Conclusion
After trauma or surgery, a patient may be locked into a vicious circle of pain, oedema, inflammation and reduced active mobilization. These phenomena, when combined with therapeutic immobilization, can lead to progressive stiffness and cortical exclusion. Electroactive exercise, by adding electrical stimulation synchronized with the patient's voluntary contraction, is one of the most efficient treatments to help a patient break this vicious circle. Mobilization produced by electrical stimulation is justified in many clinical conditions.

Electroactive exercise should be used as soon as the therapist realizes that the patient's active mobilization is insufficient to maintain range of motion. It hastens recovery time in many clinical conditions, and has improved cases that had not been helped by months of conventional hand therapy.

REFERENCES

Barclay, V., Collier, R. J. and Jones, A. (1983). Treatment of various hand injuries by pulsed electromagnetic energy (diapulse). *J. Phys. Ther.*, **69**, 9.
Campbell, D. A. and Kay, S. P. (1998). What is cold intolerance? *J. Hand Surg.*, **23B (1)**, 3–5.

Cannon, N. M. and Taylor Mullins, P. (1984). Use of electrical currents for therapeutic purposes. In: *Manual on Management of Specific Hand Problems*, pp. 79–84. American Rehabilitation Educational Network.

De Soras, T. D., Guinard, D., Guinard, D. *et al.* (1994). Utilisation d'une electrode implantable pour la reeducation des tenolyses des tendons flechisseurs. *Ann. Chir. Main*, **13(5)**, 317–27.

Dyson, M. and Suckling, J. (1978). Stimulation of tissue repair by ultrasound – a survey of the mechanisms involved. *J. Phys. Ther.*, **64**, 4.

Evans, P. (1980). The healing process at cellular level: a review. *J. Phys. Ther.*, **66**, 8.

Gracanin, F. (1972). *The Use of Functional Stimulation in the Rehabilitation of Hemiplegic Patients*. The Institute of S. R. Slovenia for Rehabilitation of the Disabled.

Johnson, C. L. (1984). Physical therapists as scar modifiers. *J. Phys. Ther.*, **64**, 9.

Kennedy, S. M., Peck, F. H. and Stone, J. T. H. (1998). The treatment of interphalangeal joint flexion contractures with reinforced Lycra fingersleeves. *J. Hand Ther.*

Kesson, M. and Atkins, E. (1998). *Orthopaedic Medicine: A Practical Approach*, pp. 52–62. Butterworth–Heinemann.

Kidd, G., Musa, I. and Lawes, N. (1992). *Understanding Neuromuscular Plasticity*. Churchill Livingstone.

Kielhofner, G. C. (1993). Occupation as the major activity of humans. In: *Willard and Spackman's Occupational Therapy* (Hopkins and Smith, eds), p. 138. J.B. Lippincott & Co.

Kleinert, H. E., Kutz, J. E., Atasoy, E. and Stormo, A. (1973). Primary repair of flexor tendon. *Orth. Cl. N. America*, **4(4)**, 865–77.

Kots, J. M. and Xvilon, V. A. (1977). Notes from Dr Kots' (USSR) lectures and laboratory periods, Canadian–Soviet Exchange Symposium on Electrostimulation of Skeletal Muscles, Concordia University, Dec 6–15. English translation by Dr Balkin and N. Timtsenko.

Liberson, W. T. (1961). Stimulation of the peroneal nerve synchronized with the swing phase of gait of hemiplegic patients. *Arch. Phys. Med. Rehabil.*, **42**, 101–5.

Macdonald, R. (1992). *Taping Techniques: Principles and Practice*. Butterworth-Heinemann.

Maslow, A. (1970). *Motivation and Personality*, 2nd edn, p. 44. Harper and Row.

Merletti, R. *et al.* (1978). Mid- and long-term variations of gross muscle force due to functional electrical stimulation in hemiplegic patients. In: *Proceedings of the Sixth International Symposium on the External Control of Human Extremities*, Dubrovnik, Yugoslavia.

Moutet, F. *et al.* (1988). *Rééducation et Appareillage de la Main Traumatique*. Masson Ed.

Otthiers, J. (1998). The technique of suction – varying experiences of application. *Br. J. Hand Ther.*, **3(3)**, 10–11.

Rancho los Amigos (1980). *Functional Electrical Stimulation: A Practical, Clinical Guide*, 2nd edn. Rehabilitation Engineering Center, Downey, California.

Sherrington, C. S. (1961). *The Integrative Action of the Nervous System*. Yale University.

Taub, A. and Kane, K. (1975). History of local analgesia. *Pain*, **1**, 125–38.

Thomas, D. (1987). L'apport de la stimulation electrique dans la reeducation de la main traumatique. In: *Les Plaies de la Main* (Y. Allieu, ed.), pp. 115–19. Sauramps Medical.

Thomas, D. (1996). Electrostimulation des muscles fléchisseurs des doigts et du poignet. Proposition d'une nouvelle cartographie. *Cah. Kinesither.*, **178(2)**, 37–42.

Thomas, D. and Frere, G. (1979). Le point sur l'electrostimulation selective dans la rééducation de la main traumatique innervee. *Cah. Kinesither.*, **76**, 45–62.

Thomas, D., Moutet, F. and Bellon Champel, P. (1993). L'interet de l'implantation d'une electrode percutanee dans la rééducation des tenolyses. *Ann. Kinesither.*, **20(8)**, 419–24.

Voss, D. E., Ionta, M. K. and Myers, B. J. (1985). *Proprioceptive Muscular Facilitation*. Harper and Row.

FURTHER READING

American Society for Surgery of the Hand. (1990). The role of hand therapy. *The Hand*, 151–163. Churchill Livingstone.

Barr, N. and Swan, D. (1988). *The Hand: Principles and Techniques of Splintmaking*. Butterworths.

Boscheinen-Morrin, J., Davey, V. and Conolly, W. B. (1992). Introduction. In: *The Hand: Fundamentals of Therapy*, pp. 1–11. Butterworth Heinemann.

Brand, P. and Hollister, A. (1992). *Clinical Mechanics of the Hand*. Mosby Year Book.

Collins, D. C. and Schwarze, L. (1991). Early progressive resistance following immobilisation of flexor tendon repairs. *J. Hand Ther.*, **4(3)**, 111–16.

Duchenne De Boulogne, G. B.(1867). *Physiologie des Mouvements*. Bailliere et fils.

FES (1998). *FES Update*, **8(1)**. FES Information Center.

Functional Electrical Stimulation of Extremities (1983). Josef Stefan Institute, Ljubljana, Yugoslavia.

Golledge, J. (1998). Distinguishing between occupation, purposeful activity and activity. Part 1: Review and explanation. *Br. J. Occ. Ther.*, **61(4)**, 100–105.

Golledge, J. (1998). Distinguishing between occupation, purposeful activity and activity, and activity. Part 2: Why is the distinction important? *Br. J. Occ. Ther.*, **61(4)**, 157–160.

Hagedorn, R (1992). *Occupational Therapy: Foundations for Practice*. Churchill Livingstone.

Horowitz, M., Wilner, N. and Alvarez ,W. (1979). Impact of event scale: a measure of subjective stress. *Psychosom. Med.*, **41(3)**, 209–18.

Licht, E. (1967). *Therapeutic Electricity and Ultraviolet Radiation*. Newhaven.

Levine, M. G., Kabat, H. *et al.* (1954). Relaxation of spasticity by physiological techniques. *Arch. Phys. Med. Rehabil.*, **35**, 214–23

Low, J. and Reed, A. (1990). *Electrotherapy Explained*, pp. 73–91. Heinemann Medical.

Mills, D. and Fraser, C. (1989). *Therapeutic Activities for the Upper Limb*. Winslow Press.

Nicholas, J. S. (1977). The swollen hand. *Physiotherapy*, **69(12)**, 285–6.

Problem Orientated Medical Records: Guidelines for Therapists (1988). Kings Fund Centre.

Rancho Los Amigos (1971). *Task Nos 1–3, Contracture Prevention, Annual Reports of Progress*. Rehabilitation Engineering Center, Downey, California.

Reid, D. C. (1992). *Sports Injury: Assessment and Rehabilitation*. Churchill Livingstone.

Roberts, M., Rutherford, J. H. and Harris, D. (1982). The effect of ultrasound on flexor tendon repairs in the rabbit. *The Hand*, **14**, 1.

Salter, M. (1987). *Hand Injuries: A Therapeutic Approach.* Churchill Livingstone.

Smith, B., Peckham, H. and Keith, W. (1987). An externally powered, multichannel, implantable stimulator for versatile control of paralyzed muscles. *IEEE Trans. Biomed. Eng.*, BME-34.

Sorensen, M. K. (1989). The edematous hand. *J. Phys. Ther.*, **69,** 12.

Stanley, B. G. and Tribuzi, S. M. (1992). *Concepts in Hand Rehabilitation.* F. A. Davis Co.

Strickland, W. J. (1989). Biological rationale, clinical application and results of early motion following flexor tendonrepair. *J. Hand Ther.*, **2(2)**, 71–82.

Vodovnik, L. (1971). Information processing in the central nervous system during functional electric stimulation. *Med. Biol. Eng.*, **9,** 675–82.

Watkins, A. W. (1972). *A Manual of Electrotherapy,* 3rd edn. Lea & Febinger.

Wilson, D. H. and Jagerdeesh, P. (1976). Experimental regeneration in peripheral nerves and the spinal cord in laboratory animals exposed to a pulsed electromagnetic field. *Paraplegia.*

Woods, Z. and Withrington, R. H. (1992). Continuous passive motion as a treatment modality in reflex sympathetic dystrophy. Proceedings from the British Society for Surgery of the Hand.

Zigmund, A. S. and Snaith, R. P. (1983). The Hospital Anxiety and Depression Scale (HAD). *Acta Psychiatr. Scand.*, **67,** 361–70.

6 Principles of joint mobilization

Sheila Crowley

Biomechanics is by definition the mechanics of movements in living bodies. This chapter will examine one aspect of biomechanics, namely arthrokinematics – the intimate mechanics of the joints.

Normal movement requires integrity of the joint surfaces, ligaments, muscle continuity and the nerve supply to these structures and the skin. The dynamics of a joint depend on the physical configuration of the joint surfaces, the architecture of the ligaments and their attachments. On close examination, it can be seen that the articular surfaces of synovial joints are never truly flat or truly spherical.

Most synovial joints can be classified either ovoid (egg-shaped) or sellar (saddle-shaped). In an ovoid joint, one articular surface is biconcave and the other is biconvex. In sellar joints, each articular surface is concave in one plane and convex in another plane, usually at approximately right angles (concavo-convex).

MOVEMENTS

When considering the movement between joint surfaces, it is seen that any changing relationship between the two can be analysed into three basic components: slide, roll and spin (Williams, 1995). Assuming that one surface is stationary whilst the other moves:

- slide is a translatory movement (Figure 6.1)
- roll is a rolling movement of the long bone (Figure 6.2), and is a physiological movement
- spin is a pure rotatory movement (Figure 6.3), i.e. adjunct or conjunct rotation.

Slide, roll and spin are combined in most physiological movements and, for therapeutic purposes, slide together occasionally with spin are the components that can be called accessory movements.

Maitland (1991) defines accessory movements as 'movements that a person cannot perform himself but which can be performed on him by someone else'. Take, for example, flexion of the proximal phalanx at the metacarpophalangeal (MCP) joint. Note how the head of the metacarpal is exposed as the proximal phalanx moves from extension to flexion.

An individual cannot perform this pure postero-anterior glide of the base of the proximal phalanx in isolation, but an operator could do so. Therefore, the glide is an accessory movement.

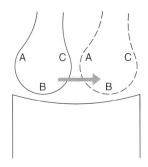

Figure 6.1 Slide is a translatory movement.

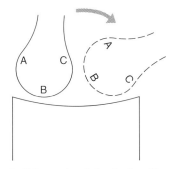

Figure 6.2 Roll is a physiological rolling movement of a long bone.

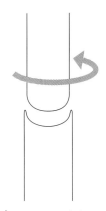

Figure 6.3 Spin is a pure rotatory movement.

1. When a convex surface is moving on a fixed concave surface, the accessory movement occurs in the opposite direction to the physiological movement and is called roll (Figure 6.4)
2. When a concave surface is moving on a fixed convex surface, the accessory movement occurs in the same direction as the physiological movement (Figure 6.5).

Because the joints are ovoid in cross-section there is no single axis of movement but several, giving a moving axis of rotation (Figure 6.6). In clinical practice it is difficult to make a lively splint completely mimic normal movement unless it has a moving axis at its motion point.

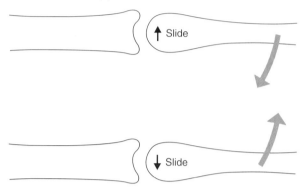

Figure 6.4 When a convex surface moves on a fixed concave surface, the accessory movement is in the opposite direction to the physiological movement.

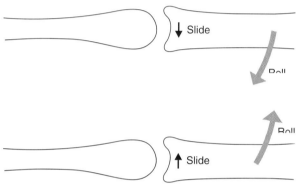

Figure 6.5 When a concave surface is moving on a fixed convex surface, the accessory movement occurs in the same direction as the physiological movement.

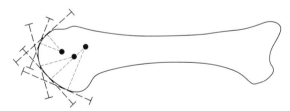

Figure 6.6 A moving axis of rotation (with permission from the *J. of Physiotherapy*).

The course of a joint's motion will also be determined by both the shape of the ligaments, whether a narrow band or fan-shaped, and where they attach on the adjacent bones.

JOINT DYNAMICS

Muscle action, the force of gravity and other external influences must all be considered when examining the dynamics of the joint.

Adjunct rotation describes a movement around a longitudinal axis that can sometimes be performed as an active movement independent of other physiological movements, e.g. medial and lateral

rotation at the glenohumeral joint. Conjunct rotation always accompanies another main movement, and occurs as an inevitable consequence of the joint mechanics – the bony profile and the position and shape of the ligaments – e.g. opposition at the carpometacarpal joint.

For many joints the opposing articular surfaces are of different sizes, and in this situation the combination of slide and roll helps to increase the overall range of movement available. It also means that the two joint surfaces only fit fully in one position, the 'close-packed' position of the joint first described by MacConaill in 1964.

In the close-packed joint position:

- the articular surfaces are maximally congruent
- the joint surfaces are compressed
- parts of the fibrous capsule and ligaments are maximally spiralized and taut
- no further physiological movement is possible
- accessory movement is minimal or nil
- when weight bearing, this position minimizes the muscular effort required to sustain the posture (Williams, 1995).

In all other positions the joint is in the loose-packed position, i.e.:

- the articular surfaces are not maximally congruent
- the joint space is larger
- all or part of the joint capsule and ligaments are lax
- this position allows maximal freedom of accessory movement.

For the hand, the close-packed positions are:

- radioulnar – semi-pronation
- wrist – extension
- metacarpophalangeal (MCP) joints two to five – full flexion
- interphalangeal joints (IP) – extension
- first carpometacarpal joint (CMC) – full opposition.

NB: It is worth noting that the close-packed joint position of MCP flexion with IP extension is the shortened position of the intrinsic muscles.

For the hand, the loose-packed positions are:

- radioulnar – supination
- wrist – semiflexion
- MCPs two to five – semiflexion and ulnar deviation
- IPs – semiflexion
- first CMC – neutral position of thumb.

Therapeutic considerations

Considerations of the close- and loose-packed positions of joints are:

1. When close-packed, all the available slack in the ligaments has been taken up. If the joint sustains trauma in this position, enormous stresses may be generated and the articular structures and ligaments are more liable to injury. It is important to try and ascertain the exact injuring mechanism and thus gain some idea of the degree of tissue damage and in which anatomical structures it has occurred.
2. In the presence of severe oedema, the joints are compelled to assume the loose-packed position and will not be able to move towards the close-packed position until some of the oedema subsides. Forcing the movement at this stage towards the close-packed position will cause pain, an increased stretch to the capsule and possibly cartilage damage.
3. Any essential immobilization of joints should be approaching the close-packed position in order to prevent shortening of the ligaments and capsule (this is usually referred to as the position of safe immobilization). The hand should rarely be immobilized in the extended position, and never in the fully flexed or claw position.

   Occasionally the position of function with a small amount of IP flexion may be considered more desirable, for example when gross oedema is present, or when it is extremely unlikely that complete full range will be regained. The position of function is with the MCP joints in 45° of flexion, the PIP joints in 30° and the DIP joints in 10° of flexion. This immobilization should be interrupted daily, if at all possible, for active or passive movement.
4. When examining a joint, nearly all the ligaments and parts of the articular surface will be put under increased tension as the close-packed position is approached. Normal stress on normal tissue should not be painful, but normal stress on already abnormally tensioned and inflamed tissues could elicit pain.
5. When assessing for ligamentous damage, the test is initially performed with the joint about 10–15° from the close-packed position. Joint laxity, when present in the close-packed position, indicates the partial or complete disruption of one or more ligaments.

THE WRIST COMPLEX

The distal radioulnar, radiocarpal and midcarpal joints will be considered here as the wrist complex.

The distal radioulnar joint

This is a triaxial ellipsoid joint. The joint surfaces are the biconcave ulnar notch of the radius with the biconvex ulnar head, and distally the ulnar head with the triangular fibrocartilage complex (TFCC –

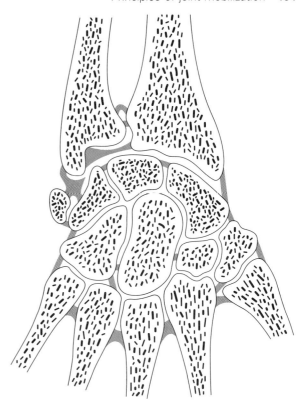

Figure 6.7 The wrist complex showing the triangular fibrocartilage.

see below; Palmer and Werner, 1984). The TFCC provides necessary stability for the distal radioulnar joint (Figure 6.7).

At the distal radioulnar joint, active forearm rotation of 140–150° occurs as the lower end of the radius and its disc slide over the ulnar head. Small movements of the ulna also occur – the ulna slides posteriorly and laterally during pronation, and anteriorly and medially during supination.

Accessory movements

These include: posteroanterior and anteroposterior movement of the head of the ulna on the radius; longitudinal movement of the radius on the ulna, either cephalad or caudad, usually by respective passive radial or ulnar deviation of the hand; and compression (i.e. squeezing the radius and ulna together) and, conversely, distraction (Maitland, 1991).

The radiocarpal joint

This is a triaxial joint. The distal end of the radius is divided by a low ridge into two biconcavities, and this articular surface continues as a triangular disc that runs from the medial border of the radius to the ulnar styloid process. The proximal surfaces of the scaphoid, lunate and triquetral and their interosseous ligaments form the reciprocal biconvexity. The two concavities of the distal end of the radius correspond to the biconvexities of the scaphoid laterally and the lunate medially (Figure 6.7).

Palmer and Werner (1981) proposed that the triangular fibrocartilage is not a discrete entity but is continuous with the dorsal and palmar radio-ulnar ligaments, the ulnar collateral ligament, the ulnar meniscus, the articular disc and the sheath of extensor carpi ulnaris. They named this unit the triangular fibrocartilage complex of the wrist. Increased movement will be possible due to the mobility of this articular disc.

Movements at the radiocarpal joint will be the same as for all ellipsoid joints: during wrist flexion there will be a posterior glide of the proximal carpal bones; during wrist extension there will be anterior glide of these bones (Figure 6.8); and rotation occurs and may be termed supination and pronation.

Accessory movements

These include anteroposterior, posteroanterior and transverse movements of the carpus on the radius, plus compression and distraction.

The midcarpal joint

This joint lies between the two rows of carpal bones. The proximal row comprises the scaphoid, lunate and triquetral, and the distal row the trapezium, trapezoid, capitate and hamate. Several authors (Kapandji, 1982; Williams and Warwick, 1989) consider the medial and lateral components separately as follows:

1. In the medial component the triquetral, lunate, and scaphoid articulate with the hamate and capitate, forming a U-shaped medial articulation with biconcave/biconvex articular surfaces.

2. In the lateral component the scaphoid articulates with the trapezium and trapezoid to form transverse lateral articulations with biconcave/biconvex articular surfaces. The axis of flexion/extension of the lateral joint is more distal than the axis for the U-shaped joint.

According to Palmer and Werner (1984):

> The radius through its articulation with the lateral carpus carries approximately 80 per cent of the axial load of the forearm and the ulna, through its articulation with the medial carpus and the TFCC, 20 per cent.

Some argue, however, that the majority of the weight is transferred via the ulna to the 'heel' of the hand and the medial carpus.

Movements at the radiocarpal and midcarpal joints

All the movements of flexion, extension, abduction and adduction involve the radiocarpal and midcarpal joints to some extent, and the total range of each physiological movement is greater than the sum of the individual joint movements. With such complexity, it is no wonder that many theories of precise action abound.

In general terms, the carpus moving on the radius and radioulnar disc is a convex surface moving on a concave surface (Figure 6.9). The *accessory* movements therefore occur in the opposite direction to the physiological movements.

For the purpose of analysis the following sequence is presented, but it should be remembered that there are simultaneous interactions among the carpal bones. The proximal carpal row (except the pisiform – see later) does not have any muscles acting directly on it, unlike the distal row; thus when moving from full flexion to full extension the movement is initiated at the distal row. The hamate, capitate and trapezoid, as the distal row, move on

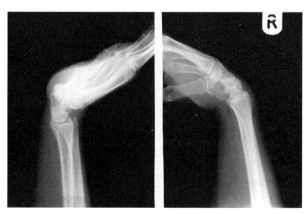

Figure 6.8 X-rays of the radiocarpal and midcarpal joints in extension and flexion.

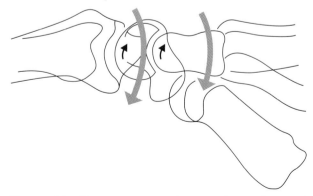

Figure 6.9 The carpus moving on the radius and radioulnar disc is a convex surface moving on a concave surface (from P. Evans, with permission from the *J. of Physiotherapy*).

the proximal row until the hand is in line with the forearm (i.e. neutral).

At this point, due to the ligaments tightening between scaphoid and lunate, the scaphoid approaches the close-packed position with the distal carpus. This unit then moves on the triquetrum and lunate. Finally, at approximately 40° extension, the majority of the carpus becomes close-packed and moves on the radius and radioulnar disc. Note that the scaphoid initially acts with the proximal row before becoming close-packed with the distal row of the carpus (Williams and Warwick, 1989; Norkin and Levangie, 1992).

The trapezioscaphoid joint is not included in the close packing of the carpus as described above. The thumb remains free to move independently even when the wrist is close-packed, which is very important functionally.

In abduction (radial deviation), the distal row moves radially on the proximal row until they are close-packed and move together as a unit on the radius and radioulnar disc. In adduction (ulnar deviation) there is a similar mechanism, but the movement is considered to be mainly radiocarpal (Williams and Warwick, 1989).

The greatest range of radial and ulnar deviation occurs in neutral flexion and extension of the wrist. Contributions to supination and pronation occur at both carpal and midcarpal joints, and this movement is adjunct rotation or 'spin'.

Accessory movements
In the loose-packed position, each of the carpal bones can be passively moved on its neighbour by the physiotherapist (Kaltenborn, 1980).

Pisitriquetral joint

This joint should not be forgotten since, among other considerations, it lies very close to the ulnar nerve as the latter enters the hand. The pisiform does not contribute to the radiocarpal movements described above. As a sesamoid bone, it acts to increase the leverage of flexor carpi ulnaris.

Accessory movements
The pisiform can be passively moved medially, laterally, cephalad and caudad with spin. It can also be compressed against the triquetral.

Intercarpal joints

This concatenation of joints has an important role in the function of the hand. For example, unless there are full physiological and slide/glide movements at the articular interfaces, the cupping of the palm and the ability to mould to differently shaped objects may be impaired. Similarly and

conversely, weight bearing on the heel of the hand could be abnormal if the relevant intercarpal movements are hypomobile.

Some of these intercarpal joints have been described above as components of the total radiocarpal and midcarpal areas, and of the base of the thumb. The following is a summary of the type of joints between the individual carpal bones

Scaphoid with	• trapezium • trapezoid • lunate • capitate	All these are ellipsoid joints
Lunate with	• scaphoid • triquetral • capitate	All these are ellipsoid joints
Trapezoid with	• trapezium • capitate	Sellar/saddle joint Ellipsoid joint
Capitate with	• trapezoid • hamate	Both these are ellipsoid joints
Triquetrum with	• lunate • pisiform • hamate	Ellipsoid joint Ellipsoid joint Sellar joint
Hamate with	• capitate • triquetrum	Ellipsoid joint Sellar joint

Carpometacarpal joints two to five

The second, third and fourth CMC joints are classed as plane joints, but on inspection are seen to be saddle-shaped. The movements are minimal flexion and extension and some spin.

The second and third CMCs are virtually immobile, and provide stability to the central hand.

The fifth CMC joint is a saddle joint and has triaxial movements – physiological flexion and extension, spin, and a small amount of physiological adduction and abduction. It has up to 20° of flexion and adduction – most important when gripping.

NB: Clinically, great care must be taken to maintain the movements of this fifth CMC joint.

Accessory movements
These are small anteroposterior and posteroanterior glides and spin.

Intermetacarpal joints

The second to fifth intermetacarpal bases and heads each articulate with those of the adjacent metacarpals. The articular surfaces for these joints appear to be biconcave/biconvex, and movement is limited mainly by the dorsal and palmar ligaments.

The intermetacarpal and CMC joints together allow cupping of the palm, and permit the palm to conform effectively to the shape of objects.

Accessory movements
These are anteroposterior and posteroanterior glides plus spin.

Metacarpophalangeal joints two to five

The head of the metacarpal is biconvex and broader anteriorly than posteriorly. The base of the proximal phalanx is much smaller by comparison, and is biconcave. This disparity in surface area allows a greater freedom of movement than would be possible if the joints had equal surface areas. However, freedom of movement often occurs at the expense of stability, and to counteract this the MCPs are each enhanced by a volar plate and collateral ligaments.

Each volar plate is made of fibrocartilage, and is attached to the base of the phalanx by a small fibrous band which acts like a hinge (Kapandji, 1982). The plates also have ligamentous attachments to the bases of the phalanges and to the collateral ligaments. On the palmar aspect they are blended with the deep transverse palmar ligament. The latter is grooved by flexor tendons and converted into a tunnel by the retinaculum.

The collateral ligaments are strong round cords from the lateral sides of the metacarpal, running obliquely to the proximal phalanx. They are under most tension in flexion, as the phalanx engages with the wider anterior aspect of the metacarpal head.

The ulnar side of the metacarpal head is also slightly larger than the radial side, and thus the fingertips move towards the scaphoid on full flexion.

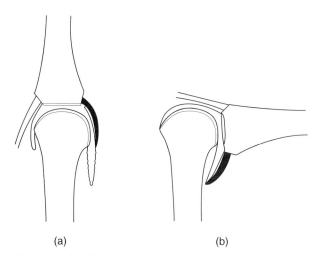

Figure 6.10 Volar plate (a) in extension, when it articulates with the metacarpal head; (b) in flexion, when it lies alongside the metacarpal neck.

In extension the volar plate articulates with the head of the metacarpal (Figure 6.10a), providing anterior joint stability and helping to restrict hyperextension. In flexion the volar plate slides over the metacarpal head until, when fully flexed, it lies alongside the neck of the metacarpal (Figure 6.10b).

This unique mechanism allows a far greater range of flexion than would be possible if the bony surfaces were of equal size.

Flexion varies from approximately 90° in the index finger to approximately 110° in the little finger. The posterior aspect of the metacarpal head is partly cartilage covered, and allows hyperextension of all the fingers. Abduction and adduction are greatest in MCP extension, i.e. when loose-packed, and virtually nil in MCP flexion, i.e., when close-packed.

Accessory movements
Anteroposterior, posteroanterior, and medial and lateral transverse glides are possible. In addition, the physiotherapist can medially and laterally rotate (i.e. spin the phalanx on the metacarpal) and distract and compress the joint.

The proximal interphalangeal (PIP) and distal interphalangeal (DIP) joints

These are saddle/sellar joints between the phalanges, with the proximal articular surfaces being convex and larger than the distal concave components. They each have a volar plate similar in construction and function to that of the MCPs, and also collateral ligaments that reinforce the joint capsule.

The proximal interphalangeal joints have minimal hyperextension, and the volar plate is liable to damage in an extension forcing injury. Flexion at the PIP is about 100–110°, being greatest on the ulnar side of the hand. The distal interphalangeal joints have a certain degree of passive hyperextension and flexion of approximately 70–90°.

Accessory movements
These are anteroposterior, posteroanterior, medial and lateral transverse glides, medial and lateral rotation, traction and compression.

The combined flexion of MCP, PIP and DIP joints
Movement is greatest in the little and ring fingers, and this is one of the reasons why the ulnar side of the hand is so powerful, even when holding small objects. Any loss of these combined flexion movements of the little finger usually results in a weaker hand.

NB: Clinically, if it is essential that the hand must be immobilized, great care must be taken to preserve these movements together with the full range of fifth CMC flexion and adduction.

THE THUMB

First carpometacarpal joint

This is a superb example of a saddle joint, both articular surfaces being clearly concavo-convex. The joint capsule is lax, allowing a wide excursion of movement, and the capsule is reinforced by two collateral ligaments, the anterior and posterior ligaments. The trapezium can be likened to the saddle on a horse and the metacarpal to the person seated in the saddle (Figure 6.11).

First CMC flexion and extension is similar to the person moving from stirrup to stirrup, i.e. concave on convex. First CMC abduction and adduction is similar to the person sliding toward the front and back of the saddle, i.e. convex on concave.

Flexion and extension occur parallel to the palm of the hand, and abduction and adduction at right angles to this. As flexion occurs there is medial (conjunct) rotation of the metacarpal. This is due to the shape of the joint surfaces and a tightening of the dorsal ligament, which fixes the ulnar side of the metacarpal but not the radial side. Extension is accompanied by lateral (conjunct) rotation.

A short, strong intermetacarpal ligament spans the bases of first and second metacarpals and checks palmar abduction (Kapandji, 1982).

Opposition brings the pulp of thumb towards the pulp of the fingers. It combines the movements of abduction, flexion and the accompanying medial rotation. Three of the four intrinsic muscles of the thumb (the opponens pollicis, abductor pollicis brevis and flexor pollicis brevis) contract together in varying degrees together with the extrinsic muscles to produce the movement of opposition. The fourth intrinsic (adductor pollicis) will also contract to produce strong pinch grip with opposition.

Medial and lateral rotation occur when an object is rolled between the thumb and an opposing finger. Here, at the first CMC joint, medial and lateral rotation occur with flexion and extension respectively.

In median nerve lesions at the wrist, the subtle movement of thumb opposition (especially medial rotation) will be lost due to the extrinsic muscle action being unopposed by the paralysed intrinsic muscles.

Muscle testing note: Opponens pollicis should be tested, by palpation and the observation of rotation, when opposing the thumb to the index finger. The conjunct rotation at the CMC joint automatically rotates the thumb medially when it opposes to the little finger.

Accessory movements

These are anteroposterior and posteroanterior, transverse movement medially and laterally, longitudinal movement caudad and cephalad, and medial and lateral rotation of the metacarpal on the trapezium.

MCP joint of the thumb

This joint is very similar to that of the fingers, with a joint capsule, volar plate and collateral ligaments. However, the articular surface of the metacarpal head is smaller, and consequently the movements available are less. It is reinforced by two cartilage-covered sesamoid bones on its volar surface – these can be considered to be an extension of the volar plate (Kapandji, 1982). They have ligamentous ties to each other and to the collateral ligaments.

The sesamoids also increase the leverage actions of the flexor pollicis brevis and adductor pollicis. Flexion is 45–50°, and there is very little hyperextension compared with the fingers. MCP abduction and adduction is extremely limited, and the ulnar side of the joint is most susceptible to trauma.

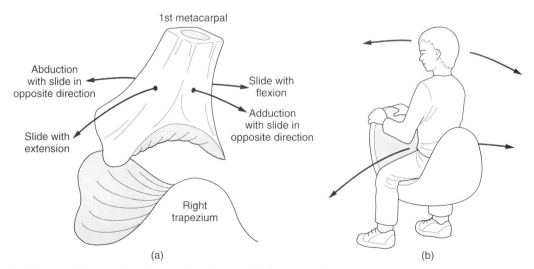

1st metacarpal

Abduction with slide in opposite direction

Slide with flexion

Adduction with slide in opposite direction

Slide with extension

Right trapezium

(a)

(b)

Figure 6.11 The saddle, or sellar, joint of the thumb (with permission from the *J. of Physiotherapy*).

Accessory movements

These are anteroposterior, posteroanterior, medial and lateral transverse glide, medial and lateral rotation, and longitudinal movement cephalad and caudad.

The IP joint of the thumb

The one IP joint of the thumb is virtually identical to those of the fingers.

ASSESSMENT AND TREATMENT CONSIDERATIONS

The following points should be considered with the assessment described in Chapter 2 and treatments in Chapter 5.

The healing time-scale

Injury of the soft tissues inevitably results in cellular damage. The enzymes released from the damaged cells increase the capillary permeability, which releases inflammatory exudate. Shortly after this the phagocytic cells begin the removal of dead and necrotic tissue (Figure 6.12).

Epithelial tissues such as skin and synovial membranes are capable of regeneration, and fibrous connective tissues such as ligaments and joint capsules are replaced but will lack the full properties of the original tissue.

Between 12 and 24 hours following injury, fibrocytes move towards the injury site. They multiply, and by the fifth day start to lay down fibrils of collagen. Initially the collagen fibres are laid down in a random fashion, but in this formation the repair is weak. Tension on the fibres seems to orientate them along the lines of stress, and this alignment, especially in response to gentle active movement, results in a stronger union.

Collagen is the fibrous tissue of the healed injury, which gradually shortens when it is fully formed. The contracting process occurs from the third week to the sixth month (Evans, 1980).

Nutrition of articular cartilage

Articular cartilage is avascular. Transport of nutrients occurs mainly from synovial fluid by diffusion, and this is particularly so for solutes of low molecular weight.

Experimental work by O'Hara *et al.* (1990) indicates that for solutes of higher molecular weight, cyclic loading may increase the rate at which they reach the cells. These authors also state that:

> loading can influence the production of synovial fluid and help to distribute it across the surface. Without movement and loading, pools of stagnant synovial fluid may be depleted of their supply of nutrients, and may accumulate acidic wastes such as lactate and CO_2. In this way lack of movement may cause inadequate 'nutrition' of cartilage.

Function of the hand

A full range of pain-free movement is in most circumstances the aim of treatment for all joints of the hand. Where it is clear that the hand cannot be returned to its pre-injury state, the most functional movements for that individual patient and his or her circumstances should be ascertained. This will involve a detailed discussion between the patient and therapist to determine the joint mechanics most necessary to maintain the patient's lifestyle.

Before fully mobilizing the joint it should be considered whether active control is likely to be regained or not, as a permanently flail joint could be a handicap. Passive range will need to be maintained for patients awaiting secondary reconstructive surgery such as tendon transfers. It is important to know whether any of the joints have suffered degenerative or pathological changes (however minor) before the trauma, as this may influence the choice of treatment and affect the prognosis and speed of progress.

Accessory movements

The foregoing description of the individual joints describes the main accessory movements accompanying the physiological ones. Due to the complexity of joint movement, it is important to test all the accessory movements available in different physiological starting positions and not just the ones associated with the painful and/or stiff physiological movement.

The findings of these tests will reveal where in the accessory range the pain and/or stiffness and/or muscle spasm begins, how it behaves, and which

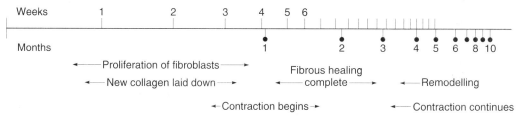

Figure 6.12 The healing process and time-scale (with permission from the *J. of Physiotherapy*).

limits the movement. It is interesting to note that in some instances an accessory glide of the distal component on the proximal may not reproduce any symptoms, but the seemingly similar accessory glide of the proximal component on the distal does so.

Comparable sign

A comparable joint sign is a specific movement that elicits the patient's symptoms. This direction can be used as a test to determine the value of the treatment technique after it has been applied.

Joint mobilization/manipulation

The subject of peripheral joint manipulation has been comprehensively discussed and practised by Maitland (1991). The Maitland concept underpins the application of passive joint mobilization techniques. Its open-minded philosophy together with the continual analytical re-evaluation of therapy makes it the ideal basis for all good clinical practice.

Maitland uses the 'two compartmental mode of thinking':

1. The theoretical compartment consists of anatomy, neurophysiology, biomedical engineering and pathology, and the diagnosis etc.
2. The clinical compartment comprises the history and behaviour of the signs and symptoms, plus any changes brought about by treatment.

The two are separated by a 'symbolic semipermeable brick wall', which allows the theoretical side to support or modify the clinical diagnosis. Where the theoretical knowledge is incomplete, it allows for incomplete clinical diagnosis (Maitland, 1991).

A positive attitude to the patient, continuing analytical assessment and reassessment are all vital and central to the concept.

Nature of the joint condition
This refers to factors that govern how the treatment is managed. The following factors must be considered:

- which tissues have been damaged
- the degree of damage
- the surgery that has been performed
- the healing achieved
- the patient's goals
- collaboration with the rehabilitation team so that maximum effect is achieved
- the presence of infection and in which tissues
- the emotional and psychological needs of the patient.

Irritability of the joint
Maitland determines irritability 'by relating the vigour of an activity that causes pain, firstly to the degree of pain that ensues and secondly to the length of time taken for this increased pain to subside to its prior level'. Thus if a simple light movement performed only once or a few times produces moderate to severe pain that continues for an hour or more, the condition is considered to be irritable.

The irritability of the condition will determine how vigorously the joint should be examined and where in the range the treatment technique should be performed.

Grades of movement
Passive movement (both physiological and accessory) is divided into four grades (Maitland, 1991):

1. Grade I – small amplitude movement performed at the beginning of the range
2. Grade II – large amplitude movement performed within the resistance-free part of the range; it may be before the onset of the symptom, up to the onset of the symptom or into a low level of the symptom
3. Grade III – large amplitude movement performed into resistance or up to the limit of the range; it will reproduce a low or high level of symptoms
4. Grade IV – small amplitude movement performed well into resistance or up to the limit of the range, reproducing some or all of the symptoms.

These gradings still apply. The treatment can be a passive physiological movement, an accessory movement, or a combination of both.

The rhythm of movement may be fast or slow, staccato or smooth. In some cases it may be advantageous to sustain the grade at a selected point. The passive movement technique may be applied with or without compression.

Joint movement may be limited by pain, stiffness, muscle spasm, or a combination of these. The joint may have a full excursion of movement, but exhibit pain, resistance or muscle spasm within or at the end of the range. It is important also to determine how each of these factors behaves and which one predominates.

Movement diagrams as described by Maitland (1991) are most helpful to clarify and record these details.

Treatment techniques

These are many and varied. The physiotherapist should apply the principles outlined above to adapt to the patient's needs.

Treatment by passive movement needs a detailed initial assessment to establish, amongst other things, the stage and stability of the disorder. Then at each treatment the effect of each technique is assessed before, during and after the application.

The physiotherapist may need to modify the grade, the position in range, the rhythm etc. to obtain the optimum effect.

Further assessment takes place from treatment to treatment, and retrospectively over the course of treatment. Treatment will mainly be directed to relieve pain or stiffness, or a combination of both. General points only will be discussed.

Joint dysfunction due to pain only
Great care must be taken for patients with pain. The treatment technique is performed in the painless part of the range when the condition is irritable.

Accessory movements are the treatment of choice when the joint has high irritability, pain early in the range, and pain that quickly increases. The joint should be positioned in a pain-free position (or as near as possible), which is usually the joint's neutral position. In these cases, by necessity the treatment will be of a smaller amplitude and the number of oscillations performed also small – i.e. ½–2 minutes in total.

On testing, improvement may be noted by any of the following:

- the pain starting at the same point in the range but rising more slowly
- the pain starting later in the range though the limit is the same
- the pain allowing a further range of movement (Maitland, 1991).

In between the treatments, improvement may be evident as:

- pain of the same frequency but less severe
- pain of the same intensity but occurring less frequently
- better still, a combination of these.

With this improvement an increased amplitude of movement is possible, the larger amplitudes being the most effective in treating pain. When the total range is almost regained (i.e. greater than 75 per cent of the normal for that individual), the treatment techniques can be taken towards the limit of the range.

For the larger joints, when the active range increases beyond 60 per cent the physiotherapist can, with careful continuous assessment, change from an accessory to a physiological movement.

Joint dysfunction due to stiffness only
Painless stiff joints need to be mobilized at the limit of the available range in all directions. Small amplitude accessory movements performed at the limit of the physiological range are the most useful. Physiological movements can also be used especially for the larger joints. A sustained period of the accessory movement repetition is very useful for the smaller joints of the hand. These techniques may produce soreness during the treatment, and to relieve this treatment soreness, large amplitude movements that gently approach the limit of pain are found to be most helpful.

When the joint's physiological movements are limited in opposite directions (e.g. both MCP flexion and extension), treatment should usually be towards one direction only at each session. A gain in MCP flexion by accessory movements at the limit of flexion may occasionally give a temporary small loss of extension, but the latter quickly recovers. Treating opposing directions at one treatment can have the effect of reducing the overall gain.

Treatment in the early stages should be daily, gradually reducing as the range increases or if soreness becomes excessive. Any gain in range will need to be consolidated wherever possible by active movements. If, however, active movements are not yet possible, the range may be maintained by passive movements. In both cases splints may be used to maintain the increased range, and patients should be supplied with a programme of auto-exercises.

Joint dysfunction due to pain and stiffness
The most commonly encountered group of patients has both pain and stiffness. For this group, the skill lies in deciding which is the prevailing component:

- if pain predominates, the treatment follows that described for pain
- if stiffness predominates, the treatment follows that described for stiffness
- if there is any doubt, it is advisable to treat the pain component first.

Careful recording of the techniques used enables accurate reassessment at each treatment session.

Dysfunction of the nervous system
Trauma to the hand is often accompanied by injury to other structures at the same time. For example:

- a person who falls onto the hand may injure the upper limb and neck
- a person who is pulled into a piece of machinery by the arm or hair may suffer traction injury to the upper limb, the cervical and/or thoracic spine.

Obviously, joints and muscles in these areas are susceptible to injury. Equally important is the nervous system (central and peripheral), which is a continuum of all the parts of the body. The nervous system interfaces with bony, fibro-osseous and soft tissues, and is capable of adapting to multiple combined joint movements whilst being supported by protective connective tissues. Normal movement is necessary to maintain normal impulse conduction and cytoplasmic flow within the axons (Butler, 1991), and injury, immobilization and surgery all impair this process. Some nervous system disorders may present with a less dramatic and more gradual onset – e.g. carpal tunnel syndrome.

The hand physiotherapist should also be familiar with the upper limb tension tests 1, 2a, 2b and 3, as described by Butler (1991). These tests and techniques have a place in the examination and treatment of patients both with and without trauma.

Acknowledgements

I would like to thank Philip Evans, Gregory Grieve, Jill Guymer and Margaret Youatt for valuable criticism of this chapter; Philip Evans for kindly allowing me to reproduce his drawings (Figs 6.6, 6.9, 6.11a and 6.12); and Angie Oliver for typing the scripts.

REFERENCES

Butler, D. S. (1991). *Mobilisation of the Nervous System*, 1st edn, pp. 30, 220. Churchill Livingstone.

Evans, P. J. (1980). The healing process at cellular level: a review. *Physiotherapy*, **66(8)**, 256–9.

Evans, P. J. (1988). Ligaments, joint surfaces, conjunct rotation and close-pack. *Physiotherapy*, **74(3)**, 105–14.

Kaltenborn, F. M. (1980). *Mobilisation of the Extremity Joints*. Olaf Norlic Bookhandel.

Kapandji, I. A. (1982). *The Physiology of the Joints, Vol. 1, Upper Limb*, 2nd edn. Churchill Livingstone.

MacConaill, M. A. (1964). Joint movement. *Physiotherapy*, **50(11)**, 359–67.

Maitland, G. D. (1991). *Peripheral Manipulation*, 3rd edn. Butterworths.

Norkin, C. and Levangie, P. K. (1992). *Joint Structure and Function: A Comprehensive Analysis*, 2nd edn., p. 268. F. A. Davis.

O'Hara, B. P., Urban, J. P. G. and Maroudas, A. (1990). Influence of cyclic loading on the nutrition of articular cartilage. *Ann. Rheum. Dis.*, **49**, 536–9.

Palmer, A. K. and Werner, F. W. (1981). The triangular fibrocartilage complex of the wrist – anatomy and function. *J. Hand Surg.*, **6(2)**, 153–62.

Palmer, A. K. and Werner, F. W. (1984). Biomechanics of the distal radioulnar joint. *Clin. Orth. Rel. Res.*, **187**, 26–35.

Williams, P. L. (1995). *Gray's Anatomy*, 38th edn, pp. 505–9, 651–3. Churchill Livingstone.

7 Specific conditions and injuries

Sue Boardman and Maureen Salter

The injuries and conditions mentioned in this chapter are discussed as separate lesions. However, it is highly likely that when trauma is experienced damage will occur in more than one type of tissue, and these additional factors will therefore complicate both assessment and treatment. An attempt has been made to identify the problems and outline the treatment of lesions both in isolation and collectively.

Assessments and treatments have already been discussed in detail in previous chapters. A description will be given of:

- the signs and symptoms that need assessment
- a brief outline of the treatment aims and their priorities
- a rationale of the rehabilitation of these injuries and conditions.

Tried guidelines are given for commencing treatment, but these may not always be applicable. Some surgeons may agree to earlier treatment than others, and the severity of injury and complications during both surgery and recovery will have a bearing on the most suitable day to commence therapy and the regime that is followed.

Some therapists find themselves supervising and treating patients whose surgery and early postoperative therapy has been carried out in specialized centres. In these cases, instructions on this later management must always accompany the patient. Particular queries or worries concerning the patient's treatment can nearly always be answered if a telephone call is made directly to the therapist involved.

FRACTURES

Crucial factors affecting the recovery of function are:

- the severity and position of the fracture
- the duration and position of immobilization.

A fracture into the joint is likely to limit recovery of movement and lead to arthritis in later years.

Whilst an unstable fracture may need longer immobilization or internal fixation, immobilization should be as brief as is necessary to achieve bony union and the joints should preferably be immobilized either in the 'safe' close-packed position or in the 'position of function'. If a fracture requires positioning in plaster in a non-functional position, it is better to fix it internally by operation (Semple, 1979).

The injury will be accompanied by some degree of soft tissue damage with release of fibrinogen into the surrounding tissues. It is therefore essential to reduce any oedema as quickly as possible, with the hand supported in elevation initially, to prevent permanent fibrosis from occurring.

Fractures of the wrist

These injuries occur most commonly from falling onto the outstretched hand, and fractures of the radius and ulna in adults will need up to 5 weeks' immobilization (fractures sustained in children are often of the greenstick type and need only a short period of protection – probably about 2 weeks). As it is usually more difficult to regain wrist extension than flexion, it is preferable for the wrist to be immobilized in a slightly extended position. The plaster must always permit full flexion of the metacarpophalangeal joints. This, however, may not be possible for some fractures that are unstable.

Severe crushing injuries can cause disruption of the carpus, but fractures of the carpal bones (with the exception of the scaphoid) occur infrequently. If pain continues in the area of the anatomical snuffbox although a fracture has not initially been diagnosed, the patient must be referred to an orthopaedic consultant. Not all scaphoid fractures can be seen on the first X-ray, and a further examination is therefore essential. A fracture of the proximal pole will need 3 months' immobilization due to the resulting poor circulation of this section of the bone. Occasionally it may require bone grafts and internal fixation (Figure 7.1).

Therapy involving supervision and sessions of treatment must be available until good function is achieved.

A check-up during the first few days, and preferably during the first 24 hours, will ensure that the plaster is not too tight. Any report by the patient of tingling must be investigated immediately.

Difficulty may be experienced when the patient is attempting to regain full movement of the wrist and particularly any loss of extension. This is most likely due to the fact that the small gliding movements at the intercarpal and carpometacarpal joints are responsible for a high proportion of wrist extension, and extension is a close-packed position. After immobilization, these joints are difficult to mobilize unless individual accessory movements are given. The capitate should be identified and all gliding motions given while the wrist is flexed (i.e. when it is in the loose-packed position). Therefore, careful assessment of joint range – and especially of the intercarpal joints – must be made. If the patient finds movement painful it is quite probable that the exact position of this pain can be located on

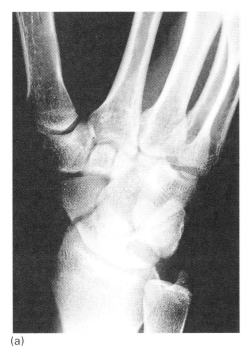

(a)

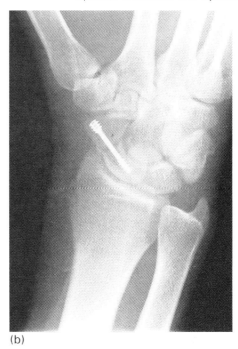

(b)

Figure 7.1 (a) Un-united scaphoid; (b) internal fixation of un-united fracture.

examination of the passive physiological and accessory movements, using Kaltenborn's 10 wrist movement plan (Kaltenborn, 1980). Gentle mobilization of the joint towards its painful range will usually, after a few sessions, totally relieve that pain, and the range of wrist movement will then automatically increase (see Chapter 6). The use of TENS can be of value in reducing pain and discomfort, allowing the mobilization techniques to be performed effectively. Active exercises and functional movements must also be given, increasing the resistance to improve power as quickly as possible. The therapist must ensure that all activities of daily living are possible and that the requirements for employment are ascertained. The patient should attend for treatment, if necessary, until it is certain that steady recovery is being made and that pain-free movement is achieved. Sessions are then reduced until treatment can cease. A review is desirable over the next few months to ensure that progress has been maintained.

During icy conditions in winter, many patients are likely to fall and sustain Colles' or Smith's fractures. This can put considerable strain on the therapy departments, and may necessitate the use of classes to ensure that some therapy is available for all. It is essential that each patient is assessed initially and that progress is re-evaluated regularly. A certain amount of group activity is excellent, but any particular problems such as persistent oedema, pain and joint stiffness must be treated individually, otherwise a satisfactory result will not be achieved.

Therapy
Early advice from a therapist at a fracture clinic can help the patient to avoid problems that might arise due to ignorance of the condition. Instruction should be given on what should and should not occur – e.g. constriction of circulation by too tight a plaster – and which exercises to carry out following injury. The patient must be taught how to exercise the proximal joints to prevent them stiffening (which can occur very quickly in the elderly) and also be shown how to exercise the fingers and thumb to maintain their mobility, if these joints are not splinted.

Patients are often confused following an accident and cannot adequately remember what they have been told to do. A written list of exercises helps to remind them once they are at home, but a check within a week as an outpatient is essential. Any oedema that may have occurred must be treated immediately, using PEME and exercises in elevation.

When the plaster is removed, a crepe bandage or Tubigrip should be applied to prevent the hand and wrist from swelling. If necessary, the arm must be supported in a high sling for the first few days.

Ice dips or contrast baths are found to be most effective in returning the circulation to normal after immobilization in plaster. Wax, which produces a vasodilatation of the capillaries, is not desirable because it tends to increase the swelling. A warm-water soak using an arm bath in which the patient actively performs hand movements is an alternative. Any dead skin can be removed after the soak, and hydrous ointment applied if necessary.

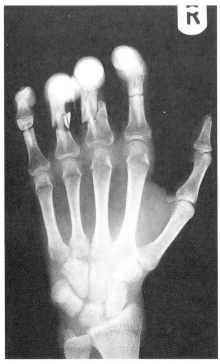

Figure 7.2 Unstable or compound fractures of the phalanges may require 3 weeks' immobilization.

Ice may also be useful for its analgesic effect prior to other treatments. If pain is a problem during mobilizing sessions, the use of TENS can be very effective and allows the range to be regained more rapidly.

Complications Complex regional pain syndrome, otherwise known as algodystrophy, post-traumatic sympathetic dystrophy (PTSD), Sudeck's atrophy or reflex sympathetic dystrophy, may occasionally result following a Colles' fracture. Immobilization with the wrist in slight extension (whenever possible), prevention of oedema and adequate instruction on the immediate use of the hand, followed by regular checks, will usually help to prevent this troublesome condition from occurring. Therapy is essential to remedy any autonomic changes that may appear. Immobilization should be for as short a time as possible if signs of dystrophy do appear, so that intensive treatment may be given.

Acute carpal tunnel syndrome may occasionally occur. Often this settles without intervention but, when severe, decompression may be necessary.

Fractures of the metacarpals and phalanges

Semple (1979) states that most fractures of the metacarpals and the distal part of the fingers heal with minimum treatment and few complications (Figure 7.2), although he indicates a problem zone consisting of the metacarpal head, proximal phalanx and base of the middle phalanx. Any fracture in this area must be diagnosed and treated by a hand specialist, otherwise deformity will occur due to the pull of muscles and tendons causing displacement at the fracture site. These fractures may need internal fixation.

A fracture of the shaft of one metacarpal will be splinted by its neighbours and usually causes few

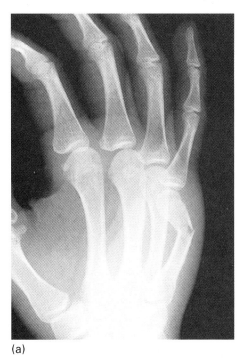

(a)

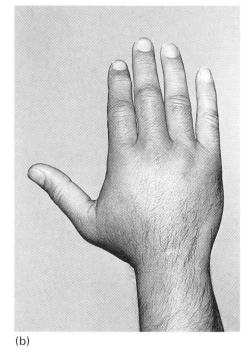

(b)

Figure 7.3 (a) Fracture of the fifth metacarpal; (b) swelling associated with metacarpal fractures.

problems. However, a fracture of the neck of the metacarpal may produce an anterior angulation, thus affecting the normal glide of the extensor mechanisms and producing joint stiffness. If the angulation is greater than 40°, the fracture is usually reduced and immobilized for 2–3 weeks using a K-wire. This type of fracture often occurs in the fifth metacarpal, and may well be a 'punching' injury (Figure 7.3).

Fractures of several of the metacarpals are likely to be accompanied by soft tissue damage and oedema with resultant stiffness of the hand. Early intensive therapy will prevent this. Occasionally the extensor tendons become bound down in the new callus and are therefore unable to glide effectively, thus preventing full extension of the fingers. Some fractures of the proximal phalanx, if not internally fixed, are easily displaced by the pull of the muscles and may therefore need careful immobilization for 2–3 weeks before active treatment commences. The immobilization of a finger in the flexed position should be avoided; full extension or very slight flexion of the interphalangeal joints with the metacarpophalangeal joints either left free or flexed in approximately 75° of flexion provides a position of function. This allows the patient to use the thumb and available fingers while in the splint and facilitates the later mobilization of the joints. Most are neighbour-strapped.

When the pain and swelling reduces, usually within 5–7 days of injury, physiotherapy for simple stable fractures of the metacarpals and phalanges can be introduced. Unstable or compound fractures and those involving dislocations may require 3 weeks' immobilization. A crepe bandage or, for the fingers, a double Tubigrip finger-stall may be useful temporarily to prevent swelling and provide a feeling of support in the early treatment stage when free active movements are given.

Mobilization of the joints by passive physiological and resisted movements can only be commenced when the fractures are united (usually after 6 weeks). Passive stretching of joints should rarely be performed when the articular structures have been involved. Active exercises, increasing the resistance gradually, will usually achieve a functional result.

DISLOCATIONS AND JOINT INJURIES

Dislocation and joint injuries are common in sport, especially in contact sports such as rugby and in 'ball' sports following failure to catch the ball correctly. The extent of ligamentous damage together with possible fracture involvement, particularly of the articular surfaces, governs the immediate treatment and length of immobilization after dislocation. An accurate diagnosis is therefore an essential requirement to ensure a good result. A simple dislocation of an interphalangeal joint, for example, which when reduced is found to be perfectly stable, will need only a short period of rest for 3–4 days followed by early mobilization. A dislocation with gross ligamentous damage, however, may need either longer immobilization in a splint or internal fixation.

A perilunate dislocation, usually caused by falling onto the hand, displaces the lunate in an anterior direction. Surgery is required to reduce and maintain the bone in correct alignment, otherwise it may press on the median nerve or cause circulatory damage. The rest of the hand must be kept mobile when the wires are removed after 3–4 weeks, and intensive treatment given.

Dislocation of all the carpometacarpal joints is rare, but if this does occur the joints may prove unstable when reduced unless pinned and immobilized for 3–4 weeks. It is extremely important during this immobilization period that the metacarpophalangeal and interphalangeal joints are exercised through as full a range as possible. If the metacarpophalangeal joints have to be immobilized they must be positioned in flexion, as it would take many weeks of intensive treatment to mobilize them if left in extension following this injury.

Dislocation of the metacarpophalangeal joints of the fingers is infrequent, but dislocation of the interphalangeal joints is common and often occurs during games such as cricket, rugby, basketball and volleyball. The joints should be examined carefully and diagnosed for bony or ligamentous damage. The possibility of a volar plate rupture should be considered, and X-rays taken to exclude its existence. Normal oblique pictures may not show a very small fragment of displaced bone, and true lateral views must therefore be taken. Preferably, both collateral ligament and volar plate damage should be repaired immediately by surgical means.

A metacarpophalangeal joint, if stable after reduction, should be rested alongside its neighbour in about 60° flexion with the interphalangeal joints in nearly full extension.

An interphalangeal joint, when stable after reduction, should be rested in nearly full extension beside its neighbours. A plaster of Paris or thermoplastic splint, made individually for two fingers and strapped on, is a more comfortable form of immobilization than a commercial splint. Three to four days' rest should be adequate for these joints before gentle active mobilization is commenced. At this stage, a double or treble finger-stall made of Lycra or double-thickness Tubigrip helps to prevent oedema, and the neighbour fingers provide lateral support during movements.

When a volar plate injury is suspected but has not been repaired, it is essential to immobilize the joint in flexion for 2–3 weeks to allow the rupture to heal. Following this, the joint should be very gradually mobilized into extension. A two-part splint of metal or thermoplastic pieces, which are

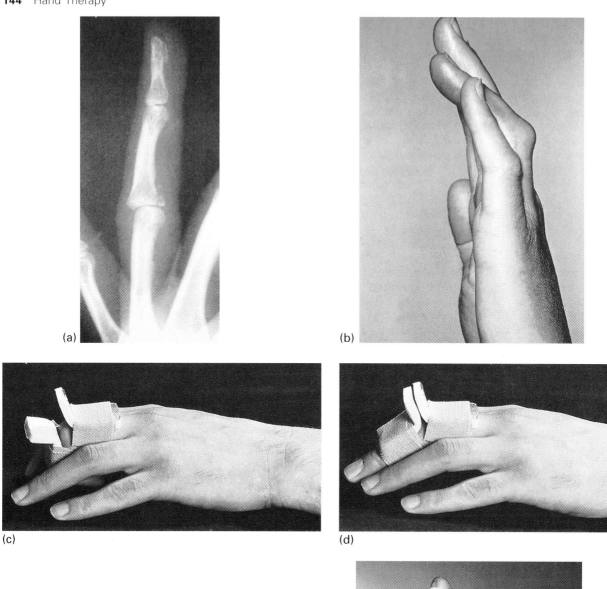

Figure 7.4 (a) Lateral X-ray showing avulsion fracture at proximal interphalangeal joint, which is often associated with a volar plate injury; (b) bruised, swollen and flexed following volar plate injury; (c) and (d) splintage for a volar plate injury; (e) Capener splint used to assist full recovery of proximal interphalangeal joint extension.

bent and fit over the dorsum of the finger, permits full active flexion of the joint but prevents full extension. The splint is easily adjusted by altering the degree of bend in the splint. If there is any residual loss of extension, which cannot be regained either by active or passive stretching, a Capener splint will usually help to stretch the contractures (Figure 7.4).

Therapy

The aims of treatment for all dislocations include:

- reduction of oedema and promotion of healing
- maintenance of those joints that are free during any immobilization period
- gentle active rehabilitation as early as possible.

Sufficient rest must be given for 3–4 days initially, in order to facilitate the process of repair. The effects of the position in which the hand and wrist are immobilized must be reviewed frequently, and the hand should be kept elevated by a sling for a few days. Ice treatment and PEME will assist in the reduction of oedema, and should be commenced immediately following injury.

After the initial rest period is over, the available joint range should be measured and monitored frequently until treatment is completed. Ice dips are found to be particularly beneficial prior to the mobilizing sessions, as they help to reduce oedema and have a slightly analgesic effect. Wax baths are not suitable because they tend to make the joint swell. Active movements given in warm but not hot water may be preferable if the patient cannot tolerate the cold.

Active (but not passive) physiological movements are commenced gradually. Resistance should be added only when:

- the range improves
- the joint is stable
- the pain allows.

Accessory movements and passive stretching are found to exacerbate both pain and swelling, and are therefore contraindicated in the early stages. Slow improvement can usually be gained in all but the most severe injuries by the gradual increase of the patient's own muscle power. The introduction of stronger functional work is therefore a normal progression.

Following fracture and joint injuries to the fingers it may be wise to strap the finger to its neighbour in order to minimize further injury, especially if the patient is taking part in sporting activities.

Thumb injuries

Fractures and dislocations of the thumb are treated similarly to those of the other digits. It is, however, worth discussing rupture of the ulnar collateral ligament of the metacarpophalangeal joint.

This injury used to be called 'gamekeeper thumb', but has been seen more frequently in recent years due to the increased popularity of skiing. It occurs when the patient catches a hand in the matting of the dry ski slope or on the ski poles. The ligament itself may be torn or may remain intact, but is pulled away at its insertion with or without a piece of bone. These injuries are treated either by immobilization in a scaphoid plaster for 4–6 weeks or, especially in the presence of an avulsion fracture, by repair and internal fixation. In cases where the thumb is extremely unstable, the metacarpophalangeal joint may have to be fused.

Without correct treatment this can be a very disabling injury, as it leaves the thumb unstable when performing the pinch or key grip.

Therapy

Active exercises of the thumb are commenced when the metacarpophalangeal joint is stable. Opposition and flexion of the joint usually return quickly, but extension and abduction, where the repaired tissues are being stretched, take longer. Careful serial splinting of the web space to regain the span may be necessary in the later stages of rehabilitation.

Support for the thumb may be required if the patient is returning to sporting activities, and strapping in the form of a thumb spica is often helpful.

TENDON INJURIES

All tendon injuries, including those with limited tendon involvement, can result in severe disability. Skin lacerations may appear very small and inconsequential on the surface, but must be examined carefully by the casualty officer to ensure a tendon injury is not overlooked.

Tendons are divided mainly as a result of lacerations from knives or glass, road accidents or severe crushing injuries and, occasionally, ruptures at the insertion. Results often depend on the type and site of injury, and the patient's compliance with rehabilitation. The final functional result is better following a clean division of one tendon only than after the involvement of several tendons and other structures, with possible haematoma formation and infection from dirty wounds combined with loss of sensation.

Flexor tendon injuries

These tendon injuries have been classified into zones by Verdan (1960); Figure 7.5):

- zone I is distal to the insertion of the superficialis and therefore affects the profundus only
- zone II (or 'no man's land'; Bunnell, 1970) is the section where the fibrous sheath is occupied by both the superficialis and profundus; this is

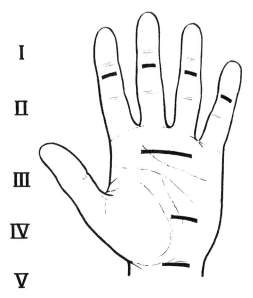

Figure 7.5 Zones for classification of flexor tendon injuries in the hand.

mainly in the finger, but is partly in the distal section of the palm also

- zone III is the palmar section where the fibrous sheath is absent
- zone IV is under the carpal tunnel
- zone V is at the wrist, proximal to the carpal tunnel, and lacerations in this area frequently sever several tendons and nerves.

Tendon repair
A primary tendon repair is performed whenever possible in order to achieve the best results. Delayed primary repair may be advisable if infection is suspected, and secondary repair may have to be undertaken either when a primary repair has failed or when there has been considerable delay between injury and surgery. In some severely traumatized hands, infection control and healing of surrounding tissue may be of prime importance before tendon surgery can be considered.

The tendon ends are located and held by transfixing needles so that the repair can be performed in the absence of tension (Smith and Boardman, 1986). The two strands of a criss-cross suture approximate and hold the ends of the tendon, while the peripheral (circumferential) suture ensures a smooth exterior to the repair. If the pulleys are damaged, an attempt should be made to repair them (to prevent later bow-stringing of the tendons).

Repair of either one or both flexor tendons in zone II, especially the repair of flexor digitorum profundus in the presence of an intact flexor digitorum superficialis, demands the best surgical expertise. In the past the results of primary suture

were poor, mainly because the suture material formed a bulky repair and this was unable to glide in the restricted space of the tendon sheath. Nowadays, with the use of the microscope together with the extremely fine suturing materials available, the improved quality of surgery fully justifies a primary repair in 'no man's land'. Kessler sutures are normally used.

Tendons receive a large part of their blood supply from the surrounding tissues and vinculae, so post-operative splinting is aimed at relieving tension to the repair site. Rest would be ideal after surgery to allow healing of the tendon, but this conflicts with the need to mobilize in order to prevent adhesions, allow the tendon to glide within its sheath and minimize joint stiffness.

Normal excursion of the flexor tendons from full finger extension to full finger flexion is approximately 5–7 cm in the profundus but slightly less in the superficialis. Flexion of the distal joint accounts for the extra excursion of the profundus, and also is responsible for the gliding that occurs between the profundus and superficialis (McGrouther and Ahmed, 1981). There is less excursion of the extensor tendons over the dorsum of the hand.

Following surgery a dorsal backslab is applied, shaped so that the wrist is held in approximately 30° flexion. The distal section of the splint should project beyond the end of the finger, and must allow the interphalangeal joints to extend fully.

Post-operative rehabilitation
The two most common post-operative regimes are:

- the early active movement regime
- the Kleinert regime.

In this and most units the early active regime is usually the regime of choice, but the Kleinert regime is still used for some zone II injuries and for patients who need extra protection.

The early active movement regime The early active movement regime is the most commonly used regime, although the Kleinert technique may still be used in zone II injuries. A dorsal backslab is used with the wrist in 30° flexion and metacarpophalangeal joints in 60–70° flexion, allowing full extension of the IP joints. The patient is instructed to:

- actively extend the fingers to the splint
- actively flex with no resistance
- passively flex fingers down to the palm.

The splint is worn continuously for 4 weeks and for protection until 8 weeks. No resistance or passive extension is allowed until the end of this period.

On the first day post-operation, with the hand in elevation, advice is given on the progression of therapy. Dressings should be removed from the palm and fingers to allow free movement.

1. From 0–4 weeks, the patient is advised not to use the hand. Exercises include:
   - passive flexion of all the fingers down to the palm
   - active flexion of the fingers towards the palm
   - active extension of the proximal interphalangeal joints with the metacarpophalangeal joints flexed at 90°
   - active extension of the fingers to the splint
   - active flexion and opposition of the thumb.
2. From 4–8 weeks, the above exercises are continued, the patient can remove the backslab for exercises, and wrist flexion and extension can commence. Light activities only may be undertaken.
3. At 8 weeks, the back slab is discarded. Passive stretching and resisted exercises may be added to the regime. Normal hand use is encouraged, but heavy lifting and contact sports must be avoided for a further 4 weeks. If contractures are a problem, static and/or dynamic splinting may be necessary at this time.

The Kleinert regime When this regime is chosen, the hand is again placed in a backslab but elastic bands are attached from the fingers to the splint (Figure 7.6). These take the place of active flexion of the fingers and reduce stress on the repaired tendon.

Following the primary suture of flexor tendons in zones I, II and III, it is safe to commence physiotherapy immediately when dynamic Kleinert splinting is used. The patient is asked to extend against the rubber band until the dorsum of the finger rests against the backslab. It may be necessary to urge the patient into this full extension, making repeated attempts until the movement is performed easily. Having achieved full extension the extensors are relaxed, thereby allowing the elastic band to flex the finger passively.

Reflex reciprocal relaxation of the flexors occurs during active extension of the fingers against resistance. Thus very little tension is applied at any time to the repaired tendon.

1. From 0–4 weeks, the elastics remain attached and the exercises undertaken are:
   - passive flexion of all the fingers down to the palm
   - active resisted extension (against the elastics) to the back of the splint, then relaxation, allowing the fingers to be brought into flexion by the elastic band
   - active extension of the proximal interphalangeal joints with the metacarpophalangeal joints flexed to 90° – this is an important exercise to try and limit flexion contractures of the interphalangeal joints, to which there is a tendency with the Kleinert regime.
2. From 4 weeks onwards, the elastics are removed and the exercise regime is the same as for the early active movement regime.

Not all surgeons, however, use this dynamic splintage method; some prefer to rest the tendon and maintain mobility by passive flexion of the finger, and only after 3 weeks is active movement introduced.

Division of several tendons in zone V at the wrist usually also involves nerves. Care has to be taken to identify the proximal and distal ends of the divided tendons for correct approximation; mistakes are not totally unknown.

Delayed primary repair may be undertaken if infection is suspected. A secondary tendon repair is the procedure performed either when a primary repair has failed or when there has been considerable delay between injury and surgery. This delay may be necessary if the surrounding tissues have been severely traumatized and become infected. Healing is essential before tendon surgery can be considered.

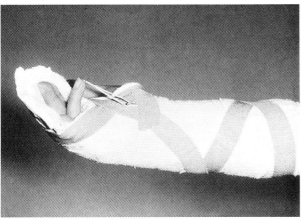
(a)
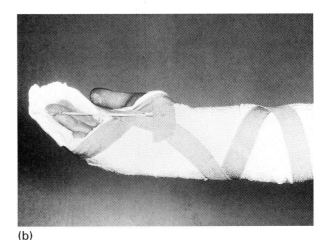
(b)

Figure 7.6 Dorsal backslab with elastic as seen in the Kleinert regime, showing the exercises.

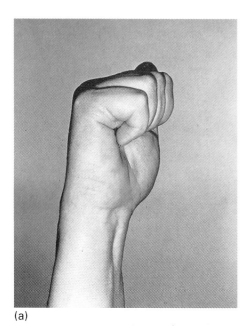

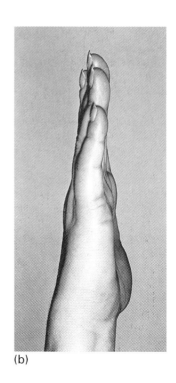

(a)   (b)

Figure 7.7 Result at 3 months post-flexor repair.

Figure 7.7 shows the results of tendon flexor repair 3 months after surgery.

Extensor tendon injuries

There are several methods of treatment following extensor tendon repair in zones I–VII (Figure 7.8). The most common are:

1. A static splint for 4 weeks and protection for a further 4 weeks
2. A dynamic extensor splint for 4 weeks and protection for a further 4 weeks (Figure 7.9)
3. A static splint for 2–3 weeks, a dynamic extension splint for the next 2–3 weeks, and protection for a further 2 weeks.

Therapy
The splintage should be checked regularly to eliminate any extensor lag. Once the period of immobilization has finished, the patient may:

- passively extend the fingers
- actively extend the fingers (or allow the splint to extend others if in a dynamic splint)
- actively flex the fingers.

Passive flexion should not commence until after 8 weeks post-surgery, and appropriate splintage may also be used at this stage (should it be necessary) to gain flexion. Heavy lifting should be avoided for a further month.

Complications following tendon surgery Complications include oedema and adhesions.

To prevent oedema from becoming a problem, elevation is required both when the patient is in bed and when ambulant.

Adhesions are liable to form between the repaired tendon, its sheath, the lacerated skin and the surrounding tissues unless preventative measures can be taken. Use of the dynamic Kleinert splint is an effective means of preventing this

Extensor tendon zones

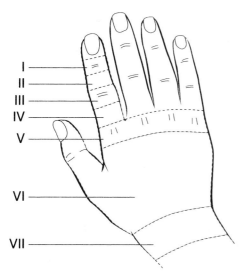

Figure 7.8 Zones for classification of extensor injuries in the hand.

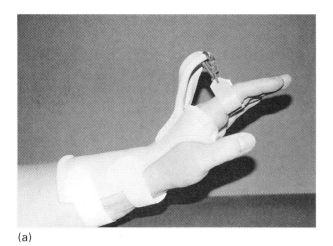

(a)

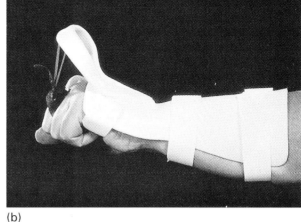

(b)

Figure 7.9 Exercises within a dynamic extension splint.

adherence following primary repairs in zones I, II and III.

Adhesions, if they form around a tendon following repair, are severely disabling and present an enormous challenge to the therapists. Some patients are unfortunate in that they react to surgery by producing a vast amount of fibrous tissue. The need for dynamic splintage is most applicable for this type of patient, but when it is not suitable the tendon must be immobilized by a resting splint for 3 weeks.

Massage using hydrous ointment a few days after surgery will help to soften any induration of tissues around the scar. Ultrasonic treatment is contraindicated for 6 weeks, as it has been shown to delay tendon healing (Roberts *et al.*, 1982). However, there is no recent research showing that low intensity pulsed waves have any detrimental effect. Deep frictional-type massage, using a bland cream (Nivea/E45) to prevent damage to the skin, should be used to stretch any adhesions that have already formed.

After 4–5 weeks a better effect can be achieved by giving this massage with the tendon on tension than with it relaxed, when skin, tendon and underlying tissues shift as one under the therapist's fingers. First, the patient should actively flex the finger (or appropriate joint) and hold the position whilst the frictional massage is given immediately over and around the tendon. It is particularly important it is applied in a caudal direction. The massage is then repeated while the patient actively extends the finger and then holds the position. Finally, when it is safe to apply a passive stretch, the finger or hand should be stretched into maximum extension by the physiotherapist, who again applies massage over the tensioned tendon. During the latter two instances, the concentration of massage should be in a cephalad direction.

Pressure applied by the physiotherapist can also enable the patient to stretch any adhesions

between skin and tendons actively for him- or herself. The therapist's firm pressure should be applied on the skin immediately proximal to the scar, and the patient actively flexes either wrist or fingers. The therapist attempts, in both directions, to prevent the adherent scar from sliding under the fingers. This can be an uncomfortable exercise, so should be performed cautiously at first.

When the tendon repair is sound, vigorous exercises can be given with repeated stretch applied by the physiotherapist to the contracting muscles. Resisted movements to the antagonists, passive stretching, and dynamic or stretch splinting may all help to free adhesions. This passive stretching of adhesions, if it is possible even in one direction only, can have the effect of improving active movement in both directions. Frequent monitoring by the therapist of excursion, range of movement and the position at rest is necessary, so that instant adjustment of treatment can be made. A gain in one direction may be at the expense of movement in the opposite direction, and this is undesirable.

At this stage, electrical stimulation (directly stimulating the muscle bellies) may help to free or stretch adhesions and increase the range of movement (see Chapter 5, Electroactive exercise).

Priorities for recovering movements are as follows:

1. *Adherence of the flexor tendons.* In this case the first priority is to regain active flexion, as this can only be achieved by the patient's own active work. Extension is easier to recover, because passive stretching and splinting can also be used to achieve movement. Therapist and patient should therefore concentrate on improving flexion and maintaining extension. Once the flexion has improved, more emphasis can be put on recovering extension, while ensuring that no flexion is lost.

2. *Adherence of the extensor tendons*. In this case the priority is to regain extension by active movement. The active power of the flexors is usually sufficient to stretch and mobilize any adherent scar on the dorsum of the hand and wrist. It is important that the hand is immobilized with the divided tendons in approximately a mid- to outer-range position when Kleinert suspension is not used. The tendons should never be positioned in the total outer range, as there is then little chance of stretching any adhesions and the patient has the daunting task of trying to regain full range by active movement only.

3. *Joint stiffness*. If adhesions are allowed to form around the repaired tendon they will inevitably have an effect on the joints, sometimes severely limiting the range of movement. The inner range may be maintained passively, as it puts no tension on the repair; however, the outer range may remain limited until the adhesions are freed. As this sometimes takes several weeks, a contracture of both ligaments and capsule may result. This is another reason why the problem of adhesions must receive prompt attention. The adherence usually has a primary effect on the joint in closest proximity and a secondary effect on those joints distal to the repair. For example, a laceration of tendons at the wrist, with both wrist and fingers immobilized in some degree of flexion, will frequently produce adhesions at the wrist. This will mainly limit wrist extension but also, to a lesser extent, wrist flexion. The effect on the more distal joints is to limit the simultaneous extension of the fingers. However, each distal joint can be mobilized individually without any strain being put on the repair. The slackening of tension at the other joints will allow the selected joint to be moved easily through its full passive range.

4. *Incorrect or lost movement patterns*. Patients may have lost the correct feeling of movement, particularly when there is sensory nerve involvement combined with tendon injury. It is important that a digital nerve, for instance, is repaired together with the tendon following injury to a finger. A patient with sensory loss will tend not to use the digit even if the tendon is functioning, and there should be liaison between the physiotherapist and occupational therapist for prompt retraining of this functional pattern. A considerable delay between tendon injury and repair may also have allowed the patient to develop a habit of altered movement. After a division of the flexors digitorum profundus and superficialis, for instance, the only intact finger flexion is at the metacarpophalangeal joints, perfumed by the intrinsic muscles. These muscles also extend the interphalangeal joints, which is the direct opposite of the action required from the flexor digitorum profundus and flexor dig-

itorum superficialis. Any altered movement will therefore need careful re-education.

Flexor tendon graft

In zone II ('no man's land'), a secondary repair may be by tendon graft. The palmaris longus is the most frequently used donor tendon when it is present in the ipsilateral limb. An extensor tendon to a toe or the plantaris tendon may otherwise be used.

If the site for the graft is scarred and fibrosed, a silastic rod is sometimes inserted and attached at one end to the profundus tendon for 3–4 weeks immediately prior to the graft. A smooth bed and sheath are formed by the passive gliding motion of the rod in the finger. It must not be used actively. The graft is then positioned without the need to re-open the finger, as it is attached to the proximal end of the rod and the rod is pulled through from the distal end, carrying the new graft with it. It is sutured into position in place of the rod. The hand and fingers are usually rested for 3 weeks in a plaster slab before early active movement commences.

A graft is dependent on receiving its blood supply from the surrounding tissues, which is why

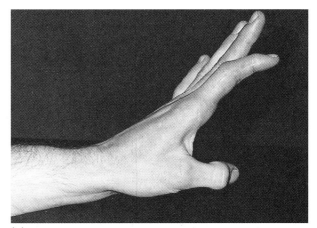

(a)

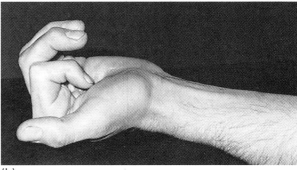

(b)

Figure 7.10 Result of a palmaris longus graft to the index finger, showing slight reduction in extension but excellent flexion.

rest is usual. Exercise is commenced immediately when conditions are particularly advantageous (Figure 7.10).

JOINT DEFORMITIES

Specific deformities in the joints of the hand and wrist occur as the result of joint tendon injury, an imbalance of muscle control, rheumatic disease or congenital deformities. Fractures that unite in poor alignment may also give the impression of a deformity at a nearby joint, and will affect the structures that pass over that joint.

Correct positioning after injury should help to prevent a deformity from either occurring or becoming fixed. Utilizing the close-packed position also ensures that the joints are in the best position of function. Fixed deformities that have already developed will need intensive treatment to regain both mobility and joint control. If this fails, surgery will need considering in order to correct the deformity and prevent its recurrence.

Stiffness of one joint, especially of either a metacarpophalangeal joint or a proximal interphalangeal joint, can cause a crippling disability because the finger sticks out and continually gets in the way. If joints of all the fingers are similarly affected, even with considerable loss of range as can occur following severe burns of the hand, the disability will in fact not be so great.

A joint replacement may be considered if only the joint itself is affected. As problems caused by trauma often involve other structures, a replacement is not always suitable and silastic replacements are not generally considered for fit, young people. The patient's own metatarsophalangeal joint may, however, be considered for the replacement of a metacarpophalangeal joint.

Corrective surgery may or may not succeed, and will inevitably be time-consuming. In a young, active person, the quickest way to return function when one finger has become an extreme nuisance may be to amputate. This is a decision that can only be made by the patient after all attempts at rehabilitation have failed. Some patients will think of this remedy for themselves, while others will not consider it at any cost.

Boutonnière or buttonhole deformity

This deformity results mainly from trauma to the dorsum of the finger at the level of the proximal interphalangeal joint, when damage is caused to the central slip of the extensor expansion. The lateral slips slide anteriorly and therefore produce a flexion deformity. Attempts at extension of the finger fail to gain full extension of the proximal interphalangeal joint, but will cause hyperextension at the distal interphalangeal joint. Due to the altered mechanics of the joints the position of the reti-

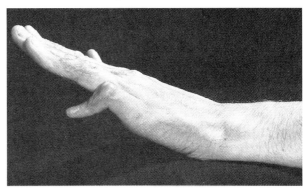

Figure 7.11 The Boutonnière deformity in the little finger and the mild swan-neck deformity in the ring finger were caused by burns.

nacular ligament is changed and it will, if allowed, contract. The resulting hyperextension contracture at the distal interphalangeal joint thus prevents both active and passive flexion from occurring and the joint quickly stiffens. If this injury is not treated urgently the resultant deformity will become extremely difficult to correct (Figure 7.11).

Direct finger injury and burns are the most common traumatic causes of this deformity and will need careful preventative positioning, splinting the proximal interphalangeal joint in full extension for 3–4 weeks and at the same time allowing active distal joint flexion. A cylinder that terminates immediately proximal to the distal interphalangeal joint or a strong Capener-style splint are both suitable as they maintain the extensor expansion in the central position, allowing it to heal, while the retinacular ligament is held on a stretch. Active movement of both metacarpophalangeal and distal interphalangeal joints must be taught and carried out. If the extensor expansion has been cleanly divided, it will need immediate surgery.

After 3 weeks of immobilization, dynamic splintage is desirable, using a weak Capener splint. This:

- allows some active but controlled flexion at the proximal interphalangeal joint
- maintains extension of the proximal interphalangeal joint at rest
- allows flexion of the distal interphalangeal joint
- protects the proximal joint during early mobilization.

Active flexion and extension of the proximal interphalangeal joint should be increased very gradually at this stage. Forced passive flexion must never be given.

A residual Boutonnière deformity is difficult to correct conservatively, especially when the joint has become stiff. The finger is vulnerable to knocks, which can result in a painful proximal interphalangeal joint. Surgery at this stage is not usually successful, and it is occasionally found that a severely deformed finger may eventually need amputation.

Swan-neck deformity

This deformity, most commonly found with rheumatic disease, can also occur as the result of trauma. There is hyperextension of the proximal interphalangeal joint and flexion at the distal interphalangeal joint. Frequently the patient has difficulty in initiating active flexion of the proximal interphalangeal joint, as the lateral slips of the retinacular ligament slide in a dorsal direction and therefore lie on the dorsal side of the fulcrum of the joint. Passive flexion of the proximal interphalangeal joint and passive extension of the distal interphalangeal joint may both be limited.

Absence or weakness of the flexor digitorum superficialis, when combined with normal profundus action, can eventually result in the same deformity, showing a volar prominence together with some hyperextension of the proximal interphalangeal joint (e.g. the long-term effect following a graft of the flexor digitorum profundus when the superficialis has been excised). One of the roles of the flexor digitorum superficialis, besides its flexor control, is to prevent this hyperextension of the proximal interphalangeal joint.

A swan-neck deformity may also result from an intrinsic contracture when the volar surface of the proximal interphalangeal joint becomes prominent. This is due to the strong inelastic pull of the ischaemic intrinsic muscles, which insert into the dorsal expansion immediately distal to the proximal interphalangeal joint.

The deformity is not easy to correct conservatively, especially when it is due to lack of full muscle control. Joint mobility must be regained and patients taught to perform the exercises for themselves. A swan-neck splint which holds the proximal interphalangeal joint in a few degrees of flexion can sometimes be helpful, as the small amount of flexion provided enables active flexion to be initiated correctly at the proximal interphalangeal joint.

The proximal interphalangeal joint may be arthrodesed in flexion with either a K-wire *in situ* for about 8 weeks or a polypropylene peg.

Mallet finger

Stubbing of the fingertip happens frequently during games such as basketball, volleyball, cricket and rugby, and occasionally during bed-making, when the extended finger is forcibly flexed, rupturing the extensor mechanism at the distal interphalangeal joint and sometimes pulling off a fragment of the terminal phalanx. This prevents active extension of the joint, with the result that the fingertip falls into a flexed position. Prompt diagnosis and treatment is essential, with immobilization in a hyperextended position using a mallet finger splint of malleable metal. The patient must understand that the tip should never be allowed to flex during this time. Gentle mobilizing to regain flexion is commenced after 6–8 weeks.

If a fragment of bone has become detached and is large enough, internal fixation with a K-wire may be used to reduce it.

The finger is immobilized in the hyperextended position for at least 6–8 weeks. After removal of the splint, gentle active exercises only are encouraged. If it appears that the DIP joint is dropping into flexion and the patient is unable to actively extend it, the splint may be re-applied for a further period of immobilization (Figure 7.12).

TENDON TRANSFERS

Transfers may be performed following the non-recovery of a peripheral nerve or cervical cord lesion in order to return active function to the hand or limb and to correct any persistent deformities

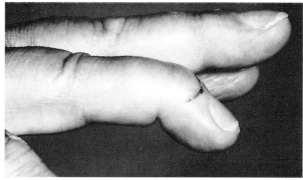

(a)

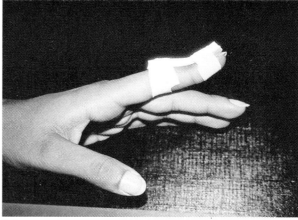

(b)

Figure 7.12 Mallet deformity following a laceration to the dorsum of the finger, and a splint used for its correction.

that result. They may also be performed after tendon division or rupture, with the inherent repair difficulties, and for ischaemic contractures or muscle necrosis.

With extensive and permanent paralysis, it may be necessary to arthrodese the wrist joint also. This then allows the donor tendons to return some movement to the fingers and thumb. It is difficult in fact for the patient to learn to control combined wrist and finger movements if only one donor is provided.

At operation, the distal end of the donor tendon is divided, repositioned and sutured to the receptor tendon. Occasionally the whole donor muscle together with its neurovascular supply is repositioned to a new site of origin before the distal tendon suture is performed. This procedure is used to improve the direction of muscle activity when in its new position.

A large variety of transfers can now be performed, but the most commonly used in the hand are for:

- the return of extension function following a radial nerve lesion
- the return of opposition to the thumb following a median nerve lesion
- the use of the extensor indicis following extensor tendon rupture in rheumatoid patients or following wrist fracture.

The effects of the transfers must be given careful thought, as the donor loses one grade on the Oxford Scale when it is repositioned. It therefore must be at least grade 4 and preferably grade 5 before transfer. Loss of power from the donor's original position must also be considered. The transfer of a muscle essential to some important activity can produce a disastrous result for an already disabled person. It must therefore be given very careful prior consideration.

Therapy for tendon transfers should include a complete assessment of the patient prior to the decision to operate. Examination of the affected muscles, the power of the suggested donors and the range of all joints should be thorough. Sensation should also be charted, together with any areas of incorrect localization. What the patient finds difficult and what activities he or she would like to perform following transfers should be ascertained. Unless well motivated and with reasonably good sensation, the patient will be unlikely to use the hand and arm.

Joints must be mobile prior to surgery, and several weeks of intensive treatment may be necessary to achieve this. It is also important that the patient can isolate or at least identify the donor muscle's contraction, as this will greatly facilitate post-operative re-education.

Following the operation the hand or limb will probably be immobilized for 2–3 weeks, during which time the free joints must be kept mobile and the available muscles exercised. Occasionally the surgeon permits gentle re-education after 1 week only. When the immobilizing splint has been removed, the transferred muscle should be re-educated with gravity eliminated at first. Usually the patient learns the desired movement remarkably easily. This is probably due to the fact that the motor unit has a particularly low ratio of nerve to muscle fibres, which enables especially good neuromuscular control.

Re-education of transfers for brachial plexus lesions is not as spontaneous as for peripheral nerve lesions due to a variety of factors (Frampton, 1986), and they will need longer and more intensive sessions of treatment. When difficulty is experienced, some time should be spent in identifying a contraction of the donor muscle and comparing it with the same muscle and normal movement of the contralateral limb. The patient is then told to think of both the movement that the donor normally makes and the desired new movement. These movements may appear to conflict; for example, flexor carpi ulnaris may have been transferred into extensor digitorum following a radial nerve lesion. As the patient is attempting to extend the fingers using the new transfer, it is undesirable to think of flexing the wrist in order to activate the donor muscle. It is, however, pertinent to think of deviating the wrist in an ulnar direction at the same time as extending the fingers.

When the transfer is from one aspect of the forearm to the other the tendons may be taken through the interosseous membrane, but some may be better passed subcutaneously (Birch and Grant, 1986). In this case the muscle bellies or tendons can usually be identified as they wind obliquely round the ulna or radius. Gentle tapping or pressure applied by the therapist's hand, and when necessary icing, brushing and electrical stimulation of those muscles, may help the patient who has difficulty in regaining a correct contraction and thereby a new movement. Biofeedback may also be useful, using EMG electrodes placed on the donor, which allows the patient to observe on a screen the correct muscle contraction.

Active movement will be of small amplitude at first and probably in the middle of the range. The primary aim should be to increase the active movement into the inner range. Only when this active inner range is improving should the outer range be increased.

Gravity must not be allowed to stretch the muscle into the outer range, and the hand, limb or digit must therefore be supported at first by the therapist's hands when exercising and by a splint or a sling as appropriate. The outer range is best regained by increasing the activity of the antagonists rather than stretching passively.

Tendon transfers most commonly used to improve hand function

1. For non-recovery of a radial nerve lesion, the pronator teres, flexor carpi ulnaris and palmaris longus (if present) are used for restoring wrist extension, finger and thumb extension, and thumb abduction respectively.
2. For non-recovery of a median nerve lesion, an opponens transfer is performed to restore opposition and palmar abduction of the thumb. The tendon of the flexor digitorum superficialis to the ring finger is detached at insertion, retracted and passed through a loop that has been formed using a section of the flexor carpi ulnaris at its insertion. The tendon of the flexor digitorum superficialis is passed under the thenar muscles and sutured into the dorsal expansion of the metacarpophalangeal joint of the thumb. The position of insertion is vital, as it ensures that the thumb not only abducts but rotates also. Re-education is helped if the patient thinks of flexing the proximal interphalangeal joint of the ring finger whilst at the same time gently abducting the thumb in a palmar direction (Figure 7.13). This operation will only succeed when sensation in the thumb is near to normal.
3. For non-recovery of an ulnar nerve lesion, if the claw deformity is pronounced, a Zancolli 'lasso'

procedure may be performed using flexor digitorum superficialis of at least grade 4. Flexor digitorum superficialis tendon is detached from its insertion and is sutured back on itself, remaining 'lassoed' through the flexor sheath pulley at the level of the metacarpophalangeal joint and preventing it from hyperextending.

A permanently abducted little finger caused by the non-recovery of the palmar interosseous to that finger can be corrected by plication of the capsule of the metacarpophalangeal joint. Extreme weakness of pinch grip can be improved by transferring extensor indicis to the first dorsal interosseous.

Problems

1. Tension of the transferred tendon is crucial:
   - If it is too slack, the donor muscle will be unable to activate inner range movement. Movement can improve with several months of exercising, as the muscle has a contractile property. Shortening by surgery, however, may eventually be advisable.
   - If it is too tight, it will prevent movement into the full outer range. Again this may improve with time, as the muscle belly is an elastic mechanism. Surgery to correct the tension when too tight may also need to be considered.
2. The transferred tendon may not always effect the desired movement because of its direction of pull.
3. If the muscle passes over more than one flail joint, it may be unable to control the proximal joint.

All likely effects must be considered carefully prior to surgery, as they will be difficult to correct later.

TENOLYSIS

Tenolysis, or the surgical excision of adhesions that surround and restrict the movements of tendons, may be necessary if active range of movement does not increase and function remains reduced. However, the surgeons are unlikely to perform a tenolysis until 6 months after injury in order to limit any exacerbation of fibrosis. It is desirable to have a full passive range of movement before surgery.

If both active and passive stretching of the adherence causes pain in a joint, and range does not increase, especially after intensive treatment has been given, it is unlikely that the adhesions will become freed without surgical intervention.

Post-operative therapy must be commenced early, usually the day after surgery. Exercises given must be gentle at first because the excision of adhesions may have reduced the blood supply to the tendon, leaving it vulnerable to excess stress. The patient is encouraged to exercise through as large a range as possible, so that full movement is

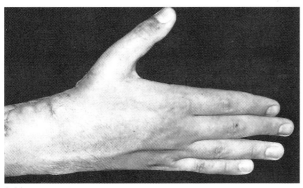
(a)

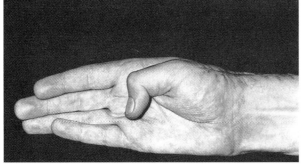
(b)

Figure 7.13 Tendon transfer of extensor carpi radialis brevis following division of extensor pollicis longus. Extensor indices may also be used.

achieved within a few days. Painkillers may be necessary initially if the movements are extremely uncomfortable. Power can be built up gradually after 2–3 weeks.

TENOSYNOVITIS AND TENOVAGINITIS

Tenosynovitis is an inflammatory condition of the synovial lining of the tendon sheaths resulting from injury. An increased amount of synovial fluid is secreted so that a swelling along the length of the sheath results. It may follow either mild trauma or some unaccustomed hard work of the hand and wrist. Tenovaginitis describes the condition when there is a painful and hard thickening of the synovium without excessive synovial fluid secretion. It can be palpated along the affected tendon sheath. It is commonly experienced as the result of repetitive and stressful work. In recent years, for instance, it has become an occupational hazard for those working in poultry processing factories.

The abductor pollicis longus and extensors pollicis longus and brevis are the tendons most commonly affected by persistent or unaccustomed trauma. Pain and crepitus are experienced on movement, and if the condition is infected or acute it may also be painful at rest.

An infected synovial sheath must be dealt with urgently by surgery, irrigation and the introduction of antibiotics, otherwise necrosis of the tendon may result (Wilson, 1983).

In some units rest is the most important aspect of conservative treatment, but this is currently being less used. Support with a crepe bandage or splint may be adequate, but frequently a cylinder that provides complete immobilization is essential. Thermoplastic is a suitable material to use, as it is rigid and can be of the perforated variety. PEME helps to reduce pain and swelling, and can be given through bandages or plaster of Paris. Resistant small areas can be massaged using ice cubes. Ultrasound, which is usually given with the splint removed, is found to be more effective if the condition has already become chronic. One or two treatments of low dosage pulsed ultrasound, or frictions, over the painful area may temporarily exacerbate the symptoms, but this technique has been more effective than other methods when the condition has become chronic. A localized painful spot can often be cured finally by a hydrocortisone injection. Exercise should then be introduced gradually to build up normal muscle power.

Surgery may be necessary if the condition is totally resistant to conservative treatment. An incision of the sheath relieves the pressure on the tendon, and very gentle exercises can be introduced 4–5 days later. It is very important to prevent adhesions from forming.

Trigger finger, with the nodular thickening of a flexor tendon, may also need an incision of the sheath when conservative treatment methods have failed, in order to allow normal tendon gliding.

Measures may have to be taken to prevent a recurrence of all these problems. These might only consist of a warning not to aggravate the condition by performing any unusually strong or repetitive activity. If the patient's occupation is the cause of tenovaginitis, however, is may be necessary to attempt to change or alter the work so that it is less repetitive. Splinting along with ergonomic advice can sometimes give support so that less stress is put on the tendons.

PERIPHERAL NERVE LESIONS

A correct diagnosis is essential when a nerve lesion is involved so that the best management may be given. Some patients will need little more than assessment, advice and reappraisal, whereas others will need surgery and intensive therapy for motor and sensory problems and for the complications arising from associated injuries.

Causes

The main causes of nerve lesions are lacerations from glass and knives, the closed injuries of fractures and dislocations, ruptures as in brachial plexus lesions, and gunshot wound and blast injuries. Crush injuries, compression from too tight a plaster or bandage or carpal tunnel syndrome, ischaemic injury and radiotherapy may all result in a nerve lesion. Drug abuse, diabetes and over-indulgence in alcohol are occasional causes of nerve damage.

Degeneration

Wallerian degeneration occurs following the division of a nerve, both to the proximal node of Ranvier and in the distal component of the nerve trunk. The debris from this degeneration is cleared away by macrophage activity, and collagen is deposited gradually in the endoneurial tube. If reinnervation does not occur, the muscle fibres also will be gradually replaced by fibrous tissue over the following 2–3 years.

Regeneration

The axons sprout at the proximal stump of the nerve and, if no repair is attempted, will form a neuroma. Regeneration takes place only if the nerve ends are in apposition.

Following a nerve repair, these sprouting axons will attempt to regenerate into their original endoneural tubes. This is rarely achieved correctly, and some crossed reinnervation to both motor and sensory end-plates will inevitably result.

The average rate of peripheral nerve regeneration is about 1.0–1.5 mm a day, but it is faster in children and usually slower in the elderly and smokers. Regeneration gradually slows when the site of the lesion is far from the skin and the muscles that need to be reinnervated. After 3 years the muscle fibres will have become irreversibly fibrosed so that, apart from some sensory recovery, very little functional ability will result.

Effects of nerve injury

The effects of nerve damage are motor, sensory and autonomic.

The motor effects of a lower motor neurone lesion are loss of tone and reflexes, and paralysis of muscles. Atrophy and deformities will develop, which if not treated will result in joint stiffness and contractures of soft tissues.

The sensory effects are loss of cutaneous and proprioceptive sensation. Some deep sensation will be saved if tendons are intact. Deafferentation may lead to problems of pain. The area of sensory loss diminishes slightly when the adjacent normal nerves expand into the affected areas. Unless patients are warned, and constant reminders given, burns are liable to result.

The autonomic effects are changes in circulation and nutrition. The limb will take on the temperature of its surroundings, and the affected skin area becomes pinkish-purple. Loss of sweating results and the skin is noticeably dry, first becoming scaly and later paper-thin and shiny.

The poor nutrition induces deformity in the hair follicles, with a resulting effect on the hairs; the nails become ridged and the pulp of the fingertips reduces in size. Any cuts or blisters suffered due to loss of sensation may become trophic lesions and take many weeks to heal.

The area of skin affected is identical to that with sensory loss. It is therefore usually possible to identify the area of anaesthesia by observing the sympathetic changes.

Types of nerve lesion

Neurapraxia, axonotmesis and neurotmesis are the main types of nerve injury.

Neurapraxia

A neurapraxia produces loss of conduction because of a block at the site of injury. The distal component does not degenerate, and when the cause of the lesion is removed there should be rapid recovery. There may be some sparing of crude sensation, and electromyographic (EMG) studies will show an absence of fibrillation potentials. Stimulation of the nerve trunk below the level of the lesion will elicit a normal muscle response, but this particular test must be delayed for 2 weeks in case any Wallerian degeneration occurs. This response differentiates a neurapraxia from an axonotmesis.

Physiotherapy for a neurapraxia should include assessment of joints, muscles and sensation and, if no EMG studies are available, the electrical stimulation of the nerve trunk distal to the site of the lesion. A neurapraxia should make an excellent recovery, and the only treatment required is to teach the patient the passive range of the joints involved, to instruct him or her on the necessary protection because of sensory loss, and to provide support to any flail joints. A description of the lesion and what to expect when recovery commences must be given and checks made frequently that the patient is maintaining the limb in good order. Spontaneous recovery should take place, with return to completely normal function usually within 6 weeks but occasionally taking as long as 12 weeks.

Axonotmesis

This produces degeneration in the axons distal to the site of the injury, but the sheath of the nerve is preserved. There is loss of conduction distal to the lesion, and an EMG test will show both lack of volitional response and the presence of fibrillation potentials. Regeneration will commence when the cause of injury is removed, and usually a good recovery results.

Physiotherapy includes assessment of joints, muscles and sensation, and instruction on the effects of the lesion and protection necessary. When there is doubt as to the type of lesion in a closed injury and an EMG is not available, the nerve trunk should be stimulated. If after 2 weeks this stimulation elicits no muscle response, it suggests that degeneration has occurred. Any additional complications of fractures and dislocations also need therapy treatment. Instruction should be given on the care of the limb, passive movements and any signs of recovery that may be expected. Flail joints should be supported, preferably with dynamic splints. At the time of motor and sensory reinnervation, an increase or some short bursts of treatment and re-education may be required for maximum results.

A mixed lesion of neurapraxia and axonotmesis

When this occurs, some axons suffer degeneration but others are spared. An EMG will demonstrate fibrillation potentials of some muscle fibres and conduction of others. A good recovery can be anticipated.

Neurotmesis

A neurotmesis involves the complete division of the nerve trunk, and is usually found in conjunction with open injuries, fractures or traction lesions of the plexus. Loss of conduction occurs, and EMG studies show similar results to those of an axonotmesis. Repair of a divided nerve is essential for regeneration, and the recovery time will again depend on the site of the lesion. The quality of recovery is frequently rather poor due to the inability of all axons to regenerate to their correct end-organs. Crossed reinnervation produces poor motor and sensory recovery with faulty localization.

Assessment must be made of joints, muscles and sensation. There are likely to be more problems from associated injuries, such as lacerations and incisions of the skin and division of tendons and arteries. These may need intensive treatment in the early stages for oedema, pain and adherence of structures. Joints must be supported, passive movements taught and instructions given, both on protection of anaesthetic skin and on the progress expected. The intensity of treatment should be increased when recovery of muscles and sensation occurs, in order to maximize function.

NB: If the lesion involves the plexus, any electrical tests performed by physiotherapists are likely to be of no significance. EMG tests are desirable to ensure an accurate diagnosis for peripheral nerve lesions, and they are essential for plexus injuries.

Nerve repair

The best results of nerve repair follow primary nerve suture, as long as the wound is clean. Dirty wounds that are liable to become infected will cause poor nerve healing and regeneration, so surgery must be delayed and a secondary repair performed. Frequently arteries will also have been divided, and these must be repaired if possible and not ligated in order to ensure an adequate circulation to the regenerating nerve.

With the advent of microsurgery, precise techniques of suturing can now be performed. Choice of technique is usually between an epineural or a fascicular repair. A gap in the nerve may necessitate the mobilization of both proximal and distal ends to prevent a stretch being put on the repair. If the gap is larger than 2.5 mm a graft may be considered, but only if the bed for the graft is well vascularized. The result of grafting is usually less effective because the regenerating axons have two suture lines through which they must pass.

Immobilization in a backslab is usually for 3 weeks, as a stretch of the repaired ends is likely to jeopardize the results. Physiotherapy is then commenced, the therapist taking care not to place a passive stretch on the repair for a further 4 weeks.

Tendon transfers, either transferring the distal portion or the whole muscle together with its neurovascular supply, are techniques that may effectively restore function when nerve regeneration is unlikely. Occasionally a joint may need fusing in order to provide stability when the nerve does not recover and no transfers are possible.

Therapy

Treatment can be divided into the early and recovery stages, although in practice they merge together. Many nerve injuries occur with tendon involvement, and in this case early active movement or the regime appropriate to the tendon injury is followed.

Early stage Physiotherapy immediately following injury and surgery, which must include chest care, should concentrate on the prevention of oedema, the prevention of pain and the maintenance of joint mobility wherever possible. It is vital that the shoulder joint is exercised, especially in the elderly. A visual assessment can be made temporarily, which includes active and passive movement as applicable, but available joints and muscles should be measured as early as possible.

Most surgeons immobilize a sutured nerve for 3 weeks in order to allow healing and to prevent any stretch on the approximated ends. To achieve some slackness of the nerve it may be necessary to position the joints in a loose-packed position, i.e. the wrist joint might be immobilized in flexion following median nerve suture. Extension is increased very gradually after 3–4 weeks.

Counselling during the first week or so allows the patient gradually to realize the severity of the injury and the likely length of time before full recovery. Emphasis must be laid on the support available and the eventual return of function so that the patient does not become too worried about the future.

After 3 weeks, when the stitches are out and the immobilizing splint has been removed, an assessment of motor, sensory and autonomic effects can be made. Occasionally a splint is still needed to limit the stretch on the nerve ends for another few days; however, the splint can usually be removed when the patient is assessed and treated in the therapy department.

The joint range is now measured and the total flexion and extension excursion of the fingers recorded. The effect that the scar has on tendon function must be observed carefully in case any adhesions prevent full flexion, full extension or possibly both. A laceration that divides a nerve will frequently have divided muscle, tendons and other tissues. The divided structures lie in layers directly one above the other, and after surgery they may have become adherent – skin to tendons, and tendons to each other and to the deeper structures such as capsules and ligaments. This problem can limit movement considerably, and will need a great intensity of treatment during early rehabilitation.

Pain, if still present after 2–3 weeks, needs urgent treatment because it is more difficult to cure when it has become longstanding. Spontaneous firing of discharges may occur at the proximal stump of the nerve, and afferent inhibition from the divided section is no longer available. In partial and recovering peripheral nerve lesions, painful paraesthesia and causalgia may result (in severe cases) in hyperpathia. If neuromata form at the proximal stump, there will also be an increase of these painful spontaneous discharges in the afferents.

TENS, if applied early after injury, is effective for pain prevention and for treatment in a large portion of cases. The electrodes must be positioned on an area where sensation is still present. Pain is frequently experienced in the anaesthetic areas, and the electrodes should therefore be placed proximal to the site of the lesion, over the nerve trunk. Several attempts may have to be made on consecutive days to find the most effective positions for the electrodes. The duration of treatment should be at least 2 hours to be beneficial, and preferably much longer. TENS can be used safely for as long as the patient desires, and stimulators should be available for the patient to use at home.

If pain is persistent, guanethidine blocks may be necessary, combined with vigorous therapy, to reduce the pain to an acceptable level. Distraction by involvement in leisure interests and games etc., when combined with more formal treatment, is one of the best ways of coping, as higher centre inhibition is produced. The patient must assess the pain daily on the 10-cm scale, recording the duration of any relief from the previous day's treatment, in order to achieve the optimum result.

Scars and their surrounding areas will need softening. Massage, pulsed electromagnetic fields (PEMF) and US are all useful. Webs must not be forgotten, as they quickly contract and must have regular stretching.

If movement is limited by adhesions, it is possible that the joints may also stiffen. Joint mobility must therefore be maintained; at the same time the therapist must ensure that the suture is not jeopardized by stretch. Tension can be slackened by flexing both the wrist and metacarpophalangeal joints, thereby allowing the interphalangeal joints to extend automatically. Similarly, by flexing both the wrist and interphalangeal joints the metacarpophalangeal joints will also extend easily. The presence of adhesions should not usually be a sufficient excuse for the development of joint stiffness.

Adhesions may usually be stretched actively (i.e. by the patient) after 3–4 weeks, as long as the stretch applied is very gentle. No passive stretch should be given to sutured structures at this stage. Active movements are gradually increased, with resistance added at 5–6 weeks. A passive stretch may be safely given at 8 weeks.

The power of the proximal muscles must be remembered. If the muscles of the hand are paralysed, the strength of the shoulder girdle, shoulder and elbow will inevitably be reduced. Similarly, the muscles that are antagonistic to those affected by the lesion will weaken unless specific exercise is

given. The use of dynamic splints helps to maintain function of these antagonists.

Joints without active control must be supported, both to prevent a prolonged stretch of ligaments and capsule, which can be very painful, and to prevent adaptive shortening of the unopposed muscles. For example, in a radial nerve injury the wrist is supported in a cock-up splint. Similarly, a recovering nerve, especially if divided and sutured, must not be left on a stretch as this will reduce recovery. Muscles will become inhibited if subjected to prolonged stretch. The normal position of rest for the wrist, fingers and thumb is suitable when support is necessary whilst awaiting nerve regeneration.

Dynamic splints form a useful adjunct during the management of nerve lesions. Their main applications are:

1. To provide support for joints and soft tissues, thereby preventing deformities and contractures
2. To improve function by:
   - placing the hand in a functional position, e.g. wrist cock-up splint
   - utilizing alternative muscle action – e.g. in a combined median and ulnar nerve lesion, if the metacarpophalangeal joints are held in very slight flexion, extensor digitorum communis (EDC) is able to extend the interphalangeal joints; this activity also prevents the claw deformity
   - directly replacing muscle function, e.g. a dynamic extension splint extends the metacarpophalangeal joints in a radial nerve lesion
   - exercising antagonist activity.

(See also Chapter 12.)

If either dynamic or static splints are used, the patient must be instructed to remove the splint regularly and mobilize the hand through the full passive range.

Counselling is essential at this stage, with instructions given to patients so that they understand the purpose of normal nerve supply, the effects of its damage, the recovery expected, and the care necessary whilst waiting for nerve regeneration. Motor and sensory effects are identified and compared with the contralateral limb. It is important that patients understand that increased wasting will occur and that there will be an inevitable time lapse before reinnervation commences. Any occupational or social problems should be discovered quickly so that action can be taken and referral to other health professionals (e.g. social worker, disabled employment advisor) can be made.

Recovery stage Assessments to discover any return of muscle activity and sensation should be increased when reinnervation is anticipated. An estimation of this event can be made by measuring the distance of the injury from the area to be reinnervated, and calculating the likely time for recovery – a millimetre a day is the average rate of regeneration. The Tinel test usually helps to indicate both the site of injury and the point of regeneration (Henderson, 1948).

Activity is first tested in those muscles expected to be normal, followed by those expected to be affected by the lesion, and all are graded on the 0–5 scale. Trick movements and anomalies should be anticipated. Sensation is charted using different colour codes for normal, anaesthetic and altered sensation, and increased treatment is given when muscle flickers are discovered. Sometimes muscles that show no activity at the time of assessment will start to contract if bombarded for several days with physiological input. The nerves have a high threshold following regeneration, which necessitates increased facilitation, and PNF techniques of treatment are therefore very appropriate. Computerized games with EMG biofeedback, using surface electrodes, are usually most helpful to the patient. Repeated sessions to maximize muscle function will be necessary for up to 3 years, depending on the distance of the lesion from the muscles needing reinnervation. After 3 years the muscle recovery is likely to be minimal, and surgery may be the only means by which function can be restored.

During this stage of recovery, observation should be made for any deterioration in the deformities. In a high-level lesion of the median and ulnar nerves, clawing will increase when the long muscles to the fingers recover. It is urgent that adequate passive movement and stretching is given, and taught to the patient, in order to prevent contractures.

Dynamic or static splinting may still be of help at this stage. Muscles that have recently recovered may tire by the end of the day, at which time the splint can be useful. At work, it may be necessary to stabilize or support a part until muscle strength improves.

Sensory return needs to be monitored by therapists at regular intervals following a median nerve lesion in order to commence re-education as early as possible and thus maximize function. Cotton wool or even the light touch of a fingertip is an appropriate means, the therapist taking great care not to produce a joint movement. Hyperaesthesia is experienced in the palm first, gradually reaching the fingertips, and thus giving some protective sensation. The pins and needles are uncomfortable for the patient, but should soon change to more normal sensation. The hyperaesthesia is due to immaturity of the myelin, and in most people this deficiency is eventually corrected although it sometimes remains a big prob-

lem in the elderly. TENS can be beneficial by lessening the pins and needles sensation, but will probably need to be used daily. These patients should ideally have their own stimulator.

Surgeons also need an assessment of the quality of their nerve repairs by the measurement of sensory regeneration. Tests, with therapists using different diameter monofilaments or a Von Frey hair, are both subjective and time-consuming, and do not address sensory function. The development of a simple EMG sensory conduction test and the measurement of skin resistance by a sweat meter may provide a rapid and more accurate answer in the future.

The static two-point discrimination test has been found to bear very little relationship to function (Wynn Parry and Salter, 1976). Static touch receptors, which are slow adapting, are the last to regenerate after nerve repair, and in fact frequently do not regenerate at all, probably due to the lack of sufficient axoplasm (Wynn Parry, 1984). The rapidly adapting mechanoreceptors, which are stimulated by a moving touch, are however likely to recover. Two-point discrimination, if included, should therefore be measured by a moving touch (Dellon, 1984). Similarly, localization should be tested with a moving finger touch and results charted.

Sensory re-education commences when there is normal sensation in the palm but some residual hyperaesthesia in the fingertips. It should start with different shapes of wood and large objects, thus mainly utilizing proprioception for recognition. When the cutaneous sensation of the fingertips becomes normal, the size of the objects is decreased and different textures and materials are introduced. Improved stereognostic ability is due to the flow of more normal sensory discharges from the recovered tactile receptors. Less information is gained from the proprioceptors when handling small objects and different textures, and the ability to recognize these is therefore dependent on cutaneous recovery. It is essential that both these aspects of sensory ability are considered during re-education. Training must also be included to correct any faulty localization in the median distribution following nerve repair.

Leprosy patients frequently suffer incurable cutaneous anaesthesia, but some proprioception may remain. This is gained from any muscles, tendons and joints that may still have a normal nerve supply, and can therefore be utilized for stereognosis training. Emphasis should be particularly on discriminating between different shapes, sizes and weights of objects. By watching and then repeating the action with the eyes closed, patients should be able to gain a more efficient idea of their hand activity. This helps to train them to protect themselves when performing activities that could be damaging to anaesthetic skin.

SPECIFIC NERVE LESIONS

Radial nerve lesions

The radial nerve supplies those muscles that extend and stabilize the elbow, wrist and fingers. Acting as fixators, they position the wrist in sufficient extension so that the finger flexors can contract strongly. Active extension movements are necessary for grasp, first to stretch the fingers round the object and later to release it. The radial nerve is responsible for this extension control.

The radial nerve is most frequently damaged by fractures of the shaft of the humerus involving it in its spiral groove. It can also be affected by pressure in the axilla. The muscles involved are the supinator, brachioradialis, extensor carpi ulnaris, extensor carpi radialis longus and brevis, extensor digitorum communis, extensors indicis and digiti minimi, extensors pollicis longus and brevis, and abductor pollicis longus. Lesions have to be close to the axilla to affect the triceps (Figure 7.14).

The trick movements include extension of the interphalangeal joints of the fingers by the intrinsic muscles when the metacarpophalangeal joints are supported and stabilized in extension by the examiner. A dipping action of the whole hand occurs when the patient is asked to extend the fingers without any support being given; this enables extension of both the metacarpophalangeal and interphalangeal joints by tenodesis action. The wrist is actively flexed downwards and held in full flexion, which has a tautening effect on the long extensors of the fingers, and a passive extension of metacarpophalangeal and interphalangeal joints therefore occurs. Conversely, some wrist extension may sometimes be produced, again by a tenodesis action, as the result of full and strong finger flexion. The tautening effect on the finger extensors will in this instance pull the wrist back into slight extension. Extension of the interphalangeal joint of the thumb can be produced by the abductor pollicis brevis, with its normal median nerve supply, because of its slip insertion into the dorsal expansion of the thumb. At the same time it pulls the thumb into abduction and rotation. If held beside the index finger, a small degree of extension of the interphalangeal joint may still be possible, and it is therefore advisable to leave the thumb free when

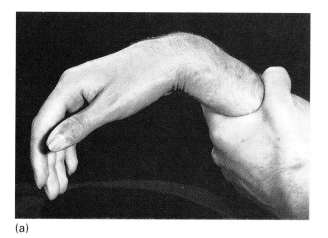

(a)

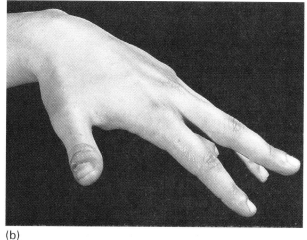

(b)

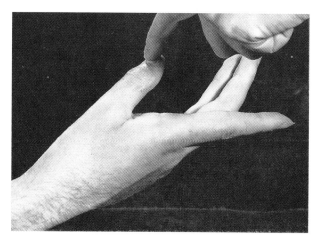

(c)

Figure 7.14 Radial nerve lesion causing:(a) a drop wrist deformity; (b) dipping of the wrist into full flexion to produce MCP and IP joint extension by tenodesis action; and (c) extension of the IP joint of the thumb by a contraction of the abductor pollicis brevis with its slip insertion into the dorsal expansion.

testing the EPL and to look for a correct movement, a contraction of the tendon and the absence of abduction. These trick movements may not be immediately apparent if the hand and forearm are in a plaster of Paris that extends slightly beyond the metacarpophalangeal joints of the fingers and thumb.

Injury at the level of the forearm can cause damage to the posterior interosseous nerve and also to the sensory nerve where it passes superficially over the shaft of the radius at the junction of mid- and lower-thirds, making it rather vulnerable. The sensory distribution is variable; it may supply the major part of the skin of the dorsum of the hand (radial side), or only a small area at the base of the thumb. Occasionally there is no sensory distribution at all from the radial nerve.

The typical posture of a patient presenting with a radial nerve lesion is with the hand held in supination, thus eliminating the wrist drop which can, after some weeks, become very uncomfortable due to the stretch on the ligaments and capsule. The effect on the function of the hand is mainly from the loss of wrist extension, combined with the difficulty of grasp and release of large objects because the fingers cannot be extended.

Therapy
Therapy is concerned with maintaining the mobility of the joints and muscles at first, followed by re-education later.

A simple cock-up splint is essential to support the wrist after a radial nerve lesion, and can be either static or dynamic. Individualized and well-made dynamic extension splints can be of enormous benefit by extending the metacarpophalangeal joints and thumb to allow grasp and release. The splint can be low profile to lessen inconveniences, and patients should be provided with one to allow them the choice of rest or function. The semi-flexed posture of the fingers, with the thumb slightly abducted and rotated, is a natural resting position for the hand, but the wrist must always be supported in some extension.

In a lesion of the posterior interosseous nerve, when activity of both brachioradialis and extensor carpi radialis longus is preserved, wrist extension remains, albeit with a bias of radial deviation due to lack of activity in the extensor carpi ulnaris. The hand can function quite efficiently if some metacarpophalangeal joint extension is provided by a dynamic extension splint.

During muscle reinnervation the brachioradialis is usually first to recover, followed by the extensor carpi radialis longus and brevis, and then the supinator. Recovery of the extensor carpi ulnaris corrects the bias of radial deviation, and is followed usually by recovery of finger extension. The metacarpophalangeal joints of the index and little fingers are frequently found to extend initially

through a greater range than the other fingers. This is because of the additional contraction of the extensor indicis, or extensor digiti minimi, with the extensor digitorum. The thumb is usually the last to recover its muscle power, and the earliest sign of recovery in the extensor pollicis longus is usually the decrease of palmar abduction when attempting to extend the terminal joint.

Splintage should be reduced when the strength improves and the patient can manage without support. This may be the case for only part of the day, but a delay in removing the splint may otherwise slow progress.

If the injury to the radial nerve is at a high level, there will be a considerable time lapse before muscle reinnervation occurs. If this is likely to be a very long time and there is some doubt over the effectiveness of recovery, tendon transfer procedures may be performed as a suitable means for returning some function to the arm. If the extensor muscles recover later, there is no real disadvantage to the patient.

Residual problems following a radial nerve lesion are mainly due to lack of reinnervation of the extensor muscles. There is usually a delay of several months between injury and recovery, so that corrective procedures should be considered when reinnervation is expected but does not actually occur. Wrist extension, and thumb and finger extension combined with abduction, are the most essential functions to restore. Sensory loss in the radial distribution only is not a very great problem to the patient.

The pronator teres, flexor carpi ulnaris and palmaris longus are commonly used as donors for tendon transfer procedures. They are sutured into the extensor carpi radialis brevis, the extensor digitorum communis and extensor pollicis longus, and the abductor pollicis longus respectively. A splint provides support for 3 weeks in order to prevent too much stretch to the donor muscles. Very gentle exercise may, with the surgeon's agreement, be commenced 1 week after surgery, but this is frequently delayed for 3 weeks. Re-education of the muscles to an altered role is not usually difficult, and most results are excellent. Lack of extension as the result of a brachial plexus lesion may, however, be more difficult to restore.

Median nerve lesions

Delicate and skilled function of the hand is achieved by the combination of an excellent motor and sensory supply, which is largely gained from the median nerve distribution. Skin receptors are particularly dense in the skin on the ulnar side of the thumb and the radial side of the index finger, and these areas are highly represented on the sensory cortex. Activities such as tying up shoelaces, doing up buttons, writing and painting are those that

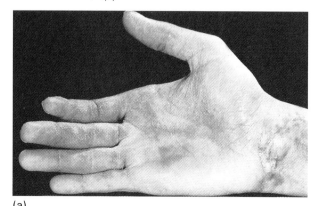

(a)

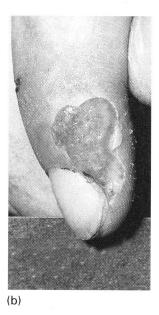

(b)

Figure 7.15 (a) A lesion of the median nerve clearly shows the cutaneous distribution; (b) a burn sustained on a lighted cigarette.

suffer most in an injury to the median nerve (Figure 7.15).

The nerve is especially vulnerable at the wrist, where it lies just below the skin and the palmaris longus tendon. It is most commonly injured by lacerations at this site, together usually with one or more tendons. It can also be affected by compression in the carpal tunnel.

With a lesion at the wrist level, the muscles affected are the abductor pollicis brevis, opponens pollicis, the superficial head of the flexor pollicis brevis, and the lateral (radial) two lumbricals. The thenar muscles become increasingly wasted so that the flat or monkey hand deformity develops, with the thumb lying lateral instead of anterior to the index finger. This is caused by the unopposed actions of the extensor pollicis longus and adductor pollicis. There may also be a very slight claw deformity of the index and middle fingers due to

inactivity of the two lumbricals, but the normal action of the interossei to these two fingers prevents this from becoming pronounced. The volar surfaces of the thumb, index and middle fingers and the radial side of the ring finger will be anaesthetic, together with the dorsal surfaces of the same digits from the level of the proximal interphalangeal joints to the tips of the digits. Autonomic changes, including loss of sweating, change of colour and change of skin texture, will be observed in the same distribution. Atrophy of the thumb web will quickly develop if not well mobilized (Figure 7.16).

Flexion of the thumb is preserved, but during attempted opposition the flexor pollicis brevis can only flex the thumb towards the base of the little finger while remaining in contact with the palm, as the rotation of the metacarpal and the normally powerful thrust of the thenar eminence muscles are both lost. This is because of the paralysis of the thenar muscles, which normally position the thumb in some abduction. An attempt to make an 'O' with index finger and thumb usually results in a very flat 'D' being formed.

The trick movement of palmar abduction may occasionally be possible due to a combined or alternating contraction of the abductor pollicis longus, with its radial nerve supply, and the deep head of the flexor pollicis brevis, with an ulnar nerve supply. It is, however, a rather weak and unstable movement.

A lesion at the level of the wrist should show signs of returning muscle activity at approximately 90 days after suture. The abductor pollicis brevis is the muscle that usually contracts first. An improvement in the position in which the thumb lies is often the first sign of recovery, before a flicker of movement can be observed. Active movement will follow, but it usually takes some weeks or months (if at all) before the thumb can perform sufficiently well to touch the little finger in a normal and strong movement pattern.

Lesions of the median nerve at the level of or above the elbow can be caused by lacerations, ischaemia, fractures and traction of the roots. The pre-mentioned muscles of the hand are involved, and also the forearm and finger flexors. These include the pronator teres, flexor carpi radialis, palmaris longus (if present) and flexor digitorum superficialis. The anterior interosseous branch, which is given off just below the elbow and is occasionally damaged in isolation, supplies the flexor digitorum profundus to both the index and middle fingers or to the index finger alone, the flexor pollicis longus and pronator quadratus.

The deformity produced by a median nerve lesion at a high level is that of a pointing finger when the nerve supplies the flexor digitorum profundus to only the index finger. If it also supplies flexor digitorum profundus to the middle finger the posture is that of benedictim. Function of

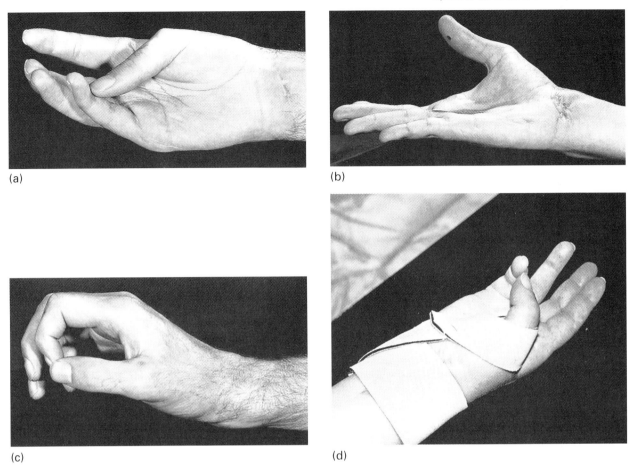

(a)

(b)

(c)

(d)

Figure 7.16 A median nerve lesion. (a) Attempted opposition involving flexion and rotation at the CMC joint is replaced by increased flexion at the MCP joint, and the little finger flexes increasingly towards the tip of the thumb. (b) Trick palmar abduction of the thumb produced by a combination of the deep head of flexor pollicis brevis and abductor pollicis longus. (c) The very flat 'D' produced when attempting to form an 'O'. (d) An opponens splint to facilitate opposition.

the other fingers (see attached list) is preserved through the supply from the ulnar nerve. Sensory and autonomic distribution is the same as in a lesion at the wrist. Adaptations or dynamic splints may be used for improving the function of an anterior interosseous nerve lesion.

Early signs of recovery at high level include:

- a slight return or pronation and wrist flexion; a contraction of the flexor carpi radialis can be felt over the tendon at the wrist
- flexion of the fingers, which follows
- flexion of the thumb, which follows
- finally, recovery of the pronator quatratus – this is the last of the forearm muscles to recover, and if the level of a median nerve lesion is at the elbow there will inevitably be a long delay before recovery can occur in both muscle power and sensation of the hand.

Therapy

Physiotherapy is important early for maintaining the passive range of joints and the suppleness of the webs, and for preventing a gross thenar eminence deformity. Provision of a dynamic splint, which pulls the thumb into some abduction and opposition, will help to prevent an excessive deformity. It also assists function, as the fingertips can be flexed towards the suitably positioned thumb. Repeated warnings must be given regarding the sensory loss.

It is more difficult to assist function if the lesion is at a high level when it involves the finger and wrist flexors. Gross deformity of the thenar eminence must be prevented, however, by the use of the above-mentioned splint.

If the webs, particularly of the thumb, have become contracted, intensive treatment must be given. Passive stretching and the use of C-splints, preferably of thermoplastic material, should improve the degree of passive abduction. It may be necessary to treat the web to increase both palmar and radial abduction, and if so, separate splints will be needed to maintain each position. Thermoplastic material is most suited for this purpose as it moulds perfectly round the digits, thus holding the required position exactly.

The wrist and finger flexors must be re-educated immediately a flicker of movement is discovered, and gradually strengthened during the following weeks. The extensors may also be found to be weak due to complete lack of hand function, and must therefore be strengthened.

Facilitation techniques are extremely important when re-educating thumb movements. The thenar muscles are exercised in the outer range at first, as recovering muscles are unable to contract through the full range in the early stages. Excursion is gradually increased as strength returns.

Sensory re-education should commence immediately there is some hyperaesthesia in the tips of the thumb, index and middle fingers, and a more normal sensation in the palm. The normal area of skin supplied by the ulnar nerve must be covered by Tubigrip or finger-stalls, otherwise the patient will only use this part of the hand. A blindfold or mask will ensure that the patient cannot see what is being felt.

Although the return of cutaneous sensation is necessary for stereognosis, a great deal of the gnostic ability is from proprioception. If a lesion of a median nerve occurs in conjunction with one of the radial nerve, particularly when at a high level, there will be an enormous disability. Proprioception from joint receptors and tendons will be greatly reduced, and patients frequently complain of dropping objects. In lesions of the median nerve alone, however, use can be made of the residual proprioceptive feedback available from the tendons, muscles and joints with a normal nerve supply. Large objects that are simple to manipulate are fairly easily recognized during early sensory recovery. Small objects and materials are recognized much later, because the proprioceptive input when handling these items is imperceptible. Stereognosis is then dependent almost entirely on feedback from the cutaneous receptors. Any incorrect localization will also need retraining in order to improve stereognostic function.

Sensation cannot be divorced from movement, so functional activities will help to improve stereognosis, and conversely practical sensory training will improve co-ordination and dexterity of movement. These facts must be utilized in all treatments, whether concentrating on muscle activity or on sensory re-education.

Residual problems of a median nerve lesion may include the permanent lack of hypothenar muscle reinnervation. The resulting loss of normal thumb movement, especially palmar abduction and opposition, may seriously handicap some patients, whilst others may manage without too much difficulty. An opponens transfer can restore function to the thumb, but only if sufficient sensation is present to ensure that an operative procedure will be worthwhile. An alternative to surgery is to make permanent use of a median dynamic splint, which provides some degree of opposition.

Failure of sensory recovery when the skin of the thumb, index and middle fingers remains anaesthetic is an extremely severe disability. At the time of injury, when the gap in the nerve is too great for local mobilization, a section of sural nerve may be used for a graft. Occasionally the ulnar or radial nerve may be sacrificed to graft into the distal portion of the ulnar, but this is an extreme decision to make.

Finally, if sensory recovery does not occur but motor function is good, some neurovascular skin island transfers may be performed using skin with ulnar nerve supply. The donor skin is taken usually from the ring finger and transposed, complete with neurovascular bundles, to thumb and index tips. Unfortunately, it has the effect of transferring the donor localization also. Intensive sensory re-education must be given to correct this localization problem, otherwise the patient will continue to feel that it is the ring finger rather than the index and thumb that is being used, and in consequence will probably not use the hand at all.

Permanent hyperaesthesia is a problem that can often be relieved by the use of TENS. However, if pain remains intense and is not helped by either TENS or guanethidine block, the patient may need to attend a pain clinic for alternative treatments to be considered.

Carpal tunnel syndrome

One of the compression syndromes is compression of the median nerve beneath the flexor retinaculum at the wrist (i.e. in the carpal tunnel). The nerve may be compressed due to a reduction in the diameter of the tunnel, occasionally due to a congenital cause, but most frequently following a fracture of the wrist (acute carpal tunnel syndrome) or from scar formation. It can also occur when the contents and pressure of the tunnel are altered – for example, in the presence of oedema, tumour or synovitis.

The patient usually complains of tingling and discomfort in the radial three digits of the hand, often worse at night, causing the patient to shake the hand to relieve the symptoms. The distribution of symptoms may vary slightly, as anomalies can occur in the median nerve supply in a small proportion of cases.

Should compression of the nerve continue, clumsiness of the hand may be noted (the patient tends to drop things and has difficulty in picking up articles). An increase in sensory loss and possible muscle weakness are also noted, especially of the thenar eminence.

Clinical diagnosis is made on the history and distribution of symptoms. It must be distinguished from symptoms arising from a neck problem or pronator syndrome. Phalan's test, which is holding the wrist in flexion, can aggravate the symptoms, and tapping over the carpal tunnel can produce a positive tunnel test. If a positive diagnosis cannot be made from the clinical picture, nerve conduction studies can be performed.

The syndrome may improve in some patients, for instance during pregnancy. In these cases, conservative treatment such as a cortisone injection and/or a wrist splint may be undertaken.

In cases when the problem persists and the symptoms become more troublesome, surgical intervention should be considered to prevent irreparable damage of the nerve and permanent sensory and muscular impairment. This consists of decompressing the median nerve by releasing the volar carpal ligament.

Post-operative treatment

The wrist is usually rested in a volar splint with the wrist in slight extension until the sutures are removed in order to prevent prolapse of the nerve and adherence to the skin. Following this, the wrist may be mobilized and strengthening exercises given. The eventual outcome is often dependent on the severity of damage to the nerve and the age of the patient, but even in the least severe of cases it is often 2–3 months before full power is regained. If sensory loss has occurred, the patient should be warned regarding protection of the hand from possible injury such as burns or cuts.

Ulnar nerve lesions

Power and stability of the hand, together with co-ordination, are gained to a great extent from the ulnar nerve distribution. Activities such as typing and piano playing are severely affected by an ulnar nerve lesion, owing to the loss of lateral movements of the fingers together with decreased sensory feedback. Inability to elevate the head of the fifth metacarpal and oppose the little finger towards the thumb impairs the power grip considerably, and objects slide through the hand. Loss of stability of the index finger and thumb severely reduces all types of pinch grip, and limits activities such as cutting meat, when the index finger normally steadies and directs the shaft of the knife. The support normally provided for the hand by resting on the little finger also is reduced because the abductor digiti minimi is paralysed and the skin anaesthetic. If patients complain of difficulty in maintaining grasp of a hammer or racquet, it may

be due not only to weakened muscles but also to poor proprioception (Figure 7.17).

The ulnar nerve is most frequently damaged by lacerations at the wrist, often by putting the hand through a window, when tendons and the ulnar artery also are liable to be severed. When the nerve and tendons are sutured it is essential that the artery is repaired and not ligated, as an adequate circulation is necessary to ensure good regeneration of the nerve.

A lesion at the wrist level affects the abductor digiti minimi, flexor and opponens digiti minimi, adductor pollicis, all the interossei, and the lumbricals to the ring and little fingers. The volar surfaces of the little and the adjacent half of the ring finger will become anaesthetic, but sensation on the dorsal aspect, except for the tips of these fingers, will be spared. This is because the dorsal cutaneous branch of the ulnar nerve is given off in the lower third of the forearm and is therefore usually proximal to the laceration. Wasting results in the hypothenar eminence and in the interosseous spaces, and is particularly noticeable in the thumb web. The claw hand deformity gradually develops with the diminishing tone of the paralysed muscles, and the arches flatten. The combined action of the long extensors and the long flexors of the fingers produce extension of the metacarpophalangeal joints and flexion of the interphalangeal joints of the ring and little fingers. As the muscles of these two fingers are unopposed, the claw or intrinsic minus deformity develops. It is the interossei that normally provide flexion of the metacarpophalangeal and extension of the interphalangeal joints. A patient with an ulnar nerve lesion can usually hold the index and middle fingers in this position by using the median-supplied lumbricals, but if their power is tested by giving even the slightest resistance, the fingers will collapse. This helps to endorse the fact that it is the interossei and not the lumbricals that produce this normally powerful intrinsic movement. When the patient is asked to extend the hand and then make a fist, it will be seen that the ring and little fingers move in a clawing fashion. Normally in flexion and extension movements the metacarpophalangeal joints flex at the same time as the interphalangeal joints, and conversely all joints extend together. This helps the fingers to reach around an object as the tips are held away from the palm by the lumbrical action. In an ulnar nerve lesion, the interphalangeal joints of the ring and little fingers flex first, followed by the metacarpophalangeal joints in a rolling movement, which is termed 'rolling flexion'. During extension the metacarpophalangeal joints of the ring and little fingers extend first, and any attempt to extend the interphalangeal joints will result in claw deformity. The normal action of the median-supplied lumbricals will prevent this clawing

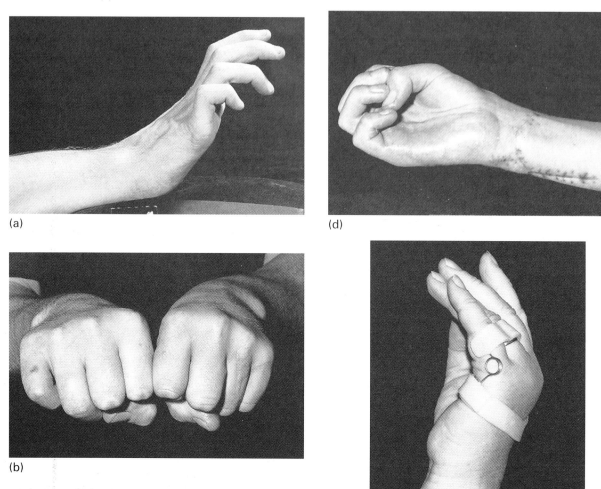

(a)

(b)

(c)

(d)

(e)

Figure 7.17 The classical ulnar nerve lesion (a) showing the claw hand deformity, with (b) flattening of the transverse arches, (c) the inability to flex the MCP joint and extend the IP joint of the ring and little fingers, and (d) the inability to raise the head of the fifth metacarpal in order to oppose the little finger towards the thumb. (e) An anti-claw splint holding the MCP joints in slight flexion, thus allowing extension of the IP joints.

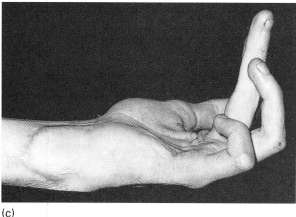

effect on the index and middle fingers. With the paralysis of the hypothenar muscles it becomes impossible to raise the head of the fifth metacarpal and to oppose the little finger towards the thumb.

The trick movements seen in an ulnar nerve lesion include a small amount of abduction and adduction of the fingers, which is possible when performing as a group. Abduction occurs in conjunction with finger extension, and is produced by the extensor digitorum. Adduction, together with some finger flexion, is provided by the flexor digitorum profundus and superficialis. Both abduction and adduction are brought about because of the angles formed by the tendons as they lie over the metacarpophalangeal joints. When the muscles contract, pulling the tendons straight, a lateral movement is produced at all the metacarpophalangeal joints except that of the middle finger. The muscles should therefore be tested not only in a

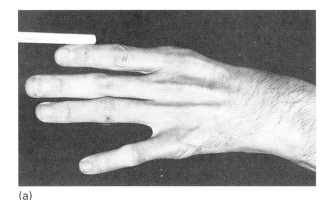

(a)

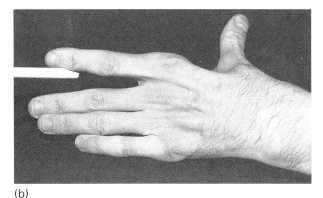

(b)

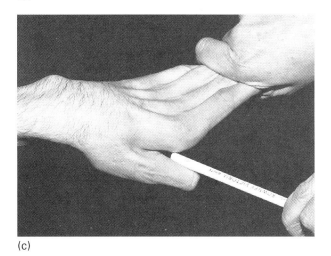

(c)

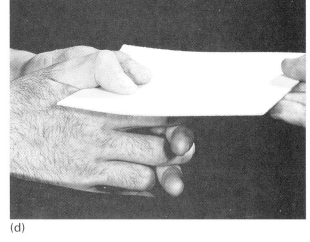

(d)

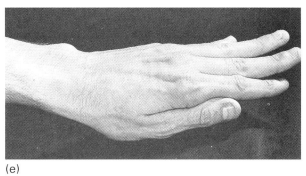

(e)

Figure 7.18 Trick movements of an ulnar nerve lesion demonstrate (and note the tendon action) (a) adduction of the index finger by extensor indicis, (b) abduction of the index finger by the extensor digitorum, and (c) adduction of the thumb by the combined action of the flexor and extensor pollicis longus (note the excessive wasting of the interosseous spaces). (d) Froment's sign demonstrates excessive IP joint flexion of the thumb in order to pinch onto a card. This patient's flexion deformities necessitate the linking of the fingers. (e) Recovery in the same patient some 5 months later, when muscle bulk has returned, the claw deformity has disappeared and thumb adduction has resumed a normal pattern.

group action but also with each finger individually. With the palm resting on the table, the patient is asked to extend and then abduct each finger in turn. In the normal hand it is simple to perform a full lateral movement, whereas with an ulnar nerve lesion it is impossible. However, the index finger may produce just a few degrees of movement by contracting first the extensor indicis followed by the extensor digitorum to the index finger, and contractions of these tendons can be seen over the dorsum of the metacarpophalangeal joint, flicking from one to the other and back again (Figure 7.18).

Any attempt to abduct and adduct the middle finger individually will produce a totally different type of trick movement. The patient will probably be able to move the tip of the middle finger first nearer to the index and then nearer to the ring finger, not by a normal movement but by a lateral shift of the whole palm. When observed carefully, it will be seen that the joints that actually move are the wrist and the metacarpophalangeal joints of the other three fingers. The same trick movement will be seen with the ring finger. In the little finger, however, the presence of two extensor tendons may enable a lateral movement to be performed similar to that seen in the index finger.

A further trick movement is seen when the patient is asked to adduct the thumb. A strong contraction at the same time of both the flexor pollicis longus and the extensor pollicis longus will abduct the thumb. This again is because of the angle of pull of the tendons. Sometimes the patient performs this movement with the thumb extended, and sometimes with it flexed. The extensor tendon jumps over the metacarpophalangeal joint as the thumb adducts, resulting in jerky movement. If pinch grip is tested by using a stiff card while the palms are placed together, normal thumb adduction is replaced by pronounced interphalangeal joint flexion. This is known as Froment's sign. Tip grip is also reduced considerably because of the paralysis of both the adductor pollicis and the first dorsal interosseous muscle; this can be illustrated when an attempt is made to form an 'O' with the index finger and thumb, and the index finger is unable to stabilize itself without fully flexing the proximal interphalangeal joint. This is different from the median nerve lesion, where it is the thumb that is unable to abduct and rotate sufficiently to form the 'O'.

A laceration of the palm may divide the deep branch of the ulnar nerve after it has given off its supply to the abductor digiti minimi and the other hypothenar muscles. The superficial branch supplying the digital nerves may also be involved. Very careful motor and sensory assessments should be performed as early as possible after this type of injury, as nerve damage may easily be overlooked. Surgery, if it is needed to repair the nerve branches, should ideally be performed before too much fibrosis can occur. Compression or constant trauma can also cause damage to both deep and superficial branches of the nerve. The cause should be removed to allow recovery to take place.

Lesions of the nerve around or above the level of the elbow will affect the flexor carpi ulnaris and flexor digitorum profundus to the ring and little fingers, and also those muscles of the hand already discussed. Sensation will be lost over both the dorsal and volar surfaces on the medial side of the hand and fingers.

Initially the claw deformity of the fingers is not so pronounced in a high-level ulnar nerve injury as in a lesion at the wrist, due to the paralysis of the flexor digitorum profundus. At the stage when the flexor digitorum profundus recovers, however, the deformity may worsen.

Recovery in the small muscles of the hand is first indicated at approximately 80 days after injury at the wrist, when the little finger starts to drift into increasing abduction. This is caused by returning activity of the abductor digiti minimi, which is unopposed by the still paralysed interossei. A contraction in the abductor digiti minimi should soon be sufficient to be palpated. Recovery of the interossei and lumbricals is often rather poor, and individual abduction and adduction of the fingers rarely fully return. The claw deformity gradually decreases, however, and a more normal flexion and extension pattern of the fingers can be observed. If the physiotherapist places the ring and little fingers with the metacarpophalangeal joints flexed and interphalangeal joints extended, the patient may be able to hold them in position for a second or two before the fingers collapse. Adduction of the thumb will take on a more normal pattern of movement, and lose its jerky trick action.

Therapy

Physiotherapy in the early stages is concerned with maintaining the mobility of the joints and soft tissues. It is important that the claw deformity is stretched out regularly, that the arches are maintained passively and the webs stretched. A dynamic splint that will prevent hyperextension of the metacarpophalangeal joints of the ring and little fingers should be worn (Wynn Parry, 1981), or a very efficient static one. If these joints are stabilized in very slight flexion, the extensor digitorum is able to pull through and extend the interphalangeal joints. The patient can thus correct their own claw deformity by means of the splint, but should not be expected to wear one that is clumsy (Figure 7.17e).

As much time as is suitable should be spent in re-educating the affected muscles when recovery is seen. Facilitation techniques help to maximize function in these small muscles, which may, until sensory feedback is applied, appear to be inactive. Approximation given through the metacarpophalangeal joints when positioning them in some flexion and through the interphalangeal joints when placing them in extension make the patient more aware of the position he or she is trying to hold. Lateral movements of the fingers and opposition of the little finger towards the thumb should be facilitated by use of stretch. At first the muscles can only contract in their outer range; the range and power will improve slowly over the following weeks. Short bursts of intensive treatment repeated fairly frequently have been found to be more effective than a continuous but minimal degree of physiotherapy.

Sensation in the ulnar distribution is regarded as far less important than that in the median distribution, and this is relevant for the cutaneous supply. Reduced proprioception from an ulnar nerve lesion can however be severely disabling; therefore, exercises and functional movements should be given with this in mind. Activities should be designed to help maximize the sensory feedback, and typing and playing of those musical instruments that need finger control are particularly suitable. Speed can be gradually increased as ability improves. Support of the hand by resting the little finger on the table enables intricate movements of the thumb, index and middle fingers to be performed, and this support is dependent on both cutaneous and proprioceptive feedback from the little finger. In the very early stages, the patient must be warned not to let the anaesthetic little finger drop onto a hot iron etc. Localization should be tested and retrained if necessary when sensation returns.

Residual problems of an ulnar nerve lesion, when regeneration is poor, include a permanent claw hand deformity affecting the ring and little fingers. This may reduce the patient's ability to perform work and leisure activities. Tendon transfers and other surgical techniques are designed to correct this deformity. If the abductor digiti minimi recovers but the interossei do not, the little finger may remain permanently abducted even when at rest and can get in the way during functional activities. This disability may also need to be corrected by surgery.

Combined median and ulnar nerve lesions

When both median and ulnar nerves are involved, the effects of each individual lesion combine to produce an extremely severe disability. The disability is more severe with the lesion at a high level, when all the flexors of wrist and digits are affected and grasp becomes totally absent. It is inevitable that when both nerves are divided at wrist level there will also be tendon injuries, combined frequently with division of arteries and possibly the joint capsule. The resulting scarring and fibrosis following bleeding will cause loss of tissue elasticity and the formation of adhesions between skin, tendons, nerves and sometimes the deeper structures of the joints. Ischaemia of the muscles may also occur following arterial damage.

The deformity that results is the totally flat claw hand (Figure 7.19). The intrinsic minus deformity will develop, with gross hyperextension of the metacarpophalangeal joints if no support is given to prevent their overmobility. This deformity can be extremely painful due to the stretch on capsule and ligaments. Forward thrust of fingers and thumb will be completely lost, and rolling flexion of the fingers will become pronounced. Sensation will be absent on the whole of the volar surface and over the dorsal surfaces of the tips of all fingers, and over the volar surface of the thumb. The autonomic effects will be visible in the same distribution, with a noticeable loss of pulp and subcutaneous tissue. Trick movements will be identical with those of the individual nerve lesions. Patients with combined lesions at a high level, however, may be able to flex the wrist, although all the muscles considered to be wrist or finger flexors are paralysed. Flexion is possible because the tendon of the abductor pollicis longus, with its radial nerve supply, lies immediately anterior to the fulcrum of the wrist joint. A tenodesis action is also demonstrated when the patient attempts to flex the fingers. The increased tension of the finger flexors produced by hyperextending the wrist will produce a small amount of passive finger flexion.

Therapy

Physiotherapy is again involved with maintaining the range of the joints, the elasticity of the soft tissues and an adequate circulation. Counselling and instruction on the care of the hand, especially of the anaesthetic areas, must be thorough. Dynamic splinting that will prevent the deformity from becoming gross, enable the patient to extend the fingers and improve function should be arranged. Pain must also be treated before it becomes intractable.

However, it is the associated problems of fibrosis and adhesions of scarring that will probably need the greatest intensity of treatment. The physiotherapist should be involved immediately after surgery in the elevation of the hand and arm to help prevent oedema, and in the movement of available joints and muscles, which will also ensure the best possible circulation in the limb. Surgeons will have differing criteria for commencement of active movement, but delay after 3 weeks will allow tissues to become extremely fibrotic. Early activity, however, must be gentle and be increased gradually, as too energetic a treatment will cause a renewed release of fibrinogen. Early passive stretching is totally contraindicated for this reason, besides putting an undesirable stretch on a sutured nerve.

The intensity of treatment must again be increased when reinnervation occurs. It is unlikely that recovery can ever be total following such a severe injury, and therefore it is imperative to maximize both motor and sensory functions. Repeated assessment of function is advisable over the following year. This applies particularly to sensory function, as it is this more than poor motor function that is likely to prove most disabling. Sessions of sensory training lasting for a week or so every 3–4 months are found to be of the greatest value until nerve recovery is complete.

The residual problems of combined lesions are the same as in the separate median and ulnar nerve lesions, further complicated by the greater degree of associated injuries. A gross hyperextension deformity of all four fingers may remain if reinnervation is poor, but this can be corrected by a superficialis transfer into the capsules of the metacarpophalangeal joints. Both the flexor digitorum superficialis and profundus must contract efficiently, however, before this procedure should be considered.

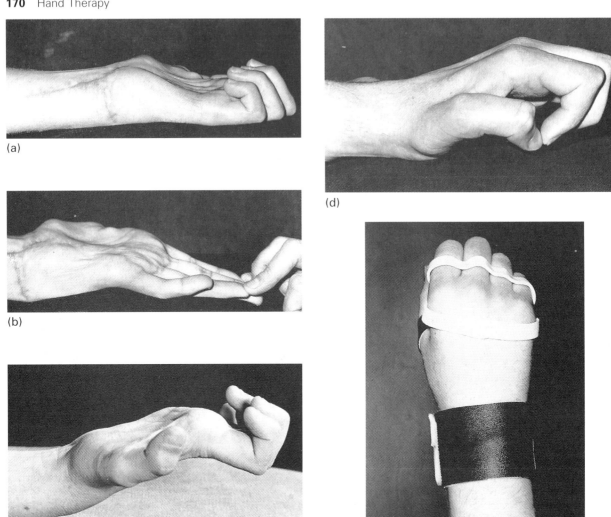

Figure 7.19 The combined median and ulnar nerve lesion (a) demonstrating a totally flat hand with claw deformity. Finger extension could be corrected passively (b) but not actively (c). (d) Total inability to thrust forward the thumb and fingertips towards one another. (e) Correction by an anti-claw splint including an opposition Kleinert for the thumb.

ISCHAEMIC CONTRACTURES

These contractures, which result from vascular impairment, may be caused by road traffic accidents, industrial injuries and gunshot wounds. Another fairly common cause is tight plasters, which constrict the arterial flow and, if not removed quickly, result in damage to the muscles and occasionally also to the nerves and skin.

A contracture may not on initial observation be instantly obvious, but nevertheless it can be severely disabling to the patient. The normal function of the hand, especially when intricate movements are involved, can only be achieved by the combined action of the long extrinisic and small intrinsic muscles. Ischaemia can cause extensive

fibrosis, when the muscles will be unable either to contract efficiently or extend fully. Moreover, there will be an impairment of proprioception, which is especially disabling when the intrinsic muscles are involved.

Volkmann's ischaemic contracture affects the muscles of the forearm, usually the flexors only, but with a severe injury it may also involve the extensors. Contractures of the long flexors will prevent full and simultaneous extension of the wrist, fingers and thumb. When the wrist is flexed, however, the fingers and thumb will usually be able to extend. Conversely, as the wrist extends, the contracture of the flexors will passively pull the fingers and thumb into a greater degree of flexion, which is a form of tenodesis action. Contracture of

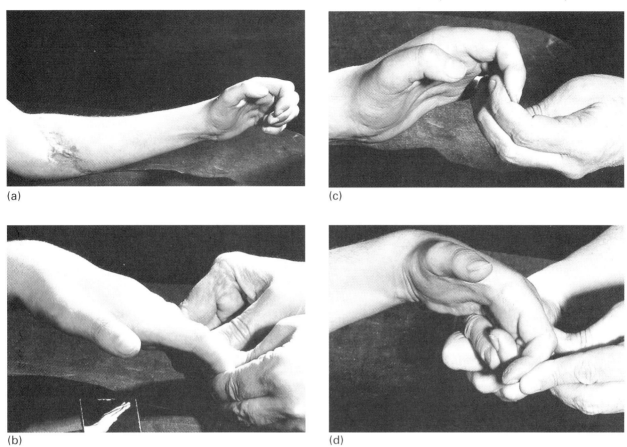

Figure 7.20 (a) Patient with severe Volkmann's contracture affecting both flexors and extensors. (b) Passive extension of the fingers is achieved only when the wrist is flexed. (c) As the wrist is extended, the fingers are pulled into flexion. (d) Neither active nor passive flexion of the wrist or fingers simultaneously is possible due to the contracture of the extensors.

the extensor muscles will prevent full flexion of wrist, fingers and thumb simultaneously. The involvement of both flexors and extensors will therefore limit function severely (Figure 7.20).

Vascular injury at the wrist or in the hand may cause ischaemia, leading to fibrosis of the intrinsic muscles and thus producing an intrinsic contracture. The muscles, when severely contracted, cause the metacarpophalangeal joints to be held in flexion together with the interphalangeal joints in extension. The reverse of this position, i.e. a combination of metacarpophalangeal joint extension and interphalangeal joint flexion, will be impossible to achieve, even with a strong passive stretch. When the thenar muscles are affected the thumb becomes clamped tightly across the palm, close to the fingers. Virtually no thumb movement may be possible, and moreover the thumb will be in the way of finger flexion; this combines to limit hand function almost entirely.

A complication of severe ischaemia may be nerve damage, causing motor and sensory loss. The circulation of the hand will therefore be affected by both the direct vascular damage and by the autonomic involvement. It is essential that the patient is warned concerning the need to protect the hand and keep it warm in cold weather.

Assessment for contractures should include an observation of the hand and forearm at rest, and of the affected hand compared with the contralateral limb. Particular note should be made of the position of the fingers and thumb and of both dorsal and volar surfaces of the joints. The following tests should then be performed to identify, or eliminate, the presence of contractures:

1. To identify a contracture of the long flexors, the patient is asked to extend the wrist, fingers and thumb as far as possible simultaneously. The Salter scale can be used to measure the excursion of movement (see Chapter 2). A mild contracture will only prevent movement into the full outer range; however, it may be sufficiently severe that it prevents the muscles from being extended further than mid-range. The physiotherapist should therefore apply over-pressure in order to

feel how much the movement is restricted and to eliminate lack of range as a result of muscle weakness or paralysis. The active movement combining wrist, finger and thumb flexion should also be examined. A comparison should be made with the range of the contralateral limb, and a note made of any restrictions that may be caused by adherent scars or stiff joints.

2. To identify a contracture of the long extensors, the patient is asked to flex the wrist, fingers and thumb at the same time. Over-pressure is then given by the physiotherapist to feel the degree of contracture. The range of wrist flexion is measured when the fingers are flexed. Adherence of scars, weakness of movement and the amount of active extension available should again be tested and compared with the contralateral limb.

3. To identify a possible intrinsic contracture, the patient is asked first to flex then extend all the metacarpophalangeal and interphalangeal joints together. A really severe intrinsic contracture will prevent full metacarpophalangeal joint extension, so this movement needs to be tested passively and in isolation by the therapist. The range should be recorded. Secondly, the patient is requested to keep the interphalangeal joints flexed whilst attempting to extend the metacarpophalangeal joints. Over-pressure should again be given by the physiotherapist to feel the extent of any contracture.

4. To identify thenar muscle contractures, the patient is asked to first extend and then abduct the thumb as fully as possible. The therapist should also apply over-pressure in order to test these movements passively.

Therapy

Scarring from the injury may have impaired the venous and lymphatic return, therefore early attention will be needed to reduce any resulting oedema. Scars, when soundly healed, should be given a stretching massage using a bland cream as the medium. Exercise with its pumping action should then follow. When oedema is present, all treatments should be given in elevation.

Contractures of the forearm flexors should be stretched, the therapist gradually increasing and sustaining the pull on the muscles and at the same time watching the effect on the patient. The physiotherapist should apply the stretch with one hand whilst supporting the mobile joints with the other to prevent any hyperextension. This procedure will probably be uncomfortable, but should never be so extreme that it is painful. The movements should never be jerky, as they might cause further damage to the fibrosed muscle fibres. During the subsequent weeks of treatment, the aim is to achieve full and simultaneous extension of the wrist and fingers.

Active exercises follow the stretch regime; the patient must be able actively to maintain the increased range obtained passively by the therapist. If the long flexor muscles have become extremely contracted, it is the extensors especially that will need strengthening. PNF techniques are a suitable means by which to achieve both lengthening and strengthening effects.

Patients should attend for several sessions a day; if these are held early and late in the morning and again in the afternoon, the contractures will be treated with sufficient intensity. After the first morning and afternoon sessions, the patient should use the hand functionally to make full use of any gained movement. After the last session, a stretch splint that will maintain the hand and wrist in the maximum stretched position should be applied for an hour. The splint should extend from mid-forearm to just beyond the fingertips. At night the patient should wear a splint that maintains a comfortable but optimum position.

For intrinsic contractures, the aim is to obtain simultaneous extension of the metacarpophalangeal joints and flexion of the interphalangeal joints. The stretch towards this claw position of the hand should be applied gradually and be followed by strong active exercise for the flexors digitorum profundus and superficialis. The metacarpophalangeal joints should be held in as much extension as possible. A palmar splint which extends distally just beyond the metacarpophalangeal joints but not as far as the proximal interphalangeal joints will allow the interphalangeal joints to be flexed over the end and be bandaged down firmly. It may also be used when exercising the long flexors of the fingers.

Because the intrinsic muscles are so small, they are less likely to respond to the stretching procedures than the forearm muscles. Any residual and disabling contractures of either the long flexors or intrinsics may need a surgical release and tendon transfer procedure to improve hand function.

CRUSH INJURIES

These injuries are probably the most severely disabling to the hand, mainly due to the resulting fibrosis of the soft tissues. Every feasible type of complication may be present, including:

1. Arterial or venous damage, needing an anastomosis or graft. A ligation is not a desirable technique, but is still frequently practised.
2. Soft tissue damage, requiring excision of any non-viable muscle and skin. The resulting oedema with its release of fibrinogen can cause extensive fibrosis and stiffness.
3. Fractures and joint disruption, requiring immobilization.
4. Skin loss and degloving, requiring coverage to prevent infection and loss of tissue fluid.

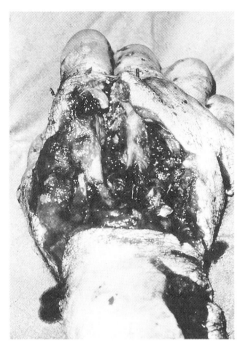

Figure 7.21 A severe crush injury affecting all tissues.

5. Nerve injury, needing repair by suture or a grafting procedure.
6. Tendon or muscle damage, requiring a primary or secondary repair or graft. Tendon transfers may be necessary later.
7. Amputation, either immediately in extremely severe cases or later because of developing necrosis.

The most urgent need is to ensure adequate vascularization, as otherwise the viability of the limb or part will be at risk. This is followed by immobilization of fractures and dislocations and provision of skin coverage (Figure 7.21).

Therapy
Active physiotherapy may be precluded during the first few days. This is usually the case when skin loss has occurred and grafts are necessary to provide skin cover.

Fractures are usually immobilized using K-wires or A-O plating techniques, and primary suture of tendons and nerves is undertaken. This often allows for early active movement or a passive motion regime, as joint mobility is of prime importance.

Should the hand or individual joints need to be immobilized, correct positioning into the 'safe' position, with the hand and arm elevated to reduce oedema, is essential. The positioning will ensure that the fingertip and thumb approximation will be functional, even though limitation of other movements may persist. The hand must never be allowed to remain fully extended, as it may well become 'frozen' in this position and be totally non-functional.

All methods should be utilized to reduce the oedema (Figure 7.22), and gentle active movements should, whenever possible, be commenced within the first 2–3 days of injury. Closed environmental therapy (CET), which blows sterile air at high pressure into the encompassing plastic bag, can be useful as it allows the hand to move inside the bag. This early active treatment must be agreed with the surgeon initially. Pulsed electromagnetic fields should be used when available; they can be given through dressings and even plaster of Paris, and are effective in reducing fibrosis and assisting the healing process. Ice and ultrasonics can also be used on accessible areas of skin.

The intensity of treatment should be increased as quickly as possible during the first few weeks, and full-time rehabilitation instituted if a stiff hand is developing. Pneumotherapy will help to reduce the oedema when the skin is healed, and massage and all active and passive treatments including accessory movements should be given with the hand in an elevated position. Treatment should continue throughout the day if a satisfactory result is to be achieved.

Passive stretching is necessary when the range remains limited, and particularly when active movement is still not possible. Initially the stretch should be applied gently and gradually. A strong stretch must be delayed until 7 or 8 weeks after injury, otherwise an exacerbation of fibrosis will result. Stretch splinting, following the physiotherapist's manual stretch, may then be introduced. Thermoplastic materials are suitable to use.

Thumb and finger webs are liable to contract, and will need active and passive stretching to prevent or correct any deformity. C-splints will help to maintain a stretch of the webs if applied when resting, together with a resting C-splint worn at night.

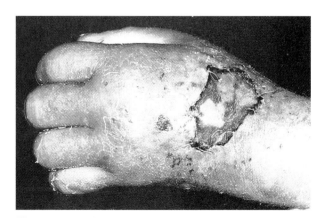

Figure 7.22 A crush injury showing severe oedema.

The priority in the plan to provide maximum hand function is to regain joint range in the following order:

1. Full metacarpophalangeal joint flexion and simultaneous interphalangeal joint extension together with palmar abduction of the thumb to ensure finger to thumb tip function and lateral pinch.
2. Flexion of the interphalangeal joints to give flexion of fingertips to palm, thus providing grasp.
3. Full and simultaneous extension of all the metacarpophalangeal and interphalangeal joints to enable the fingers to stretch and grasp around and release an object. Extension and ulnar deviation together with pronation and supination are the more essential movements of the wrist, and should be regained concurrently with movements of the fingers and thumb.

Range should be constantly monitored to ensure that a gain in one direction is not made at the expense of a loss in another. Passive range of joints is the most essential function. If active movement does not recover, there are usually surgical procedures that can be considered later and might return some function to the hand.

Severe crush injuries are likely to need several weeks or months of intensive treatment, and even then some patients are extremely unlikely to recover fully. Short-session treatments, even daily, cannot achieve a good functional result, as by the time the patient has arrived home the hand condition is usually back to where it started that morning. Full-time treatment in a rehabilitation unit is most likely to achieve the best functional result for the patient.

REPLANTATION

This term is used when the hand or digit is completely severed from the arm. If there are any structures whatsoever remaining in continuity, the term used is revascularization.

On admission, these patients should be very carefully assessed. It is essential that they understand the long-term rehabilitation and the possibility of reconstruction. Any patient unwilling to return frequently for hand therapy should be considered unsuitable.

It is not always possible to replant the severed part, especially if it has been crushed. However, to regain good function, attempts should be made to re-attach the thumb and at least one finger to create a pinch grip. If the thumb has sustained so much damage that it cannot be replaced, consideration should be given to replanting one of the fingers in its place.

When analysed, this injury is a combination of fractures with tendon, nerve and blood vessel damage. Good fixation of the fractures, leaving the joints free to be mobilized, is vital. The aim of treatment is to maintain joint mobility in the early stage whilst trying to protect the other structures that have been repaired.

Physiotherapy and splintage commences once the blood supply is stable. This may be as early as 24 hours post-surgery.

All earlier mentioned techniques for reducing pain and swelling are used and, in addition, Duran's passive motion regime, in which isolated passive motion of each joint is undertaken. Gross movements are not performed in the early stages, as both flexors and extensors have been repaired; gross flexion would result in undue tension being applied to the repair site of the extensors, thus causing the possibility of rupture, and gross extension *vice versa*. At about 8 weeks post-surgery, most repaired structures should be strong enough to allow some passive stretching and resisted exercises.

It should be remembered that soft tissue may have lost length at the time of injury and surgery, and also contracts during maturation of the scar tissue. Therefore, passive stretch and dynamic and/or serial splinting will be necessary. At this stage, the patient will start functional activities. It is interesting to note that these patients may have very good active motion, but function is limited by the nerve injury. If the replant is a just a digit the deficit will be sensory only; however, replantation around the wrist area will affect the small muscles of the hand as well as sensation.

During the later stages of rehabilitation, appropriate strengthening and sensory education should be included in the treatment regime.

Secondary surgery may be necessary if tendons rupture or become adherent, and tendon transfers are necessary due to the nerve damage. This is not usually undertaken until the hand is soft, supple and mobile.

AMPUTATIONS

Direct trauma can cause varying degrees of finger or hand amputation, and the resulting disability will depend largely on the site of amputation together with the effects of any other tissue damage. Some patients have the motivation and ability to overcome their problems better than others, and manage to achieve remarkable function despite loss of digits.

Whole hand amputation is a devastating disability for the patients. Activity may be possible to a certain extent by the use of a prosthesis, but sensory function is totally irreplaceable. With the advances in modern surgery, replantation is succeeding more frequently. Its main advantage is the retention of some sensation, besides improved function and cosmetic affect. Amputation can cause severe psychological upset.

Causes

Causes of amputation include trauma from road or industrial accidents, gunshot wounds and blast injuries. Circular saws are a particularly common cause of accidents to carpenters, resulting in loss of part of the hand or fingers. Surgical amputation may become a necessity in older people because of the effects of a circulatory disorder. It may very occasionally be considered the only solution for the total paralysis of a limb or for the residual deformity of a finger. The procedure should be implemented only when all other methods have failed and the patient particularly desires this course of action.

Sites of amputation

Loss of the thumb causes incapacitating dysfunction to the hand, and it is essential that some pollicization technique is performed if the amputated thumb cannot be replanted. In multiple amputation of digits including the thumb, it may be possible to replant one of the amputated fingers in the thumb position. Later, a great or second toe, or alternatively a ring or index finger, may be pollicized. Usually a digit from the same hand is transposed together with its neurovascular supply. Therefore, not only will the hand need retraining in movement but the location of sensation will also need intensive re-education (Figure 7.23).

Amputation of the index finger alone is not severely disabling in most cases because the middle finger has the ability to replace index function. Hand activity can be effectively retained when the patient has a normal thumb remaining, unless he or she practises such skills as typing or piano playing.

Amputation of several fingers will inevitably produce a far more serious disability, as the greater the number of amputated digits, the greater the loss of function. Little finger amputation may cause difficulty to those persons who need to use the dynamic tripod position (e.g. for writing, painting or other delicate and precise movements with the hands), as the little finger normally supports the hand during this activity.

For those needing power grasp it is better that a portion of the finger is retained, amputating, if it becomes a necessity, immediately proximal to the head of the proximal phalanx. Cosmetically this is not as noticeable as may be anticipated, as the fingers usually rest in the flexed position and the loss of the distal part of the finger is therefore not too obvious. For women who are very concerned about the cosmetic effect, the amputation of the index or little fingers may be shaped obliquely, immediately proximal to the head of the metacarpal. Removal by filleting of the whole of the metacarpal of middle or ring fingers, and the subsequent closing-in of any residual gap, will leave a slightly weakened but cosmetically improved hand. The residual disability of this procedure, especially in the early post-operative weeks, is that coins and small objects slip through the gap between the fingers.

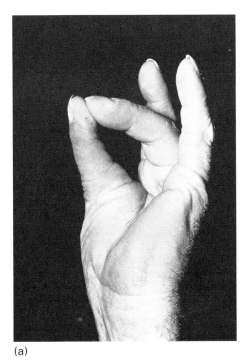

(a)

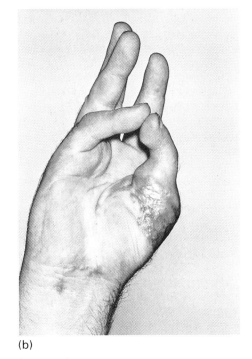

(b)

Figure 7.23 (a) Pollicization using a ring finger. (b) Toe to thumb transplant.

Therapy

A straightforward traumatic or surgical amputation should heal quickly and need relatively little early physiotherapy. However, amputations as the result of blast, crush injuries or gunshot wounds, with their extensive soft tissue damage, will need far more intensive treatment to ensure maximum mobility of the hand (see Crush injuries).

The hand and arm must be elevated to reduce oedema, whatever the extent of the amputation and whether the patient is in bed or ambulant. Adjacent joints should be kept mobile by gentle, active and, if necessary, assisted movements usually commenced the day following surgery. Early movements should be given to increase the range of the joints towards the 'safe' position in particular. Tendon activity should be aimed primarily at regaining flexion of the fingers, before extension is achieved.

Psychologically, especially initially, the loss of fingers or part or whole of the hand can be very traumatic, and for some time the patient will probably suffer a degree of shock. A sympathetic but increasingly positive approach should be made by the therapist, pointing out the ability of the hand to adapt to the situation. Photographs that demonstrate the function other patients have achieved are enormously useful at this stage. Function can become remarkably efficient, even with the loss of fingers, when the patient makes a determined effort to overcome the disability.

Tenderness of the stump is likely to be experienced following the amputation. As the healing continues and the stump settles, an increase in contact between stump and objects must be encouraged, commencing with handling and gentle tapping by the therapist's fingers. It must be ensured that the patient actually uses the end of the stump, as the sensory input will help to lessen any tender or painful sensations. The tenderness will be worse with a poor suture line, particularly when it is badly positioned, and also if the amputated nerve ends become tethered to the skin, bone or underlying tissue. Adhesions should be loosened by massage, and TENS used to reduce any pain and discomfort whilst also allowing the patient to use the stump more freely.

Phantom awareness is another symptom that most patients experience following amputation; however, only a small proportion (5–10 per cent) will suffer phantom pain for long, when it may either be continual or spasmodic. It is likely to be more severe if the hand or finger could not be saved due to the extent of primary injury. If the patient suffers pain prior to amputation, the pain patterns may continue as phantom pain after surgery. Established pain should therefore be eliminated if at all possible prior to amputation.

TENS is effective in curing longstanding phantom limb pain, and can also be used to prevent that pain from occurring. It should be commenced the day following operation to inhibit the establishment of pain patterns. The electrodes should be placed over the appropriate nerve trunk, and the optimum position may be discovered by changing the position of the electrodes during the first few days. Accurate records of positioning must therefore be kept.

Distraction by becoming absorbed in some occupation is one of the best ways of forgetting pain, and this is of particular relevance for those suffering from phantom pain. The advantage of having a good occupational therapy department for the patient with this type of problem cannot be stressed too strongly.

Temporary prostheses made in the workshop of occupational therapy departments can improve function considerably, and need not be complicated. For example, a prosthesis to provide extra length to a shortened digit can make a required activity, such as typing, possible. It is a great advantage if the patient helps to design and work on his or her own prosthesis. Thermoplastics are useful materials that can be fastened to the patient with leather and Velcro™ fastenings. Attachments for holding tools can be fixed into the material.

If there is loss of the whole hand, a prosthesis must be requested from the nearest limb fitting centre. Adequate training in its use and suitable attachments will be made available at the centre. Cosmetic hands and fingers, with excellent shape and likeness to the normal hand, are also available from the limb fitting centres. These must be offered to the patient, as appearing in public with an obvious amputation is psychologically traumatic to most people.

Complications

The main complications after amputation, besides the loss of function, usually concern the severance of peripheral nerves. The axons, following the initial Wallerian degeneration, commence to sprout in an attempt to discover their endoneural tubes. With the distal nerve amputated their search is abortive, with the result that they turn in many directions and form a demyelinated neuroma.

Most neuromata are non-symptomatic, but any problems will depend mainly on local factors. Gross scarring with contracting fibrous tissue formation is considered the most likely cause of a troublesome neuroma. Careful resection of the nerve at the time of amputation and provision of the nerve end with a good tissue bed is the best way of preventing later symptoms. Surgery, with transportation of the nerve to an adjacent site that is free of scarring and less liable to trauma, is sometimes undertaken, but the results have proved extremely disappointing.

Desensitization Gentle tapping, at first in an area surrounding the neuroma and gradually approaching the tender spot until right over it, will frequently improve and occasionally relieve all painful symptoms. Patients must be shown how to continue the tapping for themselves, as ongoing treatment may be needed. A vibrator provides a gentle method of commencing this treatment in extremely painful cases, and the use of TENS may allow the therapist to perform the vibration or tapping more comfortably. It should be used for several hours of the day, with the electrodes sited over the section of the nerve proximal to its neuroma. Patients must be encouraged to use their amputated stump as normally as possible, as pain is likely to increase if there is inadequate sensory input to the affected area. A padded splint or leather cuff may be effective in protecting a painful neuroma.

Extremely tender or hyperpathic areas adjacent to the line of incision may produce severe stump pain. TENS and pressure splinting or elasticated garments can help to reduce this problem by the input of normal sensory stimuli and utilization of the pain-gate theory. Revision of the stump may eventually have to be considered.

Severe and longstanding phantom limb pain can frequently be reduced by the use of TENS, and it has been know to completely eliminate phantom pain after 50 years of continuous duration. A determined effort must be made by the rehabilitation team not only to reduce the pain but also to return the patient to work as soon as possible. Intellectual occupation, which provides an increase of central inhibition of the pain pathways, is probably one of the most effective means of phantom pain control.

COMPLEX REGIONAL PAIN SYNDROME

This condition, known also as Sudeck's atrophy, algodystrophy, reflex sympathetic dystrophy or post-traumatic sympathetic dystrophy, can result in a severe problem that is often far worse than the initial injury itself.

Why this extreme response occurs in some people yet not in others is still not fully understood, and studies by psychologists have shown no consistent pattern of personality involvement. What is absolutely certain is that it must be treated instantly and urgently in order to prevent it from becoming an acute problem that is difficult to cure.

The main signs and symptoms include:

- oedema
- pain that is far more severe than can be anticipated for the underlying condition
- excessive sweating at first
- colour and temperature changes
- osteoporosis shown on X-ray
- unwillingness to move the hand
- excess hair growth.

At first, the hand becomes hot and swollen with pronounced sweating. The patient will probably dislike both using the hand and having it touched. These signs and symptoms worsen if the condition is not treated, becoming more acutely painful in particular. There may be two kinds of pain; a spontaneous burning pain and hyperpathia, the acutely painful response to touch.

Eventually the skin will change to become dry, shiny and cold, with a cyanosed colour (Figure 7.24). Porosis will show on X-ray, and severe pain persists; however, osteoporosis alone is not sufficient evidence to make the diagnosis of a sympathetic dystrophy, as it occurs from most severe hand injuries without any of the other signs and symptoms being present.

Stiffness will inevitably result if the oedema and pain persist and the patient over-protects and does not use the hand. This disuse will also lead to muscle weakness.

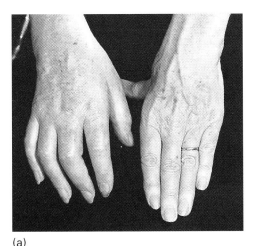 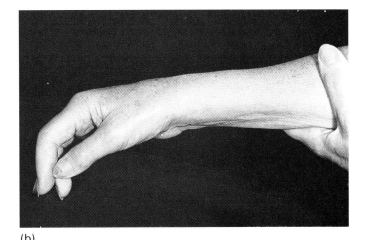

(a)   (b)

Figure 7.24 (a) Typical appearance of a hand suffering from complex regional pain syndrome, demonstrating swelling, shiny skin and the inability to fully extend the fingers, and (b) the inability to flex the fingers.

Therapy can be beneficial in reducing pain in a proportion of cases. It may need to be combined with guanethidine blocks when the pain is particularly severe or, if this does not succeed, a stellate ganglia block. A sympathectomy may eventually be necessary for those who do not respond to either form of treatment.

Therapy

Physiotherapy and occupational therapy are invaluable both in the prevention of this disorder and in its reversal during the very early stages. Later, if it has become established, it is a more difficult condition to treat successfully.

When immobilization is necessary, prevention may be possible by the correct positioning of the hand in the 'safe' position, together with immediate active exercising of all available joints. Bombardment both peripherally and centrally by performing interesting functional activities will all help to retain normal sympathetic responses. Frequent checks should be made during the first few weeks following any injury or surgery that no dystrophy is developing. The patient must be warned to report immediately if the hand develops any of the recognized symptoms.

If a dystrophy does develop, all means must be used to reverse the condition quickly. If the hand has had to be immobilized in a plaster of Paris cylinder, it is advisable, if at all possible, that the cylinder is replaced with one made from a material that can be immersed in water. As most of the initial effects of the dystrophy are sympathetic by nature, it makes sense to treat the problem as far as possible by using methods that normally affect sympathetic function – e.g. by contrast baths, which produce a vasodilation followed by a vasoconstriction in response to the changes of temperature. The cylinder should be replaced as early as possible by a splint that can be removed to allow free active exercising under supervision.

Elevation, with use of iced towels, is imperative when oedema is present, as its reduction will assist in decreasing pain and improving mobility, besides preventing the development of fibrosis. The swollen hand and digit are made rigid by the excess fluid content, which can also be extremely painful. The continuing use of contrast baths and introduction of ice dips, when found acceptable by the patient, will help to reduce the swelling.

NB: Interferential treatment has been found to increase the oedema that results from sympathetic dysfunction. PEME and ultrasound are therefore preferable when treating pain and swelling if a dystrophy is suspected.

Patients must be encouraged to touch their affected hand or finger with the normal, contralateral hand. Gentle active (but never passive) movements should be performed as fully as possible without causing extreme pain. These treatments

may be helped by the use of TENS to reduce the pain and discomfort. Electrodes should be positioned proximal to the affected part, over the appropriate nerve trunks. Dual output stimulators are therefore recommended.

When patients can touch their hand themselves, they must allow the therapist also to touch the painful area. They should then start moving their hand over different surfaces, using increasing pressure. Tapping movements onto first soft and then harder surfaces, clapping hands, playing pat-a-cake, etc. should be commenced when possible.

If guanethidine blocks are introduced because of continuing pain, they must be followed immediately (while the pain relief lasts) by similar treatment methods for reducing oedema and increasing activity. The blocks may need to be repeated several times if the effect is encouraging but short-lived. Therapists will probably need to urge and encourage patients in order to recover full range, especially if they have protected a painful hand for some time.

When the pain is under reasonable control, the strength of activity should be increased. Accessory movements of the joints and gentle passive stretching should be given within the limits of pain, when there is residual stiffness. The occupational therapy department plays a large role, as stress must be laid increasingly on functional activities.

Severely painful hands can improve suddenly and dramatically, and in the majority of these cases motivation appears to be the important factor. Patients usually explain the improvement as stemming from their own determination to use their hand. For those that do not improve, a stellate ganglia block may be necessary.

If joint range and soft tissue length can be retained during the acute period, patients usually regain good function.

DUPUYTREN'S CONTACTURE

Dupuytren's contracture is a relatively common condition in the Anglo-Saxon race (McCallum and Hueston, 1962), especially in those over the age of 65 years, and occurs 10 times more frequently in men than in women. It is a disorder of collagen, when the fascia underlying the skin becomes thickened and fibrotic, but the cause of the condition remains unknown. The fascia later contracts, thereby causing a flexion deformity to develop in the fingers and occasionally in the thumb.

Physiotherapy plays a relatively limited role in conservative management of this condition. The maximum joint range may be preserved for some time by teaching patients how to stretch their own contractures and by the application of a stretch splint, but in no way can this treatment prevent the eventual advance of the disease. It is therefore essential that patients consult an experienced surgeon before the joint contractures become irreversible. Muscle power should be maintained to facilitate activity both pre- and post-operatively.

Post-operative treatment

Following a fasciotomy, when the affected tissue has been resected, a compression bandage is applied over the dressing and the hand is elevated to prevent oedema. Surgical techniques, post-operative management, the positioning and the duration of immobilization can vary considerably. Usually the hand is placed in as full extension as possible, but sometimes the metacarpophalangeal joints are positioned in flexion for a few days with the interphalangeal joints in nearly full extension, and a night splint is made to maintain the extension gained at operation. Some surgeons prefer the open-palm technique when skin closure is difficult, as this allows drainage and prevents the formation of haematomas (McCash, 1964). Skin grafting or the transportation of a flap may be necessary; it is found that a recurrence of this disorder rarely occurs directly under the graft (Harrison and Morris, 1975).

Exercise must be given to the shoulder and elbow, as this will help to maintain both the circulation of the limb and the mobility of the joints. With the agreement of the surgeon, active movement of the hand usually commences 2–3 days after surgery unless skin grafting has been performed. The padding is removed to allow movement, and gentle active extension in particular, and flexion and abduction exercises are given to the fingers and thumb. Opposition of the thumb towards each individual finger should be gently performed. Special attention must be paid to any oedema that may have occurred. Massage to the fingers and active movements are found to be the most effective treatment to reduce any swelling.

After a few days, when the hand is redressed following exercise, a splint is applied to position the fingers in the optimum degree of extension that can be held comfortably. Stretch must not be applied at this stage. Treatment is repeated several times daily, gradually gaining a little more extension, with the splint being altered accordingly.

After 1 week, more emphasis is placed on regaining full finger flexion. The stitches are removed on about the tenth day when, if the healing is satisfactory, the tempo of treatment may be increased.

Healing of the scars may be slow, especially if the condition was advanced prior to surgery. Ultrasonics, saline soaks, massage around the area and active movements will all help to stimulate the circulation and improve healing.

After 2–3 weeks, any adherent scars should be massaged with a bland cream and treated with ultrasound. If the surrounding area is particularly thickened and indurated, a small thermoplastic splint, moulded directly to the part, should be bandaged firmly on to the healed scar and skin. When combined with exercise, it helps to loosen any structures that might be tethered, as well as softening the scarring and induration.

Webs must be stretched, as they may have become contracted prior to the operation, and stiff joints mobilized using accessory and active movements. Very gradual passive stretching may be introduced at 3 weeks, but only if absolutely necessary and after healing has taken place. The use of serial stretch splints may be needed after 4 weeks to restore extension by applying a gentle stretch for several short sessions during the day, and maintaining an optimum but comfortable position at night.

Complications

A finger that was severely contracted down into flexion pre-operatively may suffer some complications from surgery, as an excess of stretch on nerves, blood vessels and skin compromises these tissues. Pain with increasing stiffness and swelling must also be watched for carefully. Kleinert *et al.* (1982) reported that 22 per cent of 130 patients who had undergone fasciotomy developed post-traumatic sympathetic dystrophy. This condition must be recognized quickly before it becomes severe, and can be treated by TENS and as much movement as possible.

REFERENCES

Birch, R. and Grant, C. (1986). Peripheral nerve injuries – clinical. In: *Cash's Textbook of Neurology for Physiotherapists.* pp. 469–516. Faber and Faber.

Bunnell, S. T. (1970). *Surgery of the Hand*, 5th edn. Blackwell.

Dellon, A. L. (1984). Touch sensibility in the hand. *J. Hand Surg.*, **9B**, 1.

Frampton, V. (1986). Problems in managing reconstructive surgery for brachial plexus lesions contrasted with peripheral nerve lesions. *J. Hand Ther.*, **2B(1)**, 3–9.

Harrison, S. H. and Morris, A. (1975). Dupuytren's contracture: the dorsal transposition flap. *Hand*, **7**, 2.

Henderson, W. R. (1948). Clinical assessment of peripheral nerve injuries: Tinel's test. *Lancet*, **2**, 801.

Kaltenborn, F. M. (1980). *Mobilization of the Extremity Joints: examination and basic treatment techniques.* 3rd edn. Olaf Norlis Bokhandel, 60–76.

Kleinert, H. E., Leitch, I., Smith, D. J. and Lubbers, L. M. (1982). In: *Difficult Problems in Hand Surgery* (J. W. Strickland and J. B. Steichen, eds), pp. 402–8. Mosby.

McCallum, P. and Hueston, J. T. (1962). The pathology of Dupuytren's contracture. *Aus. NZ J. Surg.*, **31**, 241–53.

McCash, C. R. (1964). The open palm technique in Dupuytren's contracture. *Br. J. Plast. Surg.*, **17**, 271.

McGrouther, D. A. and Ahmed, M. R. (1981). Flexor tendon excursions in 'no-man's land'. *Hand*, **13**, 129–41.

Roberts, M., Rutherford, J. H. and Harris, D. (1982). The effect of ultrasound on flexor tendon repairs in the rabbit. *Hand*, **14**, 1.

Semple, C. (1979). *The Primary Management of Hand Injuries*. Pitman.

Smith, P. J. and Boardman, S. (1986). Primary repair of flexor tendon injuries in 'no-man's land'. *Physiotherapy*, **72**, 2.

Verdan, C. L. (1960). Primary repair of flexor tendons. *J. Bone Joint Surg.*, **42A**, 647–57.

Wilson, D. M. (1983). Tenosynovitis, tendonvaginitis and trigger finger. *Physiotherapy*, **69**, 10.

Wynn Parry, C. B. (1981). *Rehabilitation of the Hand*, 4th edn. Butterworths.

Wynn Parry, C. B. (1984). Symposium on sensation. *J. Hand Surg.*, **9B(1)**, 4–6.

Wynn Parry, C. B. and Salter, M. (1976). Sensory re-education after median nerve lesions. *Hand*, **8**, 250–56.

FURTHER READING

Adolfsson, L., Soderberg, G., Larsson, M. and Karlander, L. E. (1995). The effects of a shortened postoperative mobilization programme after flexor tendon repair in zone 2. J. *Hand Surg.*, **21B(1)**, 67–71.

Baktir, A., Turk, C.Y., Kabak, S. *et al.* (1995). Flexor tendon repair in zone 2 followed by early active mobilization. *J. Hand Surg.*, **21B(5)**, 624–8.

Ip, W. Y. and Chow, P. (1995). Results of dynamic splintage following extensor tendon repair. *J. Hand Surg.*, **22B(2)**, 283–7.

Khan, K., Riaz, M., Murison, M. S. C. and Brennen, M. D. (1996). Early active mobilization after second stage flexor tendon grafts. *J. Hand Surg.*, **22B(3)**, 372–4.

Macdonald, R. (1994). *Taping Techniques: Principles and Practice*. Butterworth Heinemann.

Reid, D. C. (1992). *Sports Injury: Assessment and Rehabilitation*. Churchill Livingstone.

Stahl, S., Kaufman, T. and Bialik, V. (1996). Partial lacerations of flexor tendons in children. Primary repair versus conservative treatment. *J. Hand Surg.*, **22B(3)**, 377–80.

Thomas, D., Moutet, F. and Guinard, D. (1996). Post-operative management of extensor tendon repairs in zones V, VI, and VII. *J. Hand Ther.*, **9**, 309–14.

8 Brachial plexus lesions

Victoria Frampton

The complex nature of a brachial plexus lesion and subsequent long period of recovery requires careful planning and a comprehensive programme for rehabilitation from initial management through to final outcome. The sudden functional loss of an arm is a traumatic concept for patients to understand, and the correct philosophy of rehabilitation must be established. The comprehensive rehabilitation programme must be administered at appropriate stages of recovery, allowing patients to continue with their life instead of sitting at home waiting for their arm to recover (Frampton, 1990).

Total management of a brachial plexus lesion may include surgery and electrodiagnosis. Therapy is an essential and vital part of rehabilitation, immediately following the initial lesion and through all stages of recovery.

CAUSES

There are several causes of brachial plexus lesions (BPL). They most commonly result from road traffic accidents (Table 8.1) and the greater proportion of these through motorbike accidents. Obstetric brachial plexus lesions (OBP) are increasing, and now represent a significant number of lesions seen.

Early exploration and surgical repair (where possible) of traumatic lesions may lead to improved outcomes of these complex injuries (Birch *et al.*, 1998). Surgical intervention does not negate the need for good clinical diagnosis, and a comprehensive examination is essential to establish diagnosis and monitor recovery, particularly when surgical exploration has not taken place.

CLASSIFICATION

Lesions of the brachial plexus can be subdivided into direct injury and traction injuries, a summary of which can be seen in Table 8.1.

TABLE 8.1
CAUSES OF BRACHIAL PLEXUS LESIONS

Direct injury	Traction injury
Stab wound	RTA majority:
Gunshot	• motor bikes
Pressure (heavy rucksack strap)	• cars
Post-mastectomy radiotherapy	Obstetric brachial
Iatrogenic	plexus lesions

Direct injuries have a better prognosis, as the extent of the injury is clearly defined on exploration and it may or may not need grafting. In any event, the proximal part of the brachial plexus and nerve roots are intact.

Traction lesions can be further subdivided into:

1. Preganglionic lesions – avulsion of the nerve roots from the spinal cord
2. Postganglionic lesions
   • traction lesion in continuity with neurapraxia
   • traction lesion in continuity with axonotmesis (nerve sheath intact)
   • traction lesion with neurotmesis (rupture of complete nerve).

In all postganglionic lesions, the nerve roots are intact.

Common clinical patterns of lesions

Diagnosis of traction lesions of the brachial plexus is complicated because a variety of different types of lesions can occur (Wynn Parry, 1981a):

• complete C5/6 in continuity
• complete C5/6/7 in continuity
• C5/6 ruptured, complete C7/8/T1 in continuity
• C5/6 ruptured, C7/8 and T1 avulsed
• avulsion of all roots.

The resultant patterns of injury affecting different parts of the plexus may be partly due to anatomical features in relation to the upper trunk and lower trunk of the brachial plexus (Wynn Parry, 1981a).

ANATOMICAL FEATURES

Upper trunk:

• C5/6/7 – roots are tethered proximally to the transverse processes and distally by the clavipectoral fascia
• roots are linked by a fibrous bridge
• C5 is strongly inclined down and twice as long as C8.

Lower trunk:

• C8/T1 – roots tethered only distally by the clavipectoral fascia
• T1 – straight direction from exit of the spinal cord.

These anatomical factors may be attributable to the variety of injuries that can occur in the upper trunk, i.e. traction in continuity, rupture or avulsion, whereas traction lesions of the lower trunk C8/T1 result in traction lesion in continuity or total avulsion.

TREATMENT – EARLY STAGE

Surgery

Early exploration facilitates early diagnosis, and identification of postganglionic ruptures will allow surgical repair and grafting. It will also allow diagnosis of any avulsion injury that may be seen at the time of exploration. Certainly if all roots are seen to be avulsed, the definitive diagnosis can be given to the patient and appropriate counselling and treatment programming with defined goals can be established. If a postganglionic rupture is seen on exploration, vascularized nerve grafts can restore continuity and hopefully function, which could not take place without the repair. A violent force sufficient to rupture the brachial plexus frequently results in vascular damage, which also has to be repaired if recovery is to be anticipated. Diagnosis may be complicated by additional traction and ruptures of nerves distal to the plexus lesion, e.g. the musculocutaneous and suprascapular nerves. Trauma to these nerves may occur simultaneously with brachial plexus injury. Clinical signs may be misleading, as a dual lesion with peripheral nerve damage may present as a postganglionic lesion and conceal a preganglionic lesion.

Surgery for avulsion lesions of the brachial plexus is limited. Intercostal nerve grafts or neurotization of thoracic roots to distal stumps of cords or nerves that have lost their proximal cord connection is the one option, e.g. the proximal root of T2 is connected to the distal stump of the avulsed roots of C5 and 6 (Birch, 1998).

Post-operative management

Patients are given a modular collar and cuff sling. The sling holds the arm so that the glenohumeral joint is supported and the arm rests with the elbow in 90° of flexion and the forearm lying across the chest wall. This position is maintained for 4–6 weeks, during which time the patient may be discharged. If necessary, the patient is readmitted for 1 week of mobilization. Intercostal nerve grafts are immobilized for 12 weeks; rehabilitation may therefore take longer (Nicola Khar – personal communication).

CLINICAL DIAGNOSIS

Not all plexus patients are explored. It may be that a patient will present with a plexus injury and a physical examination will be the only means of diagnosing the clinical injury. Characteristic signs and symptoms will help to identify a pre- or postganglionic lesion.

Preganglionic lesions

Indications include:

1. A high velocity, large impact accident
2. An unconscious patient
3. Associated injuries, e.g. fractures, head and vascular injuries
4. Horner's syndrome – avulsion of the T1 root, resulting in ptosis of the eyelid and constriction of the pupil (Figure 8.1)
5. Positive sensory action potentials on electrodiagnosis
6. Evidence of meningoceles on myelogram, indicating avulsion of the root
7. Pain in the anaesthetic limb
8. Fracture of the first rib.

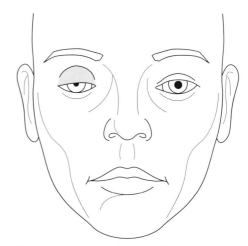

Figure 8.1 Horner's syndrome. Right eye: associated sympathetic nerve damage as a result of a T1 root avulsion leading to constriction of the pupil and ptosis of the eyelid. Left eye: normal pupil size indicating no associated sympathetic damage, or a post-ganglionic lesion.

Avulsion pain

This intense pain of a characteristic nature (Wynn Parry, 1981b)) can often be a diagnostic sign of an avulsion injury. The pain is described as constant, although insidious in onset. Burning, crushing and vice-like are common terms used to describe this pain, which is often shooting in nature, likened to an electric shock and felt in the anaesthetic arm in the dermatome of the root that has been avulsed. The paroxysms of pain gradually build up to a peak or crescendo of pain, and then gradually fade to the constant burning pain. Patients may stop an activity to grip the arm during an episode of this paroxysm of pain, and flex the head down towards the affected side until the pain eases. The pain generally does not vary with external stimulus; however, a virus or cold may make the pain worse. Sleep is usually undisturbed, but patients complain of difficulty in getting to sleep. The concept of pain in an anaesthetic limb is difficult for the patient to understand. Occasionally it is misinterpreted as a good sign, so it is important to explain to patients why they are feeling pain and how it may be controlled (see Chapter 4).

Postganglionic lesions

Indications include:

1. A slow velocity, small impact accident
2. A conscious patient
3. Absence of any associated injury
4. Negative Horner's sign
5. Negative sensory action potentials on electrodiagnosis
6. A normal myelogram
7. Neuroma sign, and/or a positive Tinel (if examined from 8 weeks post-injury) (Tinel, 1915)
8. Absence of preganglionic pain symptoms.

Neuroma sign
This is an important sign, as it indicates a rupture of the nerve root. In a regenerating nerve, tapping over the neural sprouts will reproduce a referred sensation into the part of the skin that used to be supplied by that nerve, a Tinel sign (Moldaver, 1978). A neuroma sign is distinguished from a Tinel sign in that it is exquisitely painful and the patient flinches or moves away from the stimulus. There will also be the absence of a distal Tinel, indicating a lack of nerve recovery. The presence of the distal Tinel and proximal Tinel gives an indication of the rate of growth of a regenerating nerve. A rupture in the lower trunk of the plexus is rare for the reasons previously described. Nerve growth is slow, so even if nerve growth is completed, there will be intrinsic muscle fibrosis in the hand.

ASSESSMENT

Records at all stages of recovery provide a baseline for comparative information and an ongoing record to monitor recovery. Charts devised and used at the Royal National Orthopaedic Hospital Trust, Stanmore, Middlesex consist of a summary chart, range of motion, muscle power and sensory evaluation charts (Figure 8.2, Tables 8.2–8.5).

Most occupational therapy and physiotherapy departments may see only one brachial plexus patient in a year; consequently, the use of charts will ensure a comprehensive examination and act as a checklist.

Joint range of movement

Patients with brachial plexus lesions will develop characteristic patterns of reduced range of motion if left untreated. The collar and cuff sling, while

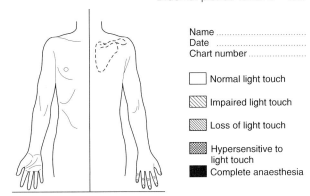

Figure 8.2 Sensory evaluation chart.

providing a support, also maintains the arm in a posture that will lead to the following limitations in movement (Figure 8.3a and b):

Joint	Loss of movement
Shoulder	Elevation, abduction and external rotation
Elbow	Extension and supination
Wrist	Dorsiflexion
Metacarpophalangeal joints	Flexion
Interphalangeal joints	Extension

Limitation of movement is due not only to joint but also to soft tissue contracture, for example:

Soft tissue contracture	Deformity
Contracture of the long flexor tendons	Clawing of the fingers
Fibrosis of the long extensors and intrinsic muscles	Loss of IP joint flexion when the MP complex joints are at 90° of flexion
Contracture of adductor pollicis	Reduction in thumb web space (Figure 8.3c)

Motor function

Motor assessment of the partially or completely paralysed arm requires specific and careful handling. The therapist tries to identify flickers of movement in individual muscles that might relate to specific nerve roots. Handling techniques must be directed at supporting the arm while at the same time leaving the therapists' other hand free to palpate the muscle so that the movement and

TABLE 8.2(A)
EVALUATION FORM FOR BRACHIAL PLEXUS INJURY – SUMMARY CHART

Assessment chart – brachial plexus lesion
Name _____   Date _____   Chart number _____   Dominant limb _____
History
Lesion   Associated injuries   Date of accident   Description of injury   Mechanism of injury   Speed of injury   Length of loss of consciousness   Treatment to date
Exploration of brachial plexus
Findings   Repair
Examination
General appearance   Horner's sign   Neuroma   Tinel   Passive joint range   Muscle power   Sensory evaluation   Other tests   Splintage   Occupation and domestic situation

TABLE 8.2(B)
EVALUATION FORM FOR BRACHIAL PLEXUS INJURY – PAIN CHART

Name _____   Date _____   Chart number _____
Pain
Onset   Increasing/static/decreasing   Nature   Distribution   Frequency of pain in a day   Daily pattern   Aggravates   Eases   Drugs   Sleep disturbance   <div align="center">Comments</div>

TABLE 8.3
EVALUATION FORM FOR BRACHIAL PLEXUS INJURY – PASSIVE RANGE OF MOVEMENT CHART

Passive range of movement chart – brachial plexus lesions

Name _____

Age _____

Chart number _____

Date _____

Shoulder girdle	Elev Retr Protr Depr	Adm	Dis	Elbow	Flex Ext	Adm	Dis
Shoulder	Elev Flex Ext Abd Add IR ER			Wrist	Flex Ext Pro Sup Abd Add		
Hand	Deformity:			Thumb web Intrinsics			

		Adm	CMC	Dis	Adm	MCP	Dis	Adm	DIP	Dis
Thumb	Flex Ext Abd Add Opp									

		Adm	MCP	Dis	Adm	PIP	Dis	Adm	DIP	Dis
Index Middle Ring Little	Ext–flex Ext–flex Ext–flex Ext–flex									

Posture

quality of muscle contraction can be assessed (DOH, 1986).

Recovery will take place proximally. If a total lesion of the plexus exists, a detailed knowledge of the shoulder girdle muscles is essential. A variation in conventional root supply is not uncommon, and must be taken into account when a particular pattern is emerging that may not be consistent with clinical findings. Paralysis of the serratus anterior (Figure 8.4a) and rhomboids indicates a very high lesion. Some consistency of root supply exists; for example, in the pectoralis major:

- upper fibres (clavicular fibres) – C5, C6 and C7
- lower fibres (sternal fibres) – C7, C8 and T1

To test for pectoralis major clavicular fibres (Figure 8.4b), support the whole arm so that the shoulder is abducted and elevated above 90°, and ask the patient to pull the arm across the body. Clearly this movement is impossible for a patient

TABLE 8.4
MUSCLE CHART – SHOULDER AND ELBOW

Right						Upper extremity			Left						
						Nerve	Roots	Muscle							
						Acc'y	$A_cC_1C_2C_3C_4$	Sternomastoid							
						Acc'y	$A_cC_2C_3C_4$	Trapezius – upper							
						Acc'y	$A_cC_2C_3C_4$	Trapezius – middle							
						Acc'y	$A_cC_2C_3C_4$	Trapezius – lower							
						Brachial plexus	$C_3C_4C_5$	Levator scapulae							
							C_4C_5	Rhomboids							
							$C_5C_6C_7$	Serratus anterior							
							$C_5C_6C_7C_8T_1$	Pectoralis major							
							C_4C_5	Supraspinatus							
							$C_4C_5C_6$	Infraspinatus							
							$C_6C_7C_8$	Latissumus dorsi							
							C_5C_6	Teres major							
						Circumflex	C_4C_5	Teres minor							
							C_5C_6	Deltoid – anterior							
							C_5C_6	Deltoid – middle							
							C_5C_6	Deltoid – posterior							
						Musc. cut.	C_5C_6	Biceps							
							C_5C_6	Brachialis							
						Radial	$C_7C_8T_1$	Triceps – long head							
							$C_7C_8T_1$	Triceps – lateral head							
							$C_7C_8T_1$	Triceps – medial head							
							C_5C_6	Brachioradialis							
							C_6C_7	Ext. carpi rad. long.							
							C_6C_7	Ext. carpi rad. brev.							
							C_5C_6	Supinator							
							C_7C_8	Extensor digitorum							
							C_7C_8	Ext. digiti minimi							
							C_7C_8	Ext. carpi ulnaris							
							C_7C_8	Abd. pollicis longus							
							C_7C_8	Ext. pollicis longus							
							C_7C_8	Ext. pollicis brevis							
							C_7C_8	Ext. indicis							

TABLE 8.5
MUSCLE CHART – FOREARM AND HAND

Right							*Upper extremity*			*Left*						
							Nerve	*Roots*	*Muscle*							
							Median	C_6C_7	Pronator teres							
								$C_6C_7C_8$	Flex. carpi radialis							
								$C_7C_8T_1$	Palmaris longus							
								$C_7C_8T_1$	Flex. dig. Sublimis							
								$C_7C_8T_1$	Flex. dig. prof. 1 & 2							
								$C_7C_8T_1$	Flex. pollicis longus							
								C_8T_1	Abd. Pollicis Brevis							
								C_8T_1	Opponens pollicis							
								C_8T_1	Flex. pollicis brevis							
								$C_7C_8T_1$	Lumbrical 1							
								$C_7C_8T_1$	Lumbrical 2							
							Ulnar	$C_6C_7C_8$	Flex. carpi ulnaris							
								$C_7C_8T_1$	Flex. dig. prof. 3 & 4							
								C_8T_1	Abd. dig. minimi							
								C_8T_1	Opp. dig. minimi							
								C_8T_1	Flex. dig. min. brev.							
								$C_7C_8T_1$	Lumbrical 3							
								$C_7C_8T_1$	Lumbrical 4							
								C_8T_1	Interossei palmar 1							
								C_8T_1	Interossei palmar 2							
								C_8T_1	Interossei palmar 3							
								C_8T_1	Interossei palmar 4							
								C_8T_1	Interossei dorsal 1							
								C_8T_1	Interossei dorsal 2							
								C_8T_1	Interossei dorsal 3							
								C_8T_1	Interossei dorsal 4							
								C_8T_1	Add. Pollicis							

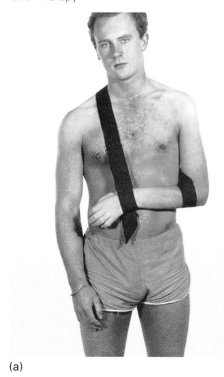

(a)

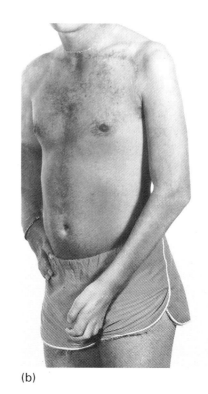

(b)

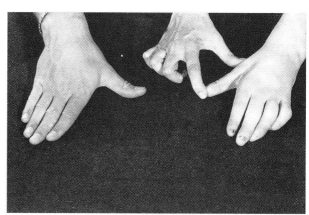

(c)

Figure 8.3 The collar and cuff sling, while providing a support (a), also maintains the arm in a posture that will lead to limitation of movement (b). Contracture of the adductor pollicis will cause a reduction in the thumb web space (c).

with a flail arm; however, with the therapist's support, any activity in this muscle will be evident.

To test the sternal fibres (Figure 8.4c), lower the patient's arm and support it in approximately 45° of abduction of the shoulder with the elbow flexed to 90°. Ask the patient to draw the elbow and arm down into the waist, and sternal fibres can be palpated if active.

Sensory function

At the early assessment stage, a sensory map of the arm to detect light touch and anaesthesia is all that is required in a total lesion of the brachial plexus. Sensory sparing of the arm will be limited to the shoulder, the tip of the acromion and the inside of

the upper arm (C4 and T2 innervation). Sensory mapping can be performed by light fingertip touch (Figure 8.2); it is important to establish whether any deep pressure can be perceived, as this may be an important factor for treatment modalities such as transcutaneous electrical nerve stimulation (TENS) for the treatment of pain.

REHABILITATION

Rehabilitation will take place over a long period, and it is important to establish short- and long-term goals. At the early stage, successful management will result from a collective team approach with contributions from the physician, surgeon, therapist, social worker, orthotist, resettlement officer and, if necessary, psychologist, all working closely

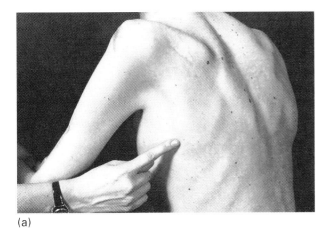
(a)

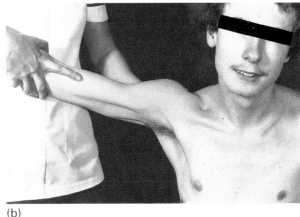
(b)

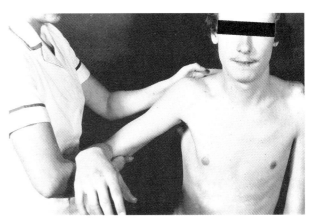
(c)

Figure 8.4 (a) Serratus anterior; (b) Pectoralis major clavicular fibres; (c) Pectoralis major sternal fibres.

together. The patient's expectations must be clearly defined at this stage.

The protracted rehabilitation must not become an impediment to patients reintegrating back into their community. They must be discouraged from sitting and waiting for the arm to recover. The absence of a defined diagnosis, either because surgical exploration has not taken place or because the lesion is in continuity and the extent of the damage from the traction force is unknown, makes the setting of long-term goals more difficult.

Early stage

Short-term goals

Short-term goals are to:

1. Maintain full passive range of movement
2. Maintain extensibility of soft tissue structures
3. Relieve pain
4. Restore function through splinting and advice on one-armed activities and ADL
5. Prevent damage to the anaesthetic arm
6. Restore social skills and reintegration into normal life

7. Re-establish the work situation or investigate alternative work opportunities
8. Establish patients' responsibility for the care and treatment programme of their own arm.

Treatment

Passive movements The priority for patients must be to maintain a full range of movement of their flail arm. Contracture or deformity will limit the functional outcome of any nerve recovery. Patients must be encouraged to perform their own passive movements, and for this goal to be achieved movements must be few, simple and effective. Combined movements of the arm must aim at restoring full joint and soft tissue extensibility (Table 8.6). A comparative movement of the uninjured arm provides a baseline for evaluation. Existing contractures must be treated, and stretching techniques, mobilization and occasionally splinting can be effective. In the totally paralysed arm, rigid splinting on the whole achieves no functional objective. Contractures should be prevented by passive movement.

TABLE 8.6
PASSIVE MOVEMENTS TO THE FLAIL ARM

Patient's position	Joint	Movement
Lying	Shoulder	Flexion, elevation
Lying	Shoulder	Elevation, external rotation
Lying	Elbow	Support upper arm with opposite hand and use weight of forearm and hand to extend flail elbow
Sitting	Elbow	Grip forearm between knees and extend elbow with the other arm
Sitting	Wrist	Flex, extend, rotate
Sitting	MP and IP joints and wrist	Flex all joints simultaneously to make a full fist
Sitting	MP and IP joints and wrist	Extend all joints simultaneously
Sitting	Thumb web	Grip hand between knees, gently stretch thumb away from palm

Pain Transcutaneous electrical nerve stimulation (TENS) provides one of the only methods of pain relief for avulsion pain of the brachial plexus (Chapter 4). One hypothesis of pain relief might be that the electrical stimulus restores an artificial afferent input to a spinal cord that has lost its normal inhibitory afferent input. Placement of electrodes has been discussed in more detail in Chapter 4, but in general they must be placed on skin that has some residual sensory sparing. Pads placed over the adjacent dermatome to the damaged dermatome and over the nerve trunk will provide the most successful placements (see Figure 4.4a). Large pads are more effective than small pads, and continued stimulation for a minimum of 8 hours a day over at least 3 weeks is recommended. As pain is relieved, the period of stimulation should be reduced gradually. A high intensity current with a wide pulse width is indicated. This is only possible due to denervation of the arm; muscle contraction would be stimulated in a normally innervated arm when using these parameters.

Flail arm splint The use of functional splinting is not always popular with a brachial plexus patient; the majority of these patients are young men, who find any form of splinting restricting. It is important to present the splint as a tool. The modular splint is a skeleton of an upper limb prosthesis that sits over the paralysed arm (Robinson, 1986; Figure 8.5a), and can be used for work or hobbies and then removed for social activities. It does require com-

mitment and practise from the patient, and undoubtedly initial training and exposure to the splint will determine its success or failure.

The full flail arm splint provides:

- shoulder support, allowing some abduction but preventing subluxation of the glenohumeral joint
- an elbow lock device with five alternative positions of flexion
- a forearm to wrist support, with a platform on the flexor aspect where standard artificial appliances can be fitted (Figure 8.5b); these are operated in the same manner as a prosthesis, and a cable running from the terminal appliance to a shoulder strap on the opposite shoulder activates the appliances (Figure 8.5c and d).

For lower trunk lesions of the brachial plexus (C8/T1) a shoulder device may not be required, and a gauntlet splint is available. This just provides the standard artificial limb appliances on the platform of the gauntlet and a cable to operate them. Similarly, for an upper trunk lesion (C5, 6, 7) the shoulder support and elbow lock splint is available. The flail arm splint is lightweight, modular, and can be assembled or disassembled depending on what part of the splint is required. It has the cosmetic advantage that it can be removed! Amputation is not as a rule encouraged; paralysis of the shoulder girdle muscles prevents good operation of a prosthetic arm, and pain frequently increases with amputation due to further deafferentation.

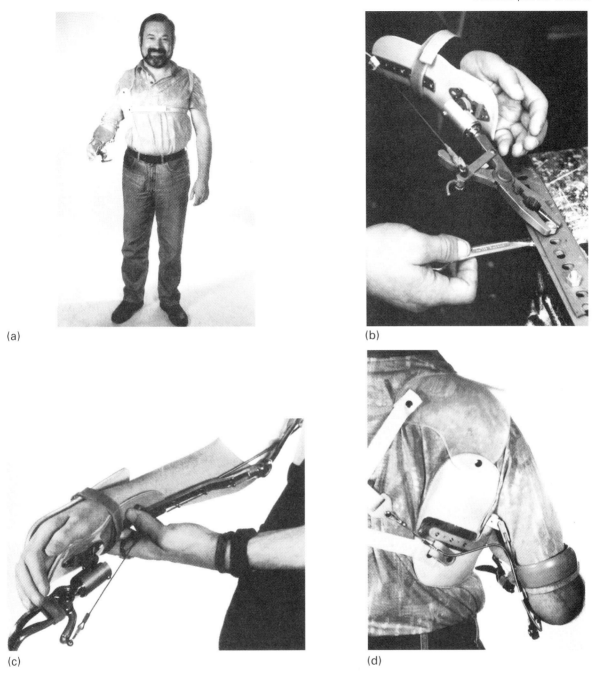

(a)

(b)

(c)

(d)

Figure 8.5 (a) and (b) Steeper's flail arm appliance; (c) and (d) Steeper's elbow lock appliance (photograph with permission of the Royal National Orthopaedic NHS Trust, Stanmore, Middlesex).

Counselling It is important that support and direction are given at the outset of the injury. The majority of traumatic brachial plexus lesions occur in young people at the beginning of their lives, many of whom have young families to support. Re-establishment of work must take place in the early stage. The options open to the patient are to return to existing employment, to return to the existing employer in a different occupation, or to retrain in an alternative skill.

Clearly, training of the patient to perform daily living activities with one arm is essential.

Summary of early stage rehabilitation
By the end of this initial episode of care:

- patients should be independent regarding daily living activities
- patients should be independent in performing a full passive exercise regime

- patients should be proficient in the use of a flail arm splint if fitted
- pain control should be established
- patients should be restored to their social environment
- the direction of work environment should be established.

Middle stage

Follow-up review is essential to monitor progress and detect early recovery. It is important to administer treatment at appropriate times of recovery and to commence intensive rehabilitation if indicated. It is also important to review the joint range and soft tissue extensibility. Following re-evaluation, goals may be reset; however, programmes should not continue for long periods if no further progress is being made. Any long-term periods of rehabilitation will disrupt the patient's life and employment status.

Middle-stage goals
Middle-stage goals are to:

1. Strengthen and re-educate reinnervating muscles
2. Restore the full joint range of movement and soft tissue extensibility
3. Re-evaluate pain and reapply TENS if appropriate
4. Review flail arm splinting, and reduce the sections if indicated.

Treatment
Re-educative techniques such as PNF (proprioceptive neuromuscular facilitation), brushing, icing and progressive resisted exercises can be employed at appropriate stages of recovery. Techniques of icing must be used with caution, depending on sensory function. Review of the patients' occupational and social situation will contribute to their full rehabilitation.

Late stage

Factors to consider in late stage management
1. Early exploration of the brachial plexus allows definitive diagnosis of poor prognostic lesions, and identification of avulsion injury may indicate reconstructive surgery at an early stage.
2. Clear assessment of the residual disability and functional loss is essential prior to consideration of reconstructive surgery. Results of reconstructive surgery for brachial plexus lesions are not as good on the whole as single peripheral nerve injuries (Frampton, 1986), and the complexity of the brachial plexus injury makes selection for reconstructive surgery more difficult. As muscles are innervated from more than one nerve root, muscles for transfer may not be of full power,

and may lack independent action and only be effective in a mass pattern of movement.
3. Poor proprioception and a reduced range of movement are more widespread problems in BPL than in single peripheral nerve injuries.
4. Following tendon transfer, pain may be another limiting factor that causes significant dysfunction. Attempted active movement by the transferred muscle (the movement of which was previously supplied by a muscle from the avulsed root) can revive avulsion pain that had previously subsided.
5. The quality of sensory function in the hand will dictate the degree of successful outcome following reconstructive surgery. Pre-operative assessment must include a full sensory evaluation. The results of the assessment may indicate that loss of function is primarily due to poor sensory stereognosis and proprioception, and that the motor loss is contributing only a small degree towards loss of function.
6. In many cases, a series of operations need to be planned to restore function to one arm. A decision has to be made regarding which function to restore first, and once the sequence of operations is set it is important to maximize the results of one procedure before attempting the next. For example, if the patient has the loss of elbow flexion and wrist and finger extension, the use of an elbow lock splint restores function to the elbow and allows surgical reconstruction of wrist and finger extension to proceed. When this procedure has been maximized, the second operation to restore elbow flexion can take place and the outcome will be improved as there is a good functioning hand to reinforce the new movement of elbow flexion.
7. If the patient has waited for 2 years for reconstructive surgery, unconventional patterns of movement may have been developed in order to achieve some degree of activity. It is therefore important to establish that tendon transfer will not compromise existing function. The assessment for tendon transfer must establish what the patient might lose as well as what they might gain, and a detailed functional assessment is therefore essential.

Fundamentally, the therapist should establish what the patient:

- can currently do
- is unable to do
- wants to be able to do.

Treatment

Pain Re-evaluation of pain must establish whether it is properly controlled, as it can seriously jeopardize the outcome of reconstructive surgery. Reapplication of TENS may be indicated.

Muscle strengthening/re-education Progressive resisted strengthening exercises may be indicated to raise the grade of a muscle to be transferred in a reconstructive procedure. Conventionally, criteria for peripheral nerve injuries dictate that muscles functionally lose a grade of power on transfer. Muscles working in a mass pattern of movement may need retraining to work independently. Techniques of PNF biofeedback and, occasionally, electrical stimulation can be helpful.

Joint/soft tissue mobilization Any soft tissue shortening must be addressed prior to reconstructive surgery. Thermoplastic splints can be used serially to gradually stretch soft tissues, particularly in adductor pollicis contractures of the thumb. Full excursion of the thumb web is essential prior to restoring thumb opposition.

Sensory re-education Desensitization programmes for hyperaesthesia and intensive stereognostic treatment to improve the sensory function may be essential prerequisites to reconstructive surgery.

Tendon transfer
Prior to reconstructive surgery, it is suggested (Omer, 1974) that it is advisable to tabulate the loss of movement, the available muscle for transfer (to restore the functional loss), and the power of that muscle and the muscles left to maintain the balance of movement following the loss of the transferred muscle. The classic tendon transfer usually performed for radial nerve lesions (Table 8.7) may be compromised by muscle weakness in an upper trunk lesion of the brachial plexus with a similar functional loss. Alternatively, muscles for transfer may be used which are full power (e.g. FDS).

1. Muscle weakness may not necessarily be a contraindication to tendon transfer in brachial plexus injuries. It may be that one muscle may have to power two actions, and that if two out of the three muscles for transfer are of adequate power then the outcome of tendon transfer, although not as good as that for a peripheral nerve injury, may be quite acceptable.

2. Co-contraction with the antagonist muscles can be another complication of tendon transfer in brachial plexus injuries.
3. The principles of tendon transfers set for single peripheral nerve injuries may have to be modified with brachial plexus lesions in an attempt to improve function. Consequently, different goals may be set for patients with brachial plexus lesions to those with peripheral nerve injuries.
4. It is vital to establish with the patient the clear expectations of surgery and the specific goals of the operation. A clear understanding of the procedure and what is required from the patient will greatly help rehabilitation and re-education.

Post-operative management Different rehabilitation goals have to be set for brachial plexus lesions as compared to peripheral nerve lesions. Re-education of a tendon transfer to restore wrist and finger extension following a BPL may take twice as long to reach the same outcome as a radial nerve injury with the equivalent functional loss.

Following a radial nerve tendon transfer, smooth co-ordinated combined wrist and finger extension movements may be expected, allowing the fingers to perform intricate tasks such as gripping a pencil while maintaining good co-ordinated control of wrist extension.

In a brachial plexus lesion, if only one muscle is powering two movements, then the re-education of finger and wrist extension may have to be performed separately. On occasion, wrist support with a splint may be necessary to allow re-education of the fingers. Expecting too much from the brachial plexus transfer will result in the tendon transfer fatiguing quickly; this will proceed to trick movements if adequate support is not provided. The following guidelines form a baseline of instruction for re-education of tendon transfers:

1. Always support the limb so that the tendon transfer is not under strain or tension
2. To stimulate the new action of the transferred muscle, imagine the old action of the same transferred muscle

TABLE 8.7
TENDON TRANSFERS TO RESTORE WRIST AND FINGER EXTENSION IN A RADIAL NERVE LESION (COMPARATIVE MUSCLE STRENGTH AND MUSCLES THAT MAY BE ABSENT C5, 6, 7 LESION SHOWN IN BRACKETS)

Loss of movement	Muscle for transfer	Power	Muscles left to balance loss of transferred muscle
Wrist extension	Pronator teres	(0) 5	(Pronator quadratus)
Finger extension	Flexor carpi ulnaris	(3+) 5	(Flexor carpi radialis)
Thumb abduction	Palmaris longus	(0) 5	Flexor digitorum profundus Flexor digitorum superficialis

3. Placement of the therapist's hands must encompass support for the transfer, palpating the muscle belly or tendon of the transferred tendon to feel the new action and at the same time provide correct proprioceptive feedback to enhance the new muscle action
4. The use of guided resistance can assist in establishing the new action of the transferred muscle
5. Peripheral joint mobilization helps restore joint proprioception and mobility to previously immobilized joints without undue stress or tension on the tendon transfer
6. Concise instruction must be given and aimed at asking for the new movement while resisting the old action of the muscle that has been transferred
7. Other proprioceptive techniques of brushing, icing and biofeedback can facilitate and encourage the new action of the tendon transfer.

Trick movements in brachial plexus lesions
These may be acceptable if it becomes evident that the tendon transfer is not sufficiently strong enough to actively restore function. They should be discouraged initially but may have to be accepted eventually; for example, following reconstruction of finger and wrist extension (Table 8.8), by flexing the wrist, passive extension of the fingers may be achieved as tension is placed on the extensor tendons (a tenodesis effect). For a patient who had no function pre-operatively, the

ability to release the grip may be a 50 per cent improvement on the pre-operative state. Post-operative splints are indicated if the patient is unable to hold the new action against gravity.

Bilateral activities and more general sports such as swimming are encouraged. When a sequence of operations is indicated, the use of video can be helpful and used as a positive comparison post-operatively. A summary of some operations performed to restore function through tendon transfer is given in Table 8.8.

CONCLUSION

Brachial plexus injuries are relatively rare and may only present infrequently. Arguably, they may best be managed in specialist centres where expertise in the management of BPL is available. However, ongoing therapy may well continue locally, and a comprehensive understanding of the full rehabilitation programme is essential.

Rehabilitation of brachial plexus injuries can be a prolonged process. It is important to establish a baseline of information from a careful and time-consuming assessment, so that appropriate treatment can be administered at all stages of recovery. A comprehensive and planned programme of rehabilitation will assist in ensuring the future independence and success of an individual's life. The role of the therapist lies not only in physical rehabilitation, but also in thorough counselling and support throughout the patient's recovery (see Chapter 3).

TABLE 8.8
CONTRASTING EXAMPLES OF SOME TENDON TRANSFERS PERFORMED IN BRACHIAL PLEXUS AND PERIPHERAL NERVE LESIONS

Functional loss	Nerve injury	Tendon for transfer		Receiving muscle/tendon
Wrist and finger extension	Radial nerve	Flexor carpi ulnaris	→	Extensor digitorum communis
		Pronator teres	→	Extensor carpi radialis brevis
		Palmaris longus	→	Abductor pollicis longus
	Brachial plexus Lesion C567	Flexor digitorum Sublimis	→	Extensor digitorum communis
Finger flexion	Brachial plexus Lesion C8T1	Brachioradialis	→	Flexor digitorum profundus and flexor pollicis longus
	Median nerve	Flexor digitorum profundus (ring and little)	→	Flexor digitorum profundus (index and middle)
Elbow flexion	Brachial plexus Lesion C567	– Steindler arthroplasty (Brooks, 1969)		
		– Latissimus dorsi	→	Biceps
		– Pectoralis major	→	Biceps
Shoulder abduction, external rotation	Brachial plexus Lesion C56	Zachary transfer (1947)		

REFERENCES

Birch, R., Bonny, G. and Wynn Parry, CB. (1998). *Surgical Disorders of the Peripheral Nerve*. Churchill Livingstone.

DOH (1986). *Aids to the Examination of the Peripheral Nervous System*. Ballière Tindall.

Frampton, V. M. (1986). Problems in managing reconstructive surgery for brachial plexus lesions contrasted with peripheral nerve lesions. *J. Hand Surg.*, **11(B)**, 3.

Frampton, V. M. (1990) Therapists' management of brachial plexus injuries. In: *Rehabilitation of the Hand: Surgery and Therapy* (J. Hunter, L. Schneider, E. Mackin and A. Callaghan, eds), pp. 47, 630–34. C. V. Mosby.

Moldaver, J. (1978). Tinel's sign, its characteristics and significance. *J. Bone Joint Surg.*, **60A**, 412.

Omer, G. E. (1974). The technique and timing of tendon transfers. *Orthop. Clin. North Am.*, **5(2)**, 377.

Robinson, C. (1986). Brachial plexus lesion. Functional splintage, Part 2. *Br. J. Occ. Ther.*, **49(10)**, 331.

Tinel, J. (1915). Le signe du 'four millement' dans les lesions des nerfs peripherique. *Press Med.*, **47**, 388.

Wynn Parry, C. B. (1981a). Peripheral nerve injuries. In: *Rehabilitation of the Hand*, 4th edn, pp. 161. Butterworth and Co.

Wynn Parry, C. B. (1981b). Peripheral nerve injuries. In: *Rehabilitation of the Hand*, 4th edn, pp. 134. Butterworth and Co.

FURTHER READING

Brooks D. (1969). Poliomyelitis: reconstructive techniques, Steindler flexorplasty. In: *Operative Surgery*, 2nd edn., Vol. 8 (R. Furlong, ed.), pp. 2, 8. Rob and Smith.

Frampton, V. M. (1984). Management of brachial plexus lesions. *Physiotherapy*, **70**, 389.

Frampton, V. M. (1988). Management of brachial plexus lesions. *Am. J. Hand Ther.*, **1(3)**, 115.

Loeser, J. D. and Ward, A. A. (1967). Some effects of deafferentation on neurons of the cat spinal cord. *Arch. Neurol.*, **17**, 629.

Salter, M. I. (1987). *Hand injuries: A Therapeutic Approach*. Churchill Livingstone.

Wells, P. E., Frampton, V. M. and Bowsher, D. (1994). *Pain Management by Physiotherapy*, 2nd edn. Butterworth-Heinemann.

Withrington, R. H. and Wynn Parry, C. B. (1984). The management of painful peripheral nerve disorders. *J. Hand Surg.*, **9B(1)**, 24.

Wynn Parry, C. B. (1980). Pain in avulsion lesions of the brachial plexus. *Pain*, **9**, 41.

Wynn Parry, C. B. and Salter, M. (1976). Sensory re-education after median nerve lesions, *Hand*, **8**, 250.

Zachary, R. B. (1947). Transplantation of the teres major and latissimus dorsi for loss of external rotation at the shoulder. *Lancet*, **2**, 757.

9 The burnt hand

Alison Davis and Annette Leveridge

The hand is particularly at risk from burn injury because of its exposed position and functional importance. As a tool at work and in the home, it comes into contact with hot objects and liquids and, in the case of fire, is instinctively used to put out the flames and to protect the face. It is not surprising, therefore, that nearly 40 per cent of all burn injuries involve the hand. In many cases it may be part of a more extensive injury.

Although the area of the burn may be small, thermal injury and the resultant scarring and contracture can greatly affect hand function. Correct management and treatment are therefore essential to maintain maximum mobility and function of the hand with minimal disfigurement and deformity.

CLASSIFICATION

There are three groups of burn injury:

1. Thermal
   - flash and flame
   - contact with hot objects and liquids
   - steam
2. Electrical
3. Chemical.

CHARACTERISTIC PATTERNS

Burns of the hand show characteristic patterns according to their cause:

1. Flash burns – the dorsum of the hand is the main area involved due to its exposed position at work and when protecting the face. These burns are usually superficial in depth.
2. Flame burns – the hand is usually held up to protect the face and therefore the dorsum of the hand is involved. If the hand is used in an attempt to extinguish the flame, the palm and fingertips may be more severely injured. This type of burn is deeper, possibly full thickness, and other areas of the body are often involved.
3. Contact burns – these result from grasping a hot object, and may cause devastating damage to the tissues in the fingers and palm (Figure 9.1). In industrial accidents, the dorsum may be involved.
4. Electrical burns – damage is due to the passage of an electrical current causing a heating effect in the tissues. There will be an entrance and exit burn, with hidden damage between the two.

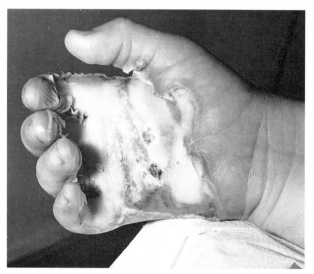

Figure 9.1   Contact burn from grasping a radiator bar fire.

5. Chemical burns – these burns will be full thickness, as the chemicals penetrate into the tissues and have a prolonged effect.

DEPTH OF BURN

The depth of tissue destruction depends on many factors, including causative agent, temperature and duration of exposure. Further tissue destruction can occur as a result of infection.

The depth of the burn will determine whether the wound will heal spontaneously or require grafting. Surviving islands of epidermis around hair follicles, sweat and sebaceous glands will provide new epidermal cells, and in time these will spread to resurface and heal the burn wound (Figure 9.2).

Burns are described as being superficial, partial or full thickness. Many burns are of mixed depth. The use of degrees to describe the depth of burn can lead to confusion, since there is more than one classification; it is therefore now seldom used.

Superficial burns are confined to the epidermis and superficial dermis, resulting in a wet burn with many blisters. They are very painful, as nerve endings remain intact, but heal quickly within 7–10 days.

In partial thickness burns, the damage extends more deeply into the dermis. There are fewer blisters, and the wound may be insensitive to pinprick due to damage to the sensory nerve endings. These burns may be converted to full thickness injury by infection. Healing should occur within 2–3 weeks, depending on the number of surviving epidermal islands. However, hypertrophic scarring and contracture are common with the deeper partial thickness or deep dermal burns, where healing takes more than 18 days.

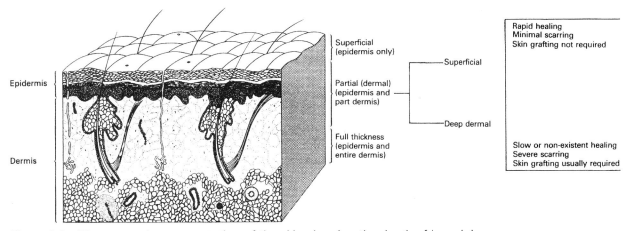

Figure 9.2   Diagrammatic representation of the skin showing the depth of burn injury.

Full thickness burns destroy the full thickness of the skin, and are characterized by a charred or white waxy appearance with visible thrombosed veins and no blisters. They are always insensitive to pinprick. Healing can only occur from the edges, as all epidermal cells are destroyed, and skin grafting will be necessary. Burn damage may be so deep that there may be destruction of muscle, fat and bone.

PATHOLOGY OF THE WHOLE BURN INJURY

Following a burn injury, the heat destroys the skin and tissue necrosis occurs. This area of necrosis is surrounded by a layer of tissue which, although affected by heat, is still viable. Pathological changes occur in this heat-affected tissue.

The main changes are due to dilation of the capillaries with an increase in capillary permeability, resulting in the passage of plasma into the extracellular spaces. This leads to blistering, exudation and gross oedema of the tissues.

This plasma loss occurs rapidly in the first few hours following injury, and diminishes over the next 2 days as the capillaries recover and the fluid within the tissue spaces is absorbed back into the circulation. Excessive fluid loss causes a decrease in circulating blood volume, resulting in hypovolaemic shock and the death of the patient if left untreated.

SIZE OF BURN

The amount of plasma loss depends on the size of the burn, and can be approximately estimated by Wallace's 'Rule of Nines'. For smaller burns, a useful measure is the patient's palm representing 1 per cent of the body surface. In assessing the size of the burn, the erythema around the burn is not included.

Any burn greater than 10 per cent of the body surface area in a child or 15 per cent in an adult will require circulatory fluid replacement via an intravenous drip to prevent hypovolaemic shock.

In smaller burns, the patient is able to compensate for the fluid loss by constriction of blood vessels in the bowel and skin and by the redistribution of fluid from undamaged extracellular spaces. Thirst results, and more fluid is taken orally.

MEDICAL AND SURGICAL MANAGEMENT OF THE BURN WOUND

In general, immediate treatment of burns consists of maintenance of the airway, assessment of the wound, analgesia, tetanus prophylaxis and fluid replacement as indicated. The wound should be treated aseptically as far as possible, since immediately following burn injury the wound surface is sterile because the heat will have destroyed the skin flora and bacteria.

Treatment of the burnt hand has two main aims:

1. The rapid healing of the wound by the most appropriate method
2. The restoration of mobility and function as soon as possible.

Infection must be minimized, as this not only delays healing but also increases the depth of injury. Delay in healing lengthens the period of impaired function and immobility, and increases the scarring, fibrosis and contracture due to the excessive formation of granulation tissue.

Superficial and partial thickness burns of the hand, especially if part of a more extensive injury, are treated conservatively, as healing should occur within 2–3 weeks.

The burnt hand is covered with an antibacterial cream (e.g. silver sulphadiazine) and placed within a polythene bag sealed at the wrist or forearm with gauze and a bandage. This bag is changed daily or more frequently in the first few days if the exudate is excessive. This hand bag method of treatment is usually preferred by the doctor, patient and therapist because it allows the wound to be viewed through the bag, is usually pain-free, permits free

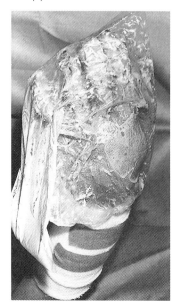

Figure 9.3 Hand bag with antibacterial cream, bandaged at the wrist.

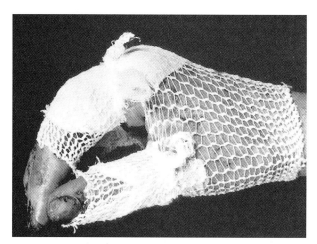

Figure 9.4 Light, non-bulky dressings covering new grafts and protecting thin epithelium.

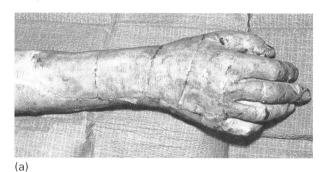

(a)

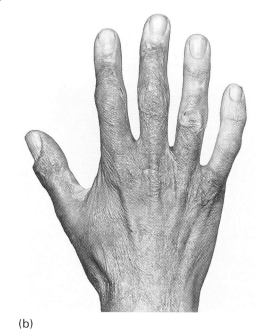

(b)

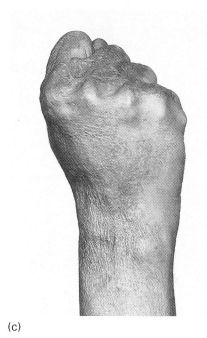

(c)

Figure 9.5 Tangential excision showing good take of grafts (a), and excellent functional and cosmetic result (b) and (c).

movement and exercise, and therefore allows some function and independence (Figure 9.3).

If healing does not occur spontaneously within 2–3 weeks, split skin grafts are applied. The bulky post-operative dressing is left intact for 5 days, allowing the grafts to adhere or take. Thereafter, light dressings permitting freedom of movement are applied until the grafts are stable and well healed (Figure 9.4).

Localized deep dermal burns of the hand may be treated by early surgery, involving tangential excision and skin grafting, at 4–5 days post-burn. The take of grafts is usually excellent, allowing early and rapid rehabilitation. There is minimal hypertrophic scarring and loss of function, as the wound is healed rapidly (Figure 9.5).

Full thickness burns of the hand require surgery. If the hand burn is part of an extensive burn injury, the surgeon's ideal choice and timing of surgery may be affected by more urgent problems in other regions.

Constricting oedema may occur following severe circumferential burns of the upper limb and hand. If left untreated, this can result in vascular compression and eventual ischaemic necrosis. Release incisions through the necrosed tissues are performed, so allowing expansion and the restoration of circulation. An anaesthetic is not required, as the sensory nerve endings are destroyed.

If the patient's condition permits, early excision is preferred to remove all the necrotic tissue so that a clean wound is produced, thus permitting early skin grafting and decreasing the risk of infection and scarring. Prior to surgery, the hand is treated either in a hand bag or in closed dressings.

Skin grafts will not take over exposed tendon or bone. In about 2–3 weeks a healthy layer of granulation tissue will form over small areas, which can then be covered with split skin grafts. However, extensive exposure of extensor tendons can be covered with a skin and subcutaneous flap that retains its own blood supply at its attachment (a pedicle flap). After 10–14 days the flap is removed, leaving a small amount of vascularized fat from the underside of the flap covering the exposed tendons and bones, to which split skin grafts can be applied. Restoration of mobility will be slow, as the hand will be relatively immobile beneath the flap, and at least a week must be allowed following grafting before commencing exercises. Vigorous physiotherapy will then be required.

In an extensive injury, coverage with a flap may be impossible and healing of exposed tendons may have to await growth of healthy granulation tissue and delayed grafting.

Full thickness injuries to the palmar surface frequently result from contact burns, and often occur in isolation. In adults, early excision and coverage with a free flap or a pedicle flap from the groin are common courses of treatment. Following inset of the flap at 2–3 weeks, aggressive physiotherapy is commenced (Figure 9.6). Surgical thinning of the flap may be indicated at a later date. In children, these contact palmar burns are best treated in hand bags. This encourages as much use of the hand as possible. Healing will be slow,

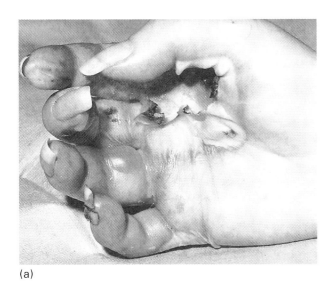

(a)

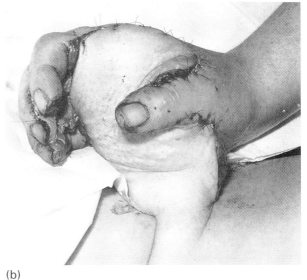

(b)

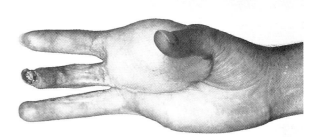

(c)

Figure 9.6 Contact burn inset into a groin flap. Good functional result, with amputation of non-viable little finger.

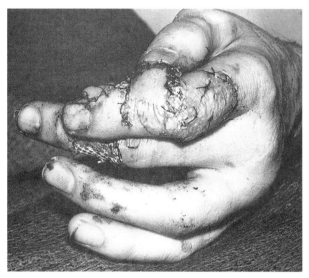

Figure 9.7 Local cross-finger flaps covering small deep burns to fingertips and thumb.

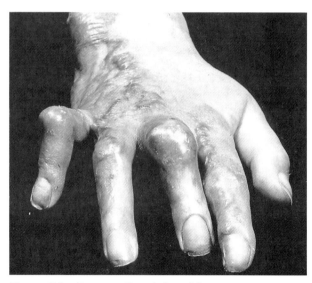

Figure 9.8 Boutonnière deformities.

usually taking 4–6 weeks. Elective resurfacing with thicker grafts, once healing is complete, will give better results than early grafting. Further surgery, regrafting and splinting is often needed as the hand grows, to correct contractures.

The small, localized full thickness skin loss on the fingers caused by electrical burns is best covered with a local flap from an adjacent finger (cross-finger flap), but limited movement is still frequently the end result (Figure 9.7). If the injury is so deep that there is permanent damage to the neurovascular bundles, even worse results can be expected.

Following full thickness burns of the dorsum of the fingers, joint surfaces may be exposed. A single exposed joint is splinted and immobilized until healing occurs, at which stage the joint can be gently mobilized and return of function encouraged. Multiple exposed joints, however, pose a major problem. Unless early healing over open joints can be achieved, internal fixation with pins should be avoided due to the risk of infection. Positioning can be provided either by splinting or, occasionally, by fusing or syndactylizing adjacent fingers and separating them at a later stage. Amputation of a non-viable digit may be indicated as a last resort.

STRUCTURAL CHANGES FOLLOWING BURN INJURY

Following burn injury, the anatomy and thus the function of the hand can be severely affected due to the soft tissue loss and damage. The fragility and adherence of the grafts to the underlying tissues and their tendency to contract will all pose problems in the rehabilitation of the hand.

The skin on the dorsum of the hand is thin, elastic and very mobile, enabling it to stretch as the joints flex. It is commonly damaged by thermal injury, which is often full thickness and requires grafting. Following injury there is often a reduction of normal elasticity and mobility, and movements become restricted. The long extensor tendons lie just beneath the dorsal skin and are thus easily damaged. If the central slip of the extensor expansion over the proximal interphalangeal joint is destroyed, a boutonnière deformity will result (Figure 9.8). Even if the central slip is intact following injury, it may subsequently rupture due to poor positioning or infection.

The skin of the palm is thick and cornified, protecting the underlying structures. Palmar burns are usually more superficial in depth and often heal spontaneously, but in the full thickness burn the thick skin no longer offers sufficient protection to the underlying structures and these may also be damaged. The long flexors of the fingers are buried beneath the palmar fascia. Only a devastating injury will involve these tendons, and such an injury will inevitably compromise the whole function of the hand.

LATER RECONSTRUCTIVE SURGERY

Despite the efforts of all concerned, some burnt hands heal with joint impairment and contracture. All free grafts tend to shrink, thin ones more so than thicker or full thickness grafts. Grafts on flexor aspects will shrink more than those on extensor aspects, since they are not put on stretch. Further surgery may then be required to improve function.

Frequently, the thumb web needs releasing and the finger webs deepening by the use of local flaps or full thickness skin grafts. Contractures of the flexor aspect of the fingers due to skin shortage, especially during the growth of the burnt hand of a child, are released by scar incision and the insertion of thicker skin grafts into the resultant defects. Adherent grafts on the dorsum may be excised and replaced by thicker or larger skin grafts.

Very little can be achieved surgically to improve tendon function following thermal injury, especially of the extensor tendons. Tenolysis or manipulation of the joint under anaesthesia may be tried. A deformed stiff digit may be fused into a more useful position, or manipulated, in order to improve use and function in the rest of the hand.

In some patients thick contracting bands of hypertrophic scar form in spite of pressure therapy, exercise and splinting, and these need releasing.

THERAPEUTIC MANAGEMENT OF THE BURNT HAND

Management of the burnt hand relies on close co-operation between all members of the Burns Team. The team consists of the burn surgeon and nurses, physiotherapists and occupational therapists, as well as bacteriologists, dieticians, psychologists, anaesthetists and social workers. Other agencies that may be called upon include the psychiatrist and resettlement officer. Regular ward rounds with an exchange of information, case conferences and comprehensive communication notes and records are needed for a good relationship between members of the team and, consequently, a quality outcome for the burn patient. It should be recognized that in many cases the hand burn may be only a small percentage of the total burn surface, and that skills to save the life of the patient may be required by the team.

Therapeutic intervention in the management of a hand burn requires close co-operation between the physiotherapist and occupational therapist, to ensure that the optimum can be achieved in the rehabilitation of the burn patient.

The aims of treatment are to:

- reduce oedema
- maintain joint range
- minimize the formation of contractures and deformities
- restore maximum function.

Therapy should start as soon as possible after the burn injury. Management of the patient will depend on the initial assessment of the hand, taking into consideration not only the type and percentage (size) of the burn, but also the circumstances of the injury, the patient's social status and family background, and any other factors (such as past medical or psychological history) that may have a bearing on the rehabilitation programme. Progressive assessments of the hand during the course of rehabilitation will indicate changes in range of movement and function, and provide guidelines for appropriate therapeutic input.

There are four stages of therapeutic management:

1. Immediate post-burn – first 48 hours
   - positioning
   - splinting
   - maintenance of movement
   - psychological support.
2. Pre-surgery/spontaneous healing
   - positional splinting
   - exercise
   - maintenance of independence
   - psychological support and liaison with the patient's family.
3. Post-operative management – first week
   - positional splinting
   - exercise of non-grafted areas
   - maintenance of independence
   - psychological support.
4. Rehabilitation – the healed hand
   - hand assessment
   - exercise
   - activity
   - management and prevention of contractures and hypertrophic scarring
   - discharge from hospital
   - work assessment and retraining
   - psychological support
   - social aspects of burn.

Immediate post-burn (first 48 hours)

Following injury oedema occurs, and the burnt hand will quickly take up a poor functional position, with wrist flexion and radial deviation, extension or hyperextension of the metacarpophalangeal (MCP) joints, flexion of the interphalangeal (IP) joints, and adduction of the thumb. This is the characteristic claw hand deformity, which can occur as early as 24 hours post-burn (Figures 9.9, 9.10).

Positioning

The burnt hand must be elevated to reduce oedema, aiding its dispersal by gravity. If the swelling is not reduced early, the hand will remain in the clawed position and normal movement patterns become more difficult.

Elevation of the hand can be achieved by using pillows, a Bradford sling, or suspension in a pillowcase or roller towel from a drip stand. It must be stressed to those patients being treated on an outpatient basis that day and night elevation is essential.

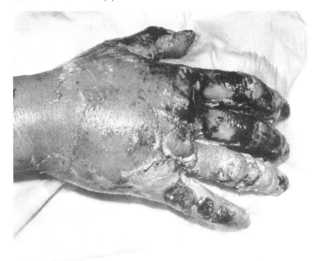

Figure 9.9   Early clawing due to oedema.

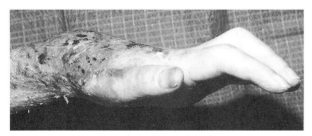

Figure 9.10   Clawed hand deformity.

Splinting
The purpose of positional splinting of the burnt hand is to prevent deformity, which is so often associated with the oedematous hand post-burn. It is imperative to start the regime of splinting as soon as possible. There is a wide range of thermoplastic materials suitable for splinting the burnt hand, including Sansplint, Orthoplast, Orfit, Aquaplast and XLite products.

Burns to the dorsum of the hand and circumferential burns should be splinted in the anti-contracture position:

- wrist in the functional position of 30–40° extension
- MCP joints in maximum flexion (70° of flexion at the MCP joints maintains the collateral ligaments at their maximum length)
- IP joints at maximum extension
- thumb in abduction.

The thumb web space and palmar arches should be maintained by conforming and moulding the thermoplastic material. This type of orthosis is known as the pan or paddle splint or volar wrist/hand orthosis (Figure 9.11).

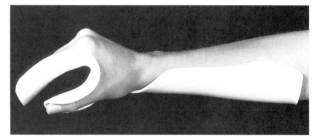

Figure 9.11   Pan or paddle splint.

For palmar burns, the wrist should be positioned in neutral. If there is evidence of palmar tightening, it may be necessary to alternate the paddle splint with one maintaining the hand with the wrist, MCP and thumb in extension.

The paddle splint can be applied over the hand bag or dressings. Initially oedema may prevent the optimum position from being achieved, but as this subsides during the first few days, so the splint can be adjusted or remade to correct the position.

Maintenance of range of movement
Exercises are performed from the day of injury, and a full range of movement is the ultimate goal. Initially pain and oedema will limit joint motion, but as these diminish, joint range will increase.

The following exercises are performed and the therapist will work with the patient several times a day until full range of movement, or the best possible range of movement, is achieved (the hand bag allows complete freedom of movement):

- wrist flexion and extension, radial and ulnar deviation
- MCP joint flexion and extension
- IP joint flexion and extension
- thumb and fingertip opposition
- finger abduction and adduction.

These contribute together to give an adequate power and pinch grip. All exercises are performed slowly and gently to minimize pain and avoid soft tissue reaction.

In deep dermal burns and full thickness burns involving the dorsum of the fingers, making a fist (gross MCP and IP flexion) and proximal interphalangeal (PIP) joint flexion are avoided as they may jeopardize the integrity of the extensor tendon.

Active and assisted active exercises are preferable, as they help to maintain muscle strength and normal movement patterns. If the patient is reluctant or unwilling to move, some gentle manual assistance through the hand bag can be given to channel the patient's efforts. Passive movements, if necessary, are performed with utmost care to prevent further damage.

The therapists will be working under strict sterile nursing procedures. Following burn injury the surface of the burn wound is sterile, and any subsequent infection is due to environmental contamination or organisms from unburnt tissue. The burn patient may be nursed in isolation, and all personnel will need to follow the Burns Unit infection control procedures, usually wearing gowns, gloves and mask.

Where the hand burn is part of a much more extensive injury, exercising may be difficult to achieve if the patient is seriously ill and saving life is the prime factor. However, elevation and splinting must still be insisted upon, thus preventing the hand from assuming the clawed intrinsic minus position.

If the burn involves the upper limb, the arm as a whole is elevated and positioned to maintain at least 90° shoulder abduction and full elbow extension, with the hand in the previously described anti-claw intrinsic plus position.

Psychological support
It is important to appreciate the common response of the patient to burn injury, especially when burns involve the hand. The hand is such a functional tool that if damaged by burn injury it can render the patient dependent on others. There may be three stages in the patient's response to injury; numbing shock, growing awareness, and final acceptance. These three stages can be recognized even in those who have only suffered burns of the hands. All affect the patient's behaviour reactions, and for this reason care and understanding is needed when treating these patients.

Initially there is the stage of acute mental shock at the loss of health and independence and the anticipation of permanent disfigurement or incapacity. Few patients have had any comparable experience of such an injury. Their fears and anxieties may be accentuated by the isolation necessary in early burn management. The response of the burn patient to acute injury may be observed either as withdrawal into personal isolation, with total passive submission and dependence, or as protest and complaint, characterized by speech obscenities, violence and non co-operation.

For the therapist, it is important to try to gain the patient's co-operation and maximum effort throughout all the stages of treatment. This can at times be difficult to achieve, and will depend on the patient's own behavioural response to injury. Much time, patience and understanding is needed, and each stage of treatment must be fully explained to the patient. The therapist's approach and attitude is all important. It must be sympathetic yet firm in order to achieve the necessary goals.

The therapists should work very closely with other members of the Burns Team, and should also work at establishing a rapport with the relatives and carers of the burn patient. Explanation of the positioning, splinting and exercise regimes should be given to the patient and family, and their active involvement in the treatment programme should be encouraged.

Pre-surgery phase/spontaneous healing
Two to three days following burn injury, the patient will be coming out of the initial acute shock phase. The circulatory changes will be resolving and oedema subsiding.

Positional splinting
Positional splinting and elevation of the hand will continue. Careful supervision is needed, as prolonged splintage should be avoided. As soon as pain and oedema allow more movement and the patient becomes more co-operative, the splint can be removed for periods during the day to allow for exercise and activities of daily living (feeding, drinking etc.). The hand is still elevated at all times when not being used or exercised.

The paddle splint will need frequent evaluation and adjustment by the therapist. In time the splint need only be worn at night, provided that the patient is freely using the hand during the day and is able to maintain MCP joint flexion and IP joint extension.

In deep dermal and full thickness burns of the dorsum of the hand, care must be taken to protect any exposed extensor tendons. The paddle splint must be worn continuously, only being removed for careful exercise under the supervision of the therapist.

Individually designed splints may also be needed during this phase; for example, a thumb web splint to maintain abduction or a small gutter splint to protect a single exposed extensor tendon.

Positional splinting of the wrist in extension
When there is a tendency for the daytime unsplinted position of the hand to be held with a dropped wrist, a volar wrist extension splint can be worn over the hand bag or dressings. This should be moulded to position the wrist in neutral to 10° of extension, but allowing functional use of the fingers and thumb. The splint must not block flexion of the MCP joints, so it must only extend to the palmar crease. The paddle splint can be applied overnight.

Exercise
As the pain and oedema decrease so joint range will increase, and exercises should become easier. Free active exercise is encouraged, with gentle manual assistance from the therapist as necessary. The exercises are progressed and repeated frequently until the maximum joint range possible is achieved. Hand use is encouraged, thus translating exercises into functional activity (Figure 9.12).

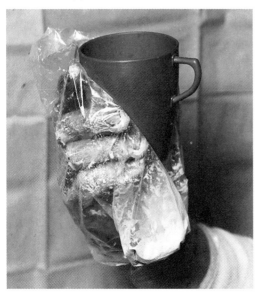

Figure 9.12 Hand bag allowing function and freedom of movement.

The exercises performed are:

- wrist flexion and extension, radial and ulnar deviation
- MCP joint flexion and extension
- IP joint flexion and extension
- thumb and fingertip opposition
- finger abduction and adduction.

Exercises in water may be performed during hand bag dressing changes, when the hand is washed in a warm water bath.

Care may still be needed to protect exposed extensor tendons over the PIP joint by excluding IP joint flexion.

Even if the burn only involves the hand, general arm exercises are encouraged; this helps to avoid a stiff shoulder or elbow, which will affect hand function. Pronation and supination must not be neglected.

Maintenance of independence

Help with daily living activities such as feeding and self-care will increase the patient's self-esteem and independence (Figure 9.13). Whilst the hand is maintained in hand bags, enlarged handles for cutlery, toothbrush, comb and pen may be required. Other ADL equipment, such as non-slip mats for stability on the bed table, can be provided. Provision of book rests, playing card holders and page turners will assist the patient to counteract the depression that often leads to idleness and regression. Any protocol for infection control must be observed, and the materials used for rehabilitation within the Burns Unit or ward should be easily cleaned or autoclaved.

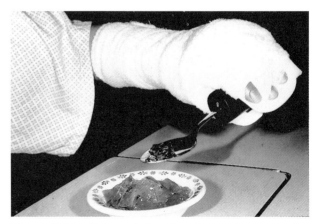

Figure 9.13 Enlarged handles for cutlery may be required (Reproduced with the permission of Nelson Thornes Ltd, courtesy of Maud Malick).

Psychological support and liaison

Explanation of the splinting, positioning and exercise regime should be reiterated to the patient, with advice to the family with regard to suitable games and hand activities in which the family can participate as well, to help improve hand function and morale.

Psychologically, the patient will be passing from the first shock phase to a growing awareness of the implication of the injury sustained and all that it entails. The patient may ask what happened and why, he or she may attempt to attach blame to others and may long to 'put back the clock'. Depression is inevitable, but should not be allowed to become a permanent feature. It is a natural response to all serious injury, the prospect of a series of dressings and surgical procedures, the feeling of uselessness and the cosmetic disfigurement that may be developing. Time must be taken by all members of the team to help the patient through this phase. If necessary, the psychologist and social worker may be called to counsel the patient and carers, and full support must be given.

Post-operative management

Following grafting, positional splinting and hand elevation will continue. Immobilization of the grafted areas will be necessary (in the correct anti-claw position), varying from 4–7 days depending upon Burns Unit protocol and the take (adherence) of the graft. After this period, exercises will recommence and night splinting will continue if full active range of movement is not being maintained with positioning and exercise.

Following the first post-operative dressing change, lighter dressings are applied and are changed on alternate days until the grafts are healed and stable. The donor site dressing is left

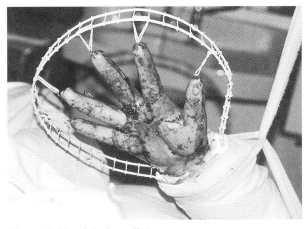

Figure 9.14 A halo splint.

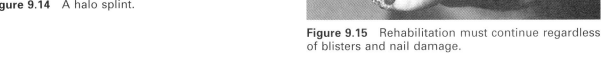

Figure 9.15 Rehabilitation must continue regardless of blisters and nail damage.

intact for 10 days, by which time it should have almost healed.

For post-skin grafting of circumferential finger burns or palmar burns, during the period of immobilization, a halo splint may be made using a thermoplastic hoop with elastic extending to finger nail hooks, Velcro loops or K-wires, thus exposing the grafted areas (Figure 9.14).

If the hand has been covered by a flap, the position of the hand is maintained by pads and strapping to prevent a kink or tension in the flap, which could jeopardize its viability by obstructing the blood flow. The mobility of the free joints should be maintained, and modified movements of the shoulder, elbow and wrist are encouraged until the flap is separated.

Rehabilitation – the healed hand

With spontaneous healing, the hand bag is discarded once the skin has epithelialized and there are no open wounds. Post-grafting, light dressings are continued until the grafts are stable and there are no open areas.

Following healing or grafting, the new skin or grafts are thin and fragile and blister easily. Careful handling and avoidance of friction is therefore required, but mobility and exercise must nevertheless be regained or maintained (Figure 9.15). Should blisters occur, a small light dressing or mefix tape is applied over the blister until dry and healed.

Hand assessment
In this healed, post-grafting phase, a full hand assessment should be carried out to highlight joint range deficits, any developing contractures, grip weakness, functional problems and specific patient needs. Structured hand assessment forms can be used, and graded exercise programmes can then be planned. A patient's fears and anxieties are often expressed during this time, and a good rapport between therapist and patient will provide an essential ingredient for successful rehabilitation.

The patient will have been treated in the ward environment until skin cover is achieved, and an introduction to the physiotherapy and occupational therapy departments may be the first time that the patient has been exposed to the reactions of persons who have not seen burns previously. Sensitive management by the therapists is important; a protected work environment may be necessary at first.

Exercise
Gentle exercise of the grafted area is recommenced once the grafts are stable, usually 5–7 days post grafting, and the patient is encouraged to use the hands functionally. Even with spontaneous healing, it is essential to restore and regain movement and function.

The new fragile skin tends to dry and crack easily. A soft cream (e.g. E45) or oil is gently applied to keep the skin moisturized and supple, and the patient is instructed to do this as often as necessary. As the skin or grafts mature, massaging can become deeper to soften fibrosis and to loosen any contracted soft tissue. Blistering must be avoided. Ultrasound to isolated tight bands can be effective unless the fibrosis is too extensive. General mobility exercises are performed, and the use of the hand in activities of daily living is encouraged. Exercising in water or silicone oil can be beneficial, and the emphasis is on MCP joint flexion, IP joint flexion and extension, thumb abduction and opposition. Heat treatment, hot water and wax baths must be avoided, as the new skin is exceedingly thin and may be insensitive to temperature. Free active exercise, manipulation of objects, squeezing a foam ball, weight and pulley exercises to strengthen the upper limb and grip, proprioceptive neuromuscular facilitation techniques and weight-bearing exercises through the hand are some of the methods that may be used to achieve hand mobility and function.

More specific techniques may be needed to restore lost joint range, including accessory and passive movements, passive stretching and serial splinting. Passive stretching must be gentle, slow and sustained in order to avoid traumatizing the joints and increasing the fibrosis, with a slow end release. Strong active exercise should follow passive stretching.

Strong resisted exercises are also part of the rehabilitation programme, to increase muscle power, strengthen the grip and provide an opposing force to potential contractures. Exercises with theraputty are most effective, as long as there is complete skin cover with no open areas or blisters.

The paddle splint may still be worn at night. The splint must be applied carefully and monitored so as to prevent skin breakdown.

Activity

Ten minutes light activity will be sufficient at the start of the work programme, and attention must be paid to prevent blistering or oedema of the delicate tissues of the hand. Light activities include large pegboard and solitaire, theraputty, dominoes, Scrabble™ (for gross pinch), pick-up sticks, small pegboard activities, puzzles and quilling (for fine pinch). To increase wrist mobility, activity can include the 'ski jump' and varying grip handles of the MULE – microprocessor upper limb exerciser (Figure 9.16). The time-span of activity should be increased as the therapist judges the patient's tolerance and as needs dictate. Activities contraindicated are those that constantly immerse the hand in water or use toxic dyes, and movements abrasive to the skin.

As the grafted area becomes settled, activities can be extended to include more resisted activities such as printing, horticulture and salt dough work. Attention should be given to equate the activity to the patient's skills and employment requirements. Graded activity will extend to include desensitization of the grafted areas. Tactile games and 'sensitivity boxes' containing lentils, polystyrene chips, marbles, dried beans etc can be used.

Contractures and hypertrophic scarring

Following healing, there is a long phase of scar maturation. For 12–18 months, or until scar maturation is complete, the scar will remain active and readily contract and thicken unless met by an equal opposing force such as that provided by exercise, stretching, splinting, the use of pressure garments and silicones. As the burn wound heals, granulation tissue spreads through the damaged area and begins to produce new connective tissue. Vascularization of this tissue is rapid and greater than in normal skin, resulting in redness of the scar tissue. There is an increase in collagen formation; fibroblasts develop contractile properties, causing the gross deformities and contractures associated with hypertrophic scarring.

Hypertrophic scarring develops in 70–80 per cent of all burn scars, especially in the deep dermal burns allowed to heal spontaneously, between grafted areas, and often in the grafts themselves, for it is the bed that becomes hypertrophic. The burn surface takes the appearance of thick, red, hard, raised scars, which are subjectively often hypersensitive, itchy and tight (Figure 9.17). Mechanical pressure with a corresponding stretch applied to a hypertrophic scar will eventually remodel it; scar maturation may take a very long time, but eventually, even without treatment, the scarring will become pale, soft and flat.

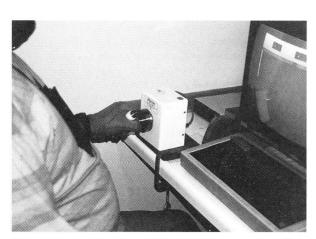

Figure 9.16 MULE – microprocessor upper limb exerciser.

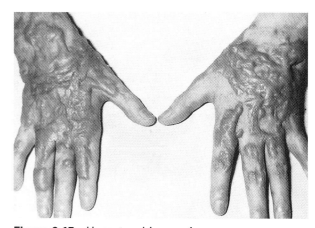

Figure 9.17 Hypertrophic scarring.

Treatment methods to alleviate contracture and hypertrophic scarring include:

- pressure therapy (gloves)
- exercise and stretching
- splinting
- elastomers and putties
- silicone gel sheets.

Pressure therapy – anti-burn scar pressure gloves
The application of pressure is one of the most effective methods of alleviating contracture and hypertrophic scarring. The Lycra/Dacron-Spandex glove, designed to put effective pressure on a hypertrophic burn scar, may be readymade or made to measure. Suppliers of these gloves include Beiersdorf/Jobst, Mainat, Beiersdorf/PanMed, Camp and Juzo. Accurate sizing or measuring is important. The glove must apply direct pressure, but allow full mobility of the hand.

The hand should be completely healed before the glove is fitted, because the dorsal skin is very thin and vulnerable to shearing forces in the early stages of burn wound healing. If necessary, the glove should be fitted with a zipper to aid application. The glove must fit correctly, with good contact in the web spaces. Open tips to the glove will make dexterity easier (Figure 9.18). The patient should wear the glove day and night; all housework, activities, sport and employment are performed wearing the glove, and it is only removed for regular washing and skin care, and

for specific physiotherapy stretching and mobilization techniques.

The direct contact pressure of the elastic glove is most effective on the convex and flat surfaces of the hand. Extra pressure may be required on the concave area of a palmar burn and on web spaces.

Instruction leaflets should be provided, and regular follow-up and checking of the hand, the fit of the glove, insets and moulds is essential. By application of pressure, the thick, gnarled, hypertrophic scarring is reduced and itching is alleviated, a more elastic and pliable scar develops, and less secondary surgery is required.

Two pairs of gloves are normally provided, and they should be remeasured and refitted every 2–3 months. The regime of pressure can last from 12–18 months, after which time the scars will be fully mature and the risk of hypertrophy over.

Exercise and stretching Regular exercise opposing the force and direction of pull of the contracture will help to lessen the formation and severity of contracture. The patient should be made aware of how important this is throughout the scar maturation phase. The potential for contractures to develop can last for many months, so exercising to stretch the new skin and grafts should be performed several times daily and continued well after healing has occurred. Strong resisted exercise is the most effective.

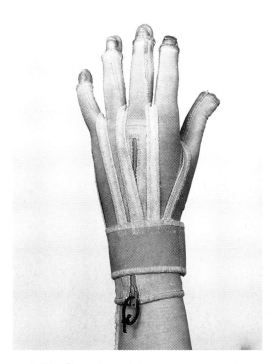

Figure 9.18 Open-tipped Lycra pressure glove with additional finger web spacers.

Splinting Splinting may reduce contractures.

1. *Web contracture.* The web between the thumb and index finger is particularly susceptible to contracture. A C-shaped night splint made from one of the thermoplastic materials will maintain the web in the optimum position required, and can be serially altered (Figure 9.19). A rubber tubing web splint allows active movement by day.
2. *Boutonnière deformity.* The boutonnière deformity occurs when the extensor slip is burnt as it crosses the proximal interphalangeal (PIP) joint, resulting in hyperextension of the distal interphalangeal (DIP) joint of the finger and flexion of the PIP joint. Careful static splinting in extension is required, initially incorporated with the paddle splint provided in the earlier stage of management with the MCP joint at 70° flexion. In the later phase of burn management, surgery may be initiated to release any contracture using K-wire fixation for 2–4 weeks followed by the use of a dynamic Capener splint to maintain extension of the PIP joint. It is the responsibility of the therapist to ensure that splints are monitored and revised as tissue changes occur and range of motion alters.

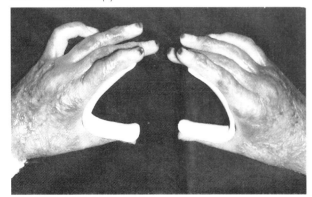

Figure 9.19 A C-shaped thumb web night splint. Reproduced with the permission of Nelson Thornes Ltd.

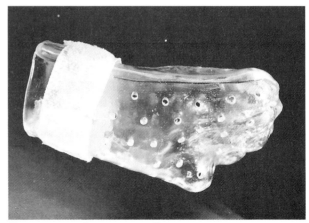

Figure 9.21 An oyster splint.

3. *Palmar burn in children.* To avoid the tightness of the palmar aspect of a child's burnt hand that can be caused by hypertrophic scarring (Figure 9.20), resulting in the clawing of the fingers and thumb, an 'oyster' splint is recommended (Figure 9.21). This is a splint in two sections clipped together in the style of an oyster, made from acrylic material or silastic elastomer. It is worn constantly for 12 weeks, only being removed for washing and exercise periods. Play should be encouraged at the exercise periods. The correct fit of an oyster splint is of paramount importance, so the splint is monitored regularly and parents are given instruction in the management. Children quickly resume and gain full movement of their hands; thus it is more important to prevent contracture at an early stage after grafting than to leave the hand free. This regime could not be used safely in adults, as the adult hand would become totally still after such prolonged splinting.

4. *Fingerweb creep.* Where burn scars cross the base of the fingers and over the MCP joints, hyper-trophic scarring produces a creep of the finger webs distally, which in turn restricts free movement of the MCP and PIP joints (Figure 9.22). Lycra web spacers may be put over a glove to give extra pressure. Web spacers to prevent creep of the scar tissue can also be made from products such as silastic medical elastomer, otoform, silicone putties or silicone sheets. They can be incorporated with splints, bandaged in place, or used with anti-burn scar Lycra gloves, providing a firm pressure that is non-abrasive to the skin.

Elastomers and putties These are made from two component silicones that vulcanize at room temperature, and are non-toxic, non-irritant and non-sensitizing. Clawing of the hand can be reduced by making a palmar mould of elastomer to fit the contours of the hand closely.

Silicone sheets Silicone sheets, made of chemically inert silicone, have been found to be a

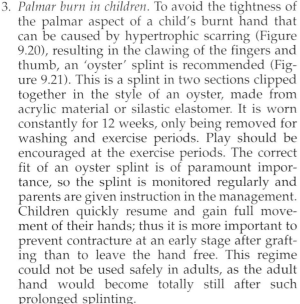

Figure 9.20 Hypertrophic scarring resulting in clawing of the fingers.

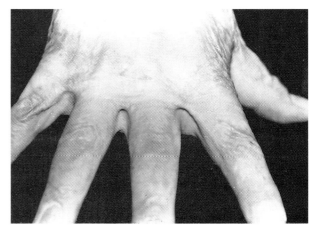

Figure 9.22 Hypertrophic scarring produces creep of the finger webs.

simple, comfortable and effective method of pressure therapy. A strip of silicone can be cut to the size of the hypertrophic scar or web space, which will drape over the skin and conform to the shape required, its elasticity allowing joint movement. This can be taped in place or is adherent to the skin and used alone, or can be incorporated within elastic gloves. As the silicone forms an effective bacterial barrier, it can be used on unhealed areas (Figure 9.23).

As a result of the use of silicone sheets, scars become softer, flatter and smoother, and change from red to the normal paler skin colour. It is recommended that the length of time the silicone sheet is worn is graded from 1–8 hours per day to prevent allergy and heat rashes forming.

Hygiene is important with the use of pressure garments, elastomers and silicone sheets. Regular cleansing and drying of the skin and pressure materials is essential, and careful instruction for the patients and their relatives is of utmost importance.

Despite early elevation, splinting, exercise and intensive rehabilitation and pressure therapy, some hands will heal with joint contractures and limitation of movement. In all circumstances, persistent contractures that limit hand function must be carefully reviewed and the possibilities of surgery may be considered and discussed with the patient and surgeon (Figure 9.24).

Discharge from hospital
Return to the home may carry with it fear and anxiety, particularly in cases where the burn resulted from an accident in the home. The patient will need considerable support from the therapists and other members of the Burns Team. Practising the activities of daily living in the sheltered environment of the occupational therapy department may be followed by a home visit prior to discharge.

Liaison with community therapists, teachers, employers and social services is most important in order that the severely burnt patient can be safely settled into the home, school and work environment. Consultation with the psychologist and introduction to local support groups may benefit the burn patient experiencing psychological problems induced by burn injury.

A thorough assessment prior to discharge is essential. Regular follow-up appointments should be arranged by the Burns Unit, and physiotherapy and occupational therapy, if required, should be organized at local hospitals for the continuity of treatment when the Burns Unit is too far away. Communication, advice and assistance between the Unit and local therapy departments should be frequent and accurate.

Work assessment and retraining
This will start in the sheltered environment of the workshop. Keyboard skills can be assessed using computer and typewriter, and clerical and domestic skills can be practised in the OT department. Grip retraining can be supervised.

The heavy workshop, using activities involving lifting weights, repetitive lifting and carrying relating to the weight required at the work place, will enable appropriate patients to be assessed with regard to suitability to return to work. Woodwork or light metal work can be utilized. Protective gloves may be necessary (Figure 9.25).

Contraindications to work – for instance occupations where high dirt or dust levels are likely, or exposure to chemicals occurs – should be noted. Where tools are likely to be abrasive to freshly healed skin, attempts should be made to produce

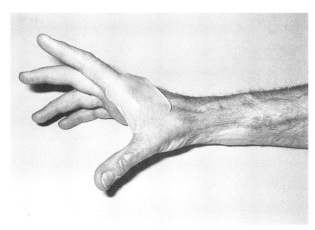

Figure 9.23 Silicone forms an effective bacterial barrier.

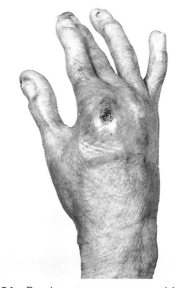

Figure 9.24 Persistent contractures which limit hand function.

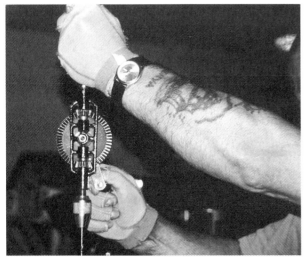

Figure 9.25 Woodwork or light metalwork can be utilized.

alternative protective grips for the tools. The assessment of muscle power and range of movement and hand function should be accompanied by an assessment of stamina, noise tolerance, anxiety level and concentration, for the burn patient may display low tolerance levels after discharge from the Burns Unit. Liaison with employers may be necessary, and the disablement officer may be involved.

Psychological support

Rehabilitation and the recovery of independence and self-respect cannot be achieved until the patient finally accepts what has occurred. This is the third and final phase of the patient's response to injury. In this phase, complete frankness is essential to assist the patient in coming to terms with the injury. Possible future treatment plans and the procedures involved, what to expect and what can be achieved, the long-term prospects of physical recovery, disfigurement and scarring, and the return to the family and to the job are all carefully and accurately explained and discussed with the patient. Not all patients will have passed smoothly from one stage to the next. A few will demonstrate true psychiatric disturbances, but this depends primarily on the pre-burn personality.

Social aspects of burns

If the burnt patient requires a long stay in hospital, then further practical problems such as finance, housing and childcare are generated. Attention must be paid to any outside stresses in order to optimize the patient's emotional recovery and focus his or her energies on rehabilitation. Adapting to a different self-image is not so much a phase as an ongoing process. A patient may be left with scars that cause stress-inducing reactions from new contacts every day. In time, the patient is encouraged to take risks by confronting issues and people in order to pursue plans made before the injury – regarding relationships, career or social activities.

CONCLUSION

Clearly, the most effective form of treatment is prevention. There is an ongoing need for education in burns prevention, especially within the domestic environment.

Treating the burnt hand is a real challenge. With effective early management leading to rapid healing, correct positioning, splinting, exercise, pressure therapy and prolonged aftercare, mobility of the hand can be maintained and contractures reduced to a minimum so that the hand can remain a functional tool with minimal deformity and disfigurement.

Acknowledgement

Figures 9.1–9.12, 9.15, 9.17, 9.18, 9.20 and Fig 9.24 are reprinted from Salter (1987), by permission of the publisher Churchill Livingstone.

FURTHER READING

Clark, J. A. (1992). *A Colour Atlas of Burn Injuries*, pp. 2–24. Chapman and Hall Medical.

Larsen, D. L. (1973). *The Prevention and Correction of Burn Scar Contracture and Hypertrophy*. Texas Shriner's Burn Institute.

Leveridge, A. C. (1991). *Therapy for the Burn Patient*, Chapters 3, 4, 7 (pp. 51–3), 10. Chapman and Hall.

Nadel, E. (1987). Rehabilitation of the burnt hand. Top acute care. *Trauma Rehabil.*, **1(4)**, 50–61.

Perkins, K., Bruce Davey, R. and Wallis, K. A. (1982). Silicone gel, new treatment for burns, scars and contractures. *Adelaide J. Burns*, **9(3)**, 201.

Salter, M. (1987). *Hand Injuries: A Therapeutic Approach*, pp. 173–87. Churchill Livingstone.

Wynn Parry, C. B. (1981). *Rehabilitation of the Hand*, 4th edn., pp. 254–62. Butterworths.

10 The prevention and management of occupational hand disorders

Jeffrey Boyling

INTRODUCTION

Occupational injuries and disorders of the upper limb are not a new phenomenon. In 1717 in his treatise *De Morbis Artificum Diatriba* (*The Diseases of Workers*, translated by Wright in 1940), Bernardo Ramazzini, the father of occupational medicine, clearly showed that common musculoskeletal disorders were associated with eighteenth century occupations. What has developed since the reporting of his work is a refinement in the terminology and management of the injuries and disorders. However, there is still confusion about the existence of certain clinical problems such as repetitive strain injuries (RSI) and even tenosynovitis (Tindall, 1993). This confusion will continue until such time as adequate research has provided definitive answers.

It is worth noting that books on the hand for physiotherapists (e.g. Boscheinen-Morrin *et al.*, 1985; Salter, 1987) do not include chapters on occupational hand conditions. This chapter examines the extent of occupational hand disorders, but it should be noted that only disorders and not injuries are considered. The terminology used is examined to highlight some of the problems facing clinicians. Consequently, a simple classification is used in presenting the various occupational hand disorders. Symptoms and signs are reviewed in relation to the numerous clinical disorders, and management, both clinical and ergonomic, is presented along with guidance for return to work.

EXTENT OF OCCUPATIONAL INJURIES AND DISORDERS

There is no universal system for the reporting and/or recording of occupation-related conditions affecting the upper limb and the hand in particular. Together with the plethora of government agencies, health providers and insurers, this means that data collection and interpretation is fraught with difficulties. However, the following data do provide a small basis from which to progress.

In the United Kingdom (UK), the Health and Safety Executive (HSE, 1993) has published data on self-reported work-related illness collected in a trailer questionnaire on the 1990 Labour Force Survey. The Labour Force survey is a survey of households living at private addresses in Great Britain, and it was carried out by the Office of Population Censuses and Surveys (OPCS) on behalf of the Employment Department.

In 1990, a trailer questionnaire was administered to the sample in England and Wales only. One of the conditions reliably reported in the survey was vibration-induced white finger (VWF). Vibration-induced white finger became a prescribed disease in 1985, and from then until September 1990, 7340 cases were diagnosed under the compensation scheme. A diagnosis of VBF effectively defines the case as occupational, and in the survey there were 15 respondents who reported that work had caused their VBF. Nine cases came from the processing (metal and electrical) occupational group, while the other cases arose in construction, farming, fishing and forestry processing (other) and transport groups.

In the same questionnaire, repetitive strain injury (RSI, including tenosynovitis, bursitis, carpal tunnel syndrome, tennis elbow and frozen shoulder) was reported with an estimated prevalence of 50 000 cases. This was classified separately from the 67 000 cases affecting the upper limbs and neck. The occupations with significantly raised rates were repetitive assembly, inspection and packing (mainly female cases), and construction (all male cases). Self-reported work-related illness in 1995 (HSE, 1998a) utilized different methodology, and as a result only the broadest of comparisons can be made. In that regard, the results show little variation.

In terms of cost, the Health and Safety Executive (1994a) reported that for RSI, 555 000 days were lost at an average of 19 days per case. This was reduced to 293 000 and 17 days respectively for cases caused by work. Unfortunately the data do not provide more detailed analysis, in particular regarding the impact of occupational factors on hand conditions. In the same report VWF alone was responsible for 10 000 days lost, with an average of 12 days lost per case. To put a financial figure on this VBF loss is difficult, but the recently agreed United Kingdom government compensation is reported to be in the region of £500 000 000.

With regard to prescribed upper limb diseases in the United Kingdom, the number of new cases assessed in 1995/96 indicated that the majority were vibration white finger (75 per cent), followed by tenosynovitis (14 per cent), carpal tunnel syndrome (7 per cent), cramp of the forearm and hand (3 per cent) and beat hand/elbow (1 per cent) (Health and Safety Commission, 1997).

More recently the Health and Safety Executive (1998b) has reported statistics in the area of manual handling, which is typically thought to be lifting but in fact includes putting down, pushing, pulling, carrying or moving by hand or by bodily force. Although sprains and strains account for 73.1 per cent of all manual handling accidents, it should not be forgotten that fractures (3.3 per cent) and lacerations (8.8 per cent) are some of the other injuries. Not all of these apply to the hand; 49 per cent apply to the back, but it is worth noting that 14.3 per cent involve the finger and thumb, followed by 8.5 per cent for the hand and wrist, and 10.3 per cent for the arm (HSE, 1998b).

Data for countries other than the UK (HSC, 1997) are available, but once again the difficulty lies with the terminology used and in making meaningful comparisons. Recently, Mital (1999a, 1999b) reported data for non-fatal occupational injuries in the United States.

If anything, the statistics highlight the problem of which diagnostic labels or descriptions are applied to the various symptoms and signs experienced by those workers with hand complaints, as well as the difficulty in quantifying the size of the problem.

CLASSIFICATION AND DEFINITIONS

How should occupational hand disorders be classified? The great variety of traumatic hand injuries makes it practically impossible to make an aetiological classification. However, Simmons and Koris (1992) presented only those disorders that most commonly cause workers to seek medical attention. This was in contrast to Terrono and Millender (1992), who grouped the disorders into either radial- or ulnar-sided wrist pain. Another approach was taken by Cailliet (1994), who considered disorders of nerve, tendon and bone, amongst other issues. The HSE (1990) took a similar approach. In the case of work-related upper limb disorders (WRULDs), Hutson (1997) classified them as Type 1 and Type 2, although Boyling (1996) had previously reported this based on early discussions with Pheasant who, in 1994, had described an additional four types.

Type 1 WRULDs include well-established diagnostic labels, which can be subdivided into two main groups. The first subgroup deals with inflammation of soft tissue, and it is worth remembering the basic definitions found in any medical dictionary. The definitions in Table 10.1 are from Osol (1973).

The second subgroup deals with nerve entrapments. Some authors (e.g. Macnicol and Lamb, 1984) simply listed the conditions based on which nerves are implicated; however, tunnel syndromes in the upper extremities are numerous (Pecina *et al.*, 1997). The list in Table 10.2 shows the disorders, extending distally from the spine to the tip of the upper extremity. This chapter will only deal with those nerve entrapments found in the wrist and hand; however, referral from a distant site should not be overlooked when dealing with symptoms reported in the wrist and/or hand.

TABLE 10.1
DEFINITIONS FOR TYPE 1 WORK-RELATED UPPER LIMB DISORDERS

Bursitis	Inflammation of a bursa
Epicondylitis	Inflammation of an epicondyle, or of tissues near an epicondyle
Ganglion	A cystic, tumour-like localized lesion in or about a tendon sheath or joint capsule
Synovitis	Inflammation of a synovial membrane
Tendonitis	Inflammation of a tendon
Tenosynovitis	Inflammation of a tendon and its sheath
Tenovaginitis	Inflammation of the sheath of a tendon

TABLE 10.2
NERVE ENTRAPMENTS OF THE UPPER QUADRANT

Thoracic outlet syndrome

Anterior scalene syndrome

Costoclavicular syndrome

Hyperabduction Syndrome

Scapulacostal syndrome

Suprascapular nerve syndrome

Lateral axillary hiatus syndrome

Supracondylar process syndrome

Pronator teres muscle syndrome

Supinator syndrome

Anterior interosseous syndrome

Sulcus ulnaris syndrome

Flexor carpi ulnaris muscle syndrome

Syndrome of the musculocutaneous nerve at the elbow

Carpal tunnel syndrome

Ulnar tunnel syndrome

Syndrome of the deep branch of the ulnar nerve

Syndrome of the tendinous arch of the adductor pollicis muscle

Syndrome of the superficial branch of the radial nerve

Collateral digital nerve syndrome

With respect to the Type 2 disorder, Ferguson reported as early as 1984 that:

> the majority of cases of repetition injury are not of localized syndromes but of a more diffuse disorder, apparently of muscles. The disorder, whose symptoms are those of aching, weakness and tenderness of muscles (with or without induration, swelling and heat), is variously termed muscle strain if acute or, if more chronic, occupational myalgia, myositis, myopathy, fibrositis, fibromyositis, muscular rheumatism, non-articular rheumatism, myofascial syndrome or tension myalgia. This syndrome has also been confused and may coexist with occupational cramp ('craft palsy') which should be considered a major variant of repetition injury. Although ill defined muscle aching is extraordinarily prevalent, little is known of its aetiology, pathogenesis and pathology (whether the symptom is of occupational or other origin), nor, if well established, why it appears to persist despite prolonged rest of the affected part.

Type 2 WRULDs include the broad descriptive terms as previously reported by Boyling (1994a, 1994b) and expanded in Table 10.3. The problem with these terms is well-illustrated with upper limb disorder (ULD), which, according to the HSE (1990), is used to encompass a range of different conditions affecting the soft tissues of the hand, wrist, arm and shoulder – i.e. Type 1 disorders plus those of a diffuse nature. In the United Kingdom this is not a new phenomenon, as the term RSI was incorrectly used to encompass a variety of conditions as early as 1987 (Huskisson and Dudley Hart, 1987).

In this chapter, the non-traumatic occupational hand disorders will be classified as Type 1 and Type 2, with subclassifications used where necessary. However, variation in the use of the terms in both Type 1 and Type 2 WRULDs associated with the inaccuracies of examination and treatment has led to confusion amongst clinicians as well as patients. For this reason, a key principle is to use diagnostic labels (Type 1) in preference to the broad descriptive terms.

A further aspect to the debate on terminology has been whether the reported conditions/disorders are caused by occupation. Barton *et al.* (1992) examined the issue of occupational causes of disorders in the upper limb, and concluded that:

> The terminology used in published work on repetitive strain injury is most unsatisfactory and should be discarded. No condition should be prescribed as an industrial disease unless it can be unambiguously defined both clinically and pathologically. At present there is insufficient conclusive evidence of occupational causation to prescribe any further types of 'repetitive strain injuries'.

However, the evidence of work-relatedness is growing (Kuorinka and Forcier, 1995).

ASSESSMENT AND DIAGNOSIS

According to Boscheinen-Morrin *et al.* (1985), assessment is the foundation of management of any occupational injury that involves the hand. Tindall (1993) stated that diagnosis should have regard for the clinical and occupational history, a physical examination as well as consideration of non-occupational causes (see Chapter 2). However, it is worth noting that, in the case of the individual with an occupational injury, it is important that functional assessment relates to the tasks undertaken at work. This will facilitate the rehabilitation process.

TYPE 1 OCCUPATIONAL HAND DISORDERS

These include soft tissue inflammation, nerve entrapments and other disorders.

TABLE 10.3
DESCRIPTIVE TERMS USED FOR TYPE 2 WRULDs*

CTD	Cumulative trauma disorder	United States
OCD	Occupational cervicobrachial disorder	Sweden, Japan
OOS	Occupational overuse syndrome	Australia, New Zealand
RMI	Repetitive motion injury	Canada
RSI	Repetitive strain injury	Australia and Canada
RSI	Repetition strain injury	Australia
TMS	Les troubles musculo-squelettiques	France**
ULD	Upper limb disorder	United Kingdom
WMSDs	Work-related musculoskeletal disorder	World-wide

*Most of the terms (e.g. ULD) have also been used to include Type 1 disorders
**There are approximately 10 terms used in the French language.

Soft tissue inflammation

Radial-sided wrist disorders

Here, there are dorsal carpal tendon sheaths, palmar carpal sheaths and palmar digital tendon sheaths (Kahle *et al.*, 1992). The tendons of the extensor pollicis brevis (EPB) and abductor pollicis longus (APL) run through the first dorsal compartment of the wrist (Lamb and Hooper, 1984). Inflammation of the sheath for the tendons of the abductor pollicus longus and the extensor pollicis brevis occurs frequently, and causes pain in the region of the styloid process of the radius; this is known as de Quervain's tenosynovitis (Figure 10.1).

According to Terrono and Millender (1992), the onset of this condition can be acute or gradual after performing a new job task or a stressful activity. Pain is localized to the area and is exacerbated by use (e.g. active medial abduction of the thumb and passive stretch of the abductor pollicis longus) and improved with rest.

Lamb and Hooper (1984) reported that on palpation, the thickened fibrous sheath may be noted along with crepitis with movement. Finkelstein's test, which involves passive ulnar deviation of the wrist with the thumb gripped in the palm, often

reproduces the pain. Standard conservative treatment involves splintage or injection of hydrocortisone into the affected compartment.

Kendall *et al.* (1993) described the action of the EPB and APL. The extensor pollicis brevis extends the metacarpophalangeal joint of the thumb, extends and abducts the carpophalangeal joint and assists in radial deviation of the wrists. The abductor pollicis longus abducts and extends the carpophalangeal joint of the thumb, radially deviates the wrist and assists in flexing it.

According to Clark *et al.* (1993), the treatment goals are:

1. Restoration of normal painless use of the involved hand
2. Resolution of the chronic inflammatory process
3. Prevention of recurrence.

To achieve these goals, they advocated splinting, anti-inflammatory medication and the reduction of demands on the affected tissues.

It is the current author's opinion that not all cases of pain over the radial styloid are full-blown cases, due to the absence of crepitis. In these cases, avoidance of activities that may involve wrist radial deviation (and flexion) associated with thumb extension should be implemented along with a stretching programme to restore length to the muscles involved. Other treatment modalities to reduce inflammation may be required, but splinting alone is ill advised.

Other radial-sided wrist disorders reported by Terrono and Millender (1992) include abductor pollicus longus tenosynovitis, intersection syndrome and tenosynovitis of the extensor indicis or extensor digitorum. Abductor pollicus longus

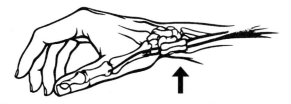

Figure 10.1   de Quervain's tenosynovitis.

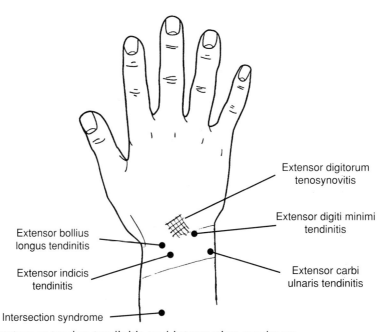

Figure 10.2   Sites of extensor tendon tendinitis and intersection syndrome.

Extensor digitorum tenosynovitis

Extensor digiti minimi tendinitis

Extensor bollius longus tendinitis

Extensor indicis tendinitis

Extensor carbi ulnaris tendinitis

Intersection syndrome

tenosynovitis is less common, and a key point to note is that the tenderness is located where the tendon inserts into the base of the first metacarpal. Intersection syndrome is tendonitis or tenosynovitis of the extensor carpi radialus longus and brevis, which insert into the dorsal surface of the base of the second and third metacarpals respectively (Kendall *et al.*, 1993). Tenosynovitis of the extensor indicis or extensor digitorum can be another presentation, although the pain should be less radially located and associated with active finger extension (Figure 10.2).

Ulnar-sided wrist pain: volar aspect
The palmar carpal tendon sheaths pass through the carpal canal, which is completed by the flexor retinaculum (Kahle *et al.*, 1992). Flexor carpi ulnaris (FCU) tendonitis can result from inflammation of the tendons passing through this region. The work by Kendall *et al.* (1993) reminds readers that the flexor carpi ulnaris inserts into the pisiform and, by ligaments, attaches to the hamate as well as the fifth metacarpal. It flexes and ulnar deviates the wrist, and may assist in flexion of the elbow.

Terrono and Millender (1992) stated that flexor carpi ulnaris tendonitis is frequently seen among workers whose tasks include excessive wrist flexion or heavy lifting. Clinically, there is acute or chronic pain on the volar aspect of the ulnar side of the wrist, and tenderness is present when the FCU tendon is palpated. Pain with resisted wrist flexion and passive wrist extension are other signs to note. The treatment advocated by these authors is splinting and non-steroidal anti-inflammatory medication (NSAIDs). Occasionally a steroid injection may be required, but no mention is made of restoration

of muscle length, which, in the opinion of this author, is essential if further problems are to minimized (refer to Figure 10.2).

Ulnar-sided wrist pain: dorsal aspect
The dorsal synovial sheaths lie in six tendon compartments formed by the extensor retinaculum (Kahle *et al.*, 1992). Extensor carpi ulnaris tendonitis can result from inflammation of the tendons passing through this region. The work by Kendall *et al.* (1993) reminds readers that the extensor carpi ulnaris inserts into the base of the fifth metacarpal on the ulnar side. It extends and ulnar deviates the wrist.

Haj and Wood (1986) stated that the patient may report acute or chronic pain over the ulnar aspect of the wrist, which is exacerbated by active extension and ulnar deviation. Pain may be present when the supinated wrist is stressed in flexion. The cause may be a recent change in activity or hyperflexion of the extended wrist. Once again, Terrono and Millender advocated splinting and NSAIDs. Occasionally a steroid injection may be required. For recurrent problems, tenosynovectomy and release of the extensor carpi ulnaris compartment may be necessary. No mention is made of restoration of muscle length, which again, in the opinion of this author, is essential if further problems are to minimized.

Locking or triggering of a finger (or thumb) is known as stenosing tenosynovitis. This is a common condition in which a finger or thumb sticks in the flexed position, and may be because the fibrous flexor sheath may be narrowed or the tendon enlarged. Normally the patient passively straightens the digit and there may be some associated discomfort (Lamb and Hooper, 1984).

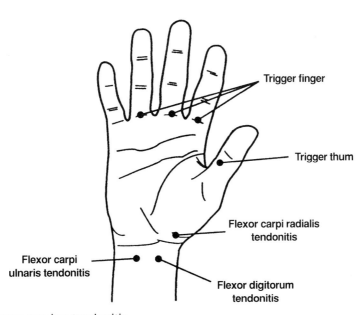

Figure 10.3 Sites of flexor tendon tendonitis.

Macnicol and Lamb (1984) have listed various causes for this condition, including repetitive trauma and excessive use. Simmons and Koris (1992) reported that triggering occurs more frequently in workers who have to perform multiple repetitive motions and/or grasp hard, cylindrical objects firmly. The same authors reported the thumb and ring finger to be the most commonly involved, whereas Macnicol and Lamb (1984) stated that typically it involves the middle finger.

If the condition persists, treatment usually involves surgical release (Lamb and Hooper, 1984). This is in contrast to Frieberg and Levine (1989) and Marks and Gunther (1989), who reported that non-steroidal anti-inflammatory medication (NSAIDs) rarely yields significant results, whereas a steroid injection alleviates complaints in 92–97 per cent of cases.

Ganglions

Lumps can appear on the hand for a variety of reasons, and consequently Macnicol and Lamb (1984) have defined a classification system for them. Their system considers characteristics, types and differentiation.

The most common hand tumour is a ganglion, which is a cystic lesion with a fibrous capsule (Lamb and Hooper, 1984) and contains viscous material similar to synovial fluid. It may be a form of mucoid degeneration of fibrous tissue, or it may be caused by herniation of synovial tissue in the joint.

Ganglions can be work and non-work related. The most common site is the dorsal aspect of the wrist, with a peak incidence in young adults. Terrono and Millender (1992) stated that these cystic masses vary in size, but usually arise from the dorsal scapulolunate interosseous ligament. The patient may have dorsal wrist pain, and the condition is often associated with lax wrists and positive scaphoid instability.

Lamb and Hooper (1984) reported that 50 per cent of ganglions disappear spontaneously. However, recurrence is often a problem where the ganglion ruptures as a result of pressure, whereas surgical excision is more successful. Terrano and Millender (1992) also suggested surgical excision, but listed other treatment options including splinting, job modification, aspiration and cortisone injection.

Terrono and Millender (1992) also described a volar wrist ganglion, which protrudes from the radiocarpal joint, the trapeziometacarpal joint or the scapho-trapezial-trapezoid joint. The onset is often after wrist injury or a change of activity, and treatment is as for a dorsal ganglion.

Nerve entrapments

This chapter will only deal with those nerve entrapments found in the wrist and hand. How-

TABLE 10.4
COMMON FEATURES OF COMPRESSION NEUROPATHIES

Pain worse at night with paraesthesiae in the distribution of the compressed nerve

Pain may be felt proximal as well as distal to the site of compression

Paraesthesiae is only experienced distally

Only symptoms in the early stages, with sensory changes later

Motor weakness and wasting are unusual, late and often irreversible

Site of compression demonstrated by nerve conduction studies

ever, referral from a distant site should not be overlooked when dealing with symptoms reported in the wrist and/or hand (Table 10.4; Figure 10.4).

Median nerve

Carpal tunnel syndrome Carpal tunnel syndrome (CTS) was originally described by Phalen in 1966. Subsequently, the experienced hand surgeons Lamb and Hooper (1984) have described CTS as a disorder caused by compression of the median nerve in the carpal tunnel beneath the flexor retinaculum at the wrist. It is common, especially in middle-aged workmen. However, it may be associated with rheumatoid arthritis, fluid retention during pregnancy, or any anatomical abnormality or tumour-occupying space in the carpal tunnel.

The typical clinical features include the patient being woken during the night by a pain described as 'burning' or 'bursting'. This is not confined to the median nerve distribution, and may often involve the whole hand and forearm. Activities such as shaking the hand or running cold water over it frequently relieves the discomfort. Only in advanced cases is median nerve paresis detectable clinically. Phalen (1966) reported that with a motor deficit in carpal tunnel syndrome, the muscles involved are those of the thumb (opponens pollicis, abductor pollicis brevis) and the first and second lumbrical muscles.

Phalen's test, which involves unforced flexion of the wrist for about a minute, reproduces the symptoms in about 75 per cent of cases. This test has been reported as being reliable by Kuschner et al. (1992).

Louis (1992) reported that CTS is related to excessive use of the hand in highly forceful and repetitive activities in the workplace, and suggested that a conservative approach is indicated if no other medical problem complicates the syndrome. Con-

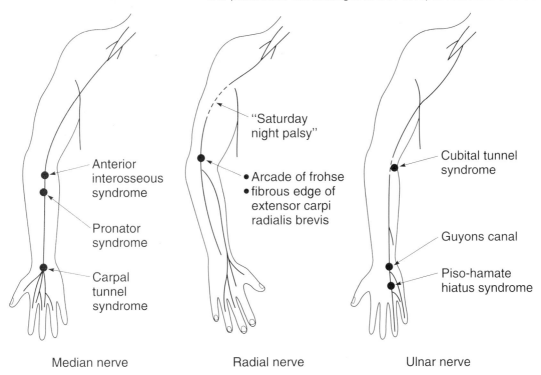

Figure 10.4 Sites of nerve entrapment.

servative treatment involves time away from work, light duties, splinting, steroid injection and NSAIDs. Clark *et al.* (1993) provided a more defined programme of management of this condition.

The author's experience of splinting is that far too often it is poorly applied, with inadequate advice given to the patient. The result is a compressive splint, which complicates the symptoms and enhances the static posture that may have contributed to the symptoms in the first place.

What has not been mentioned in most textbooks is the role of exercise. Research undertaken by Thomas *et al.* (1993) investigated the effect of increasing upper extremity flexibility, strength and circulation on symptoms of carpal tunnel syndrome. The small numbers involved in this research may explain why the outcome was not significant.

Lamb and Hooper (1984) reported that surgical decompression is very successful in the management of CTS. This is in contrast to the views of Louis (1992), who stated that aggressive surgery frequently does not restore the worker to an asymptomatic state. It is the author's experience that surgery for CTS where occupation is a primary cause is not as successful as surgery for CTS where occupation is not a causative factor.

Prevention is the key principal in avoidance of this condition in the workplace. The key tips are listed below:

1. Adopt a neutral wrist position
2. Avoid ulnar deviation
3. Avoid repetitive tasks
4. Use properly designed tools.

Pronator teres median nerve compression Sensory disturbances in the hand may not be confined to carpal tunnel syndrome (Cailliet, 1994). In particular, sensory disturbances of the forearm indicate that compression of the median nerve is proximal to the tunnel, as the median nerve normally gives off the palmaris branch prior to entering the tunnel. It is also worth noting that in the pronator teres syndrome, the muscles of the thenar eminence as well as the flexors of the wrist and fingers are involved. In particular, the patient's complaints relate to thumb, index finger and middle finger flexion.

Treatment should be directed at releasing those structures that are tight and causing compression of the median nerve. However, attention should also be given to those activities involving pronator teres activity, particularly static activity of the muscle.

It is worth noting that typists require the forearm to be pronated, and this can lead to static activity in the pronator teres muscle. This action is influenced by the extent of flexion at the elbow. A key tip is to return the forearms to a neutral position in terms of supination/pronation when not typing.

Anterior interosseous syndrome The anterior interosseous nerve is a motor branch of the median nerve, and it can be subjected to compression in the cubital tunnel. This can result in impaired function of the distal phalanges of the thumb and index finger. The main complaint of the patient is the inability to pinch between the thumb and the index finger (Cailliet, 1994).

Since the nerve is located under the deep fascial layer of the flexor digitorum superficialis, it is worth investigating this particular muscle. According to Kendall *et al.* (1993), the muscle flexes the proximal interphalangeal (PIP) joint of the second to fifth digits. Therefore, the muscle should be checked for any tightness or over-activity, especially in cases where the task requires PIP flexion (e.g. gripping). A key tip is to check the length and/or activity of the flexor digitorum superficialis.

Ulnar nerve
The ulnar nerve may be compressed at a number of sites, and each will result in symptoms and signs in the hand.

The first potential compression site is the cubital canal. Cailliet (1994) reported that, depending on the degree of motor involvement, clumsiness of hand activity may be a complaint. This, in association with an aching pain on the medial site of the elbow near the medial epicondyle and shooting pains in the ulnar aspect of the little finger, should alert the therapist to compression of the ulnar nerve in the cubital tunnel.

Butler (1991) described tests for neural mobility for this and other upper limb nerves, but Vanderpool (1968) reported a provocative test, which involved flexing the elbow fully and extending the wrist for 3 minutes. Motor evaluation should involve assessment of the first dorsal interosseous and abducti digiti minimi. In extreme forms, atrophy of the hypothenar region and in the first web space becomes apparent.

The next site of ulnar nerve compression is in the wrist (Cailliet, 1994). Here, the ulnar nerve enters the hand in a shallow trough formed between the pisiform bone and the hook of the hamate bone, which is known as Guyon's canal. Trauma to the nerve can result from a direct blow or repeated blows – a good example would be the forceful use of pliers. Apart from a fractured hook of hamate or pisiform, other causes can be non-traumatic, and Terrano and Millender (1992) listed a number, including masses, lipoma or aberrant muscles.

The palmar branch of the nerve innervates the hypothenar muscles as well as the two lateral lumbricals, all the interosseous muscles, the adductor pollicis and the deep head of the flexor pollicis brevis muscle.

A further site of compression is close by. In piso-hamate hiatus syndrome, only a motor branch of the ulnar nerve is compressed and therefore it is similar to Guyon's syndrome. Due to the anatomical arrangement, the adductor digiti quinti minimi muscle is not affected (Cailliet, 1994).

Treatment in all cases is by removal of the compressive force affecting the nerve. This may involve surgery, but prevention should not be overlooked in the industrial setting.

A key tip is to avoid nerve compression, irrespective of whether it is direct (i.e. external; e.g. repeated blows) or indirect (i.e. internal; e.g. static muscle activity) compression.

Hand–arm vibration syndrome

According to the Health and Safety Executive (1994b), hand–arm vibration syndrome (HAVS) is a widespread industrial disease that affects tens of thousands of workers. Its best-known effect is vibration-induced white finger (VWF).

For the worker, HAVS can result in painful attacks and the loss of the ability to grip properly. The cause is any vibrating tool or process that causes tingling or numbness after 5–10 minutes of continuous use (Table 10.5). For the therapist, there are a number of components to hand–arm vibration syndrome, and these are vascular, neurological, skeletal, muscular and soft tissue.

The vascular component typically manifests itself as episodic finger blanching. Normally it starts with a tip of a finger, and as the condition progresses, so does the area affected. The sequence of colour change seen in the finger is often white, purple and red. Naturally, with the return of circulation to the area there is an increase in throbbing and this can be uncomfortable. The main trigger for the symptoms is exposure to cold, and during attacks the sufferer may complain of pain, numbness and cold as well as reduced manual dexterity and loss of finger co-ordination.

Tingling, numbness, loss of sensation and manual dexterity are some of the neurological symptoms of HAVS. The skeletal component comprises disorders of the bones (cysts and vacuoles). Casual relationships with muscle fatigue and carpal tunnel syndrome have been reported.

TABLE 10.5
CAUSES OF HAZARDOUS VIBRATION

Percussive metalworking tools

Percussive tools used in stone working, quarrying, construction etc.

Grinders and other rotary tools, e.g. pneumatic tools

Timber and wood machining tools, e.g. chain saw

Other processes and tools, e.g. pounding machines

Symptoms include tingling and numbness, which are persistent and occur without provocation. Other symptoms are blanching, pain and flushing. (Simmons and Koris, 1992). The classification of symptoms has been based on a number of scales. Originally the Taylor and Pelmear classification was used, although more recently the Stockholm workshop scales tend to be invoked (Gemme *et al.*, 1987). Diagnosis ultimately depends on the judgement of the medical examiner, taking into account both reported symptoms and the findings on clinical examination, including objective testing where appropriate. The use of a standardized questionnaire can assist in this routine assessment.

According to Simmons and Koris (1992), once the disease becomes irreversible the worker no longer has the potential to return to the old job and may become permanently unable to work. There is little effective treatment for the vascular symptoms of HAVS, and there is no treatment for its neurological component. In the United Kingdom, VWF is a compensatable condition. Naturally, the management of hand–arm vibration syndrome is by prevention. This involves identifying hazardous jobs, vibration control, information and training for workers and their supervisors, and routine health surveillance (Pelmar *et al.*, 1992).

A key tip is to isolate the worker from any sources of vibration, especially those involving the hand.

Further disorders

In the absence of inflammatory conditions, compression of nerve tissue, ganglions and hand–arm vibration syndrome (HAVS), there are numerous other musculoskeletal disorders that can occur. The reader is reminded of those disorders in Table 10.6, and advised to refer to Millender *et al.* (1992) for further details.

TYPE 2 OCCUPATIONAL HAND DISORDERS

In 1984, Ferguson described the Type 2 disorder with its widespread distribution of symptoms and minimal signs. Since then, there have been few studies that have clearly detailed normal examination findings. Associated with this has been the problem of diagnosis, especially amongst the medical community. Their preoccupation with correlating symptoms and signs with a specific entity leaves little room for a condition where the presentation may vary. There is an unwillingness amongst the medical profession to accept that multiple factors may coexist, resulting in neuro-musculoskeletal dysfunction. This can then be compounded by psychological factors. What then are some of the common factors seen in the Type 2 presentation? Table 10.7 provides an answer, but it is by no means fully inclusive.

From the perspective of the medical profession, treatment is not covered in great detail. In the text edited by Millender *et al.* (1992), specific detail for treatment of the Type 2 disorder is not listed, although rehabilitation is recommended as the option of choice for returning an injured worker to the workplace. Interestingly, when discussing prevention, management and outcome, Huskisson (1992) set out the approaches to avoid, including surgery, drugs, injections and the quest for compensation. Only general therapeutic objectives were

TABLE 10.6
OTHER DISORDERS/INJURIES OF THE WRIST AND HAND (ADAPTED FROM MILLENDER *ET AL.*, 1992)

Ulnar-sided wrist symptoms	*Radial-sided wrist symptoms*
Volar aspect: • pisotriquetrial arthritis • ulnar artery thrombosis • hypothenar muscle strain	Trapezio-metacarpal joint • instability • arthritis
Dorsal aspect: Extensor carpi ulnaris-tendonitis-subluxation	Scapho-trapezial-trapezoid arthritis
Distal radio-ulnar joint (DRUJ) disorders • chondromalacia of DRUJ • DRUJ instability	Wrist joint • scapholunate dissociation (static/dynamic) • scapholunate advanced collapse • Keinbock's disease
Injuries of triangular fibrocartilage complex (TFCC) • traumatic tears of TFCC • degenerative tears of TFCC • ulnar impaction syndrome	
Disabilities of the ulnar carpus • tears of lunotriquetral ligament • mid-carpal instability	

TABLE 10.7

COMMON FACTORS SEEN IN THE TYPE 2 PATIENT

Initial symptoms are usually distal (e.g. wrist or hand)

Delayed reporting

Delayed clinical management

Poor clinical management

Rest leading to the avoidance of all activities

Loss of physical condition

Stiffness

Compensatory limb and trunk actions

Muscle imbalance of the neck shoulder region

Muscle imbalance of the forearm

Minor peripheral neuropathies

Fear, anxiety and/or depression

TABLE 10.8

GENERAL THERAPEUTIC OBJECTIVES IN THE TREATMENT OF WMSDs (ADAPTED FROM KUORINKA AND FORCIER, 1995)

Promote rest for the affected anatomical structures

Diminish spasms and inflammation

Reduce pain

Increase strength and endurance

Increase range of motion

Alter mechanical and neurological structures

Increase functional and physical work capacity

Modify the work and social environment

listed by Kuorinka and Forcier (1995), and these objectives are set out in Table 10.8. On the other hand, Hutson (1997) provided guidance on the management of the Type 2 disorder when seen early or when in an established state, and the key elements are summarized in Table 10.9. Interestingly, little is said about the established Type 2 disorder in terms of detail. This is in contrast to Hadler (1993), who does make reference to the diffuse Type 2 disorders but considers that cumulative trauma disorder (CTD) is an iatrogenic concept promulgated in the face of a contrary body of information, which he supports with six discrete bodies of information. Consequently, treatment of the diffuse category was not supplied.

The importance of accurate examination has been stressed elsewhere (Boyling, 1996), but what treatment options exist for the patient? Pascarelli and Quilter (1994) listed these as rest, splinting, drug treatment, surgery and alternative treatments. Brennan (1985) also stated that 'If your pain comes from RSI, then the most useful thing your physiotherapist can do for you is to recommend *rest, rest and more rest*'. Brennan did advocate the use of other physiotherapy modalities to supplement the rest.

In a series of 74 women seen in 1982/83 and reported by Brown and Dwyer (1987), the majority had multiple conditions and as such could be considered to be in the Type 2 classification. The main treatments reported were rest (62 per cent), graded arm activity supervised by an occupational therapist (47 per cent), physiotherapy (44 per cent), removable splints individually moulded and fitted by an occupational therapist (36 per cent), and work modification (33 per cent). The physiotherapy was not specified. However, the outcome reported was that only 26 per cent of patients recovered; 38 per cent were permanently impaired, and the outcome in the remainder was unknown.

TABLE 10.9

MANAGEMENT PRINCIPLES FOR TYPE 2 DISORDER (ADAPTED FROM HUTSON, 1997)

Early presentation	*Established presentation*
Containment (prevention of progression) Modification of work risk factors Symptomatic relief Physical treatment of underlying dysfunction Relaxation Psychological	1. Neuropathic arm pain • education of patient and employer • ergonomic improvements • relaxation therapies • symptomatic relief • tricyclics • rehabilitation counselling 2. Neuropathic arm pain (NAP) and abnormal illness behaviour (AIB) • cognitive–behavioural therapy

From all of these works it is evident that the term 'rest' needs clarification, since it is still being advocated (Kuorinka and Forcier, 1995). Pascarelli and Quilter (1994) defined rest as avoiding the activities that lead to the RSI. However, rest could also be considered as a prelude to rigor mortis and, in the author's opinion, it is a term that should be removed from medical terminology and replaced by 'controlled activity programme (CAP)'. Too often it has been the author's experience to see patients where all activity has ceased, and this has compounded the patient's initial problem both physically and mentally.

Associated with the use of the term rest has been the provision of splints to immobilize an affected joint. For example, Putz-Anderson (1988) advocated splinting, heat and cold, medication, stretching and exercise in the treatment of CTD. According to Rempel *et al.* (1992), 'Immobilization should be instituted judiciously and monitored carefully to prevent muscle atrophy'. It is often overlooked that the symptoms reported may be due to maintaining a fixed position of a joint, and immobilizing that same joint suggests an absence of clinical reasoning on the part of the person who supplied the splint. With the Type 2 disorder it will usually compound the underlying problem, and for that reason is not strongly advocated by the author.

In terms of physiotherapy, a variety of approaches have been reported. In the case of Pascarelli and Quilter (1994), aggressive physical therapy (deep tissue massage) should be provided 1–3 times a week during the rest phase. On the other hand, Duff (1997), despite being a physical therapist, does not really deal with the diffuse symptom presentation of the Type 2 disorders.

However, the contribution from other physiotherapists in the treatment of upper limb disorders should not be overlooked. Elvey and Quinter (1986) examined 60 patients complaining of arm and hand symptoms, often associated with neck pain. Their symptoms were reproduced with brachial plexus tension (and other orthopaedic) tests that compromised neural tissue in the neck. Clinical examination failed to identify any recognizable pathological condition in the arms and hands of any of the patients. In view of this, the focus of treatment was moved to neural tissue. Butler (1991) further raised awareness of the role of nerve tissue. Studies by Cohen *et al.* (1992) led them to report that refractory cervicobrachial pain syndrome may be of neuropathic pathogenesis. The symptoms and their behaviour were then explained in terms of centrally and spinally mediated processes.

The author (Boyling, 1994b, 1996) has already stated the importance of accurate examination as a foundation in the treatment of the Type 2 disorder. However, there are a couple of aspects that warrant mention, namely neural tissue and muscle balance.

With regard to neural tissue, its role in the production of symptoms has been highlighted by several published reports. Grant *et al.* (1995) highlighted the impact of screen-based keyboard operation on the extensibility of the radial nerve. A separate study of 29 office subjects and 17 patients by Greening and Lynn (1997) identified the presence of a polyneuropathy in the patient group, and suggested early evidence of the same existing in the office group. Once again nerve tissue has been implicated, but details of the brief clinical examination did not state the extent to which muscle function was investigated apart from examining range of movement and muscle power. In a second paper, Greening and Lynn (1998) suggested that, in patients with diffuse limb pain, there may be a contribution from nerve injury – i.e. a neuropathic component. They went on to suggest that manual techniques and exercises to relieve compressive effects and restore normal neural dynamics should be effective in management of these conditions.

Unfortunately, with any new approach there is a swing of the pendulum. With few exceptions, patients with positive responses to mobility testing of the neural tissue as outlined by Butler (1991) have been subjected to stretching of the same neural tissues in the erroneous belief that it was necessary. Greater attention should have focused on the interface of the nerve tissue to ascertain what was responsible for the loss of neural mobility in the first place. Attention directed at those tissues would then allow the test of neural mobility to be used for reassessment purposes.

A number of authors have studied the role of muscle balance. Grant *et al.* (1997) reported a single case study dealing with active stabilization training for screen-based keyboard operators. Although this study dealt with stability of the cervical spine, it should not be forgotten that referral from the neck to the wrist and hand is anatomically possible. Mottram (1997) also investigated the subject of stability, but in relation to the scapula. It is worth remembering that poor proximal stability limits the control of distal elements such as the hand. As such, dynamic control of the scapula is essential for optimum upper limb function.

Perhaps the only detailed clinical manual for physiotherapists dealing with the assessment and treatment of industrial over-use syndrome (upper limb) was that produced by Lucas (1986) with contributions from two other physiotherapists (Atkinson and Rogerson). What is surprising about this manual is the areas covered. For example, the brachial plexus is specifically mentioned, along with posture (particularly dynamic stability of the scapula) and the use of tape. Specific muscles are listed for examination and techniques of stretching outlined. Mobilization and manipulation is not overlooked, nor is the return to work of the worker. A return to basics in terms of treatment is not always a bad choice.

To summarize, key tips for the management of Type 2 disorders are as follows:

1. Early referral to physiotherapy
2. Accurate examination
3. Patient education
4. Use of appropriate treatment modalities
5. Restoration of fitness
6. Graded return to an ergonomically sound workplace.

ERGONOMICS

Predisposing work conditions

Pheasant (1991) reported that, for production line workers, 'the worst problems are often associated with repeated forceful gripping and turning actions executed with the wrist in a deviated position'. According to the HSE (1990), the majority of occupational factors associated with the increased risk of ULD can be grouped into three general areas – force, frequency and duration, and posture (Figure 10.5).

Force was considered to be the application of undesirable manual force. Frequency and duration related to movement, including unsuitable rates of working or repetition of a single element. Posture referred to awkward positions of the hand, wrist, arm or shoulder. Other work-related factors such as cold and vibration were mentioned (HSE, 1990). Other authors (Pheasant, 1991; Kuorinka and Forcier, 1995) have also reported these risk factors. These predisposing work conditions are considered in relation to the hand, but reference should also be made to Table 10.10.

Force

Neutral wrist postures have been reported to permit maximal power grip (Kraft and Detels, 1972). Furthermore, a pinch grip requires approximately five times greater tendon and joint loads than a power grip (Chao *et al.*, 1976). However,

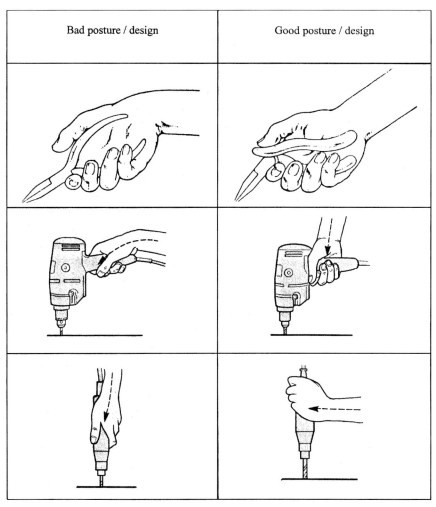

Bad posture / design	Good posture / design

Figure 10.5 Good and bad wrist positions influenced by equipment design and/or grip.

TABLE 10.10
MUSCULOSKELETAL DISORDERS OF THE WRIST AND HAND: ERGONOMIC RISK FACTORS (ADAPTED FROM PHEASANT, 1991)

Task demands	Disorder
Repeated 'clothes wringing' action (flexion/extension with supination/pronation and power grip)	Tenosynovitis, especially De Quervain's
Repeated radial and ulnar deviation, especially with forceful grip, e.g. using a spanner	Tenosynovitis, especially De Quervain's
Repeated pronation/supination with ulnar deviated wrist, e.g. twisting with pliers	Tenosynovitis, especially De Quervain's
Repeated gripping actions with flexed wrist	Tenosynovitis of finger flexors (trigger finger)
Repeated flexion/extension of wrist, especially if combined with pinch grip or power grip	Carpal tunnel syndrome
Repeated application of force with hand, with wrist in extended position	Ulnar nerve entrapment at wrist
Tools with triggers – especially if handle is too large so that proximal interphalangeal joint is extended	Tenosynovitis of finger flexors (trigger finger)

clinical factors can influence grip force, as reported by Lowe and Freivalds (1999). The primary finding from this latter study was that individuals with CTS lose some ability to co-ordinate efficient grip force on hand tools and exert higher grip forces on tools, at equivalent application forces, than controls. This is believed to be a result of tactile sensibility deficits associated with CTS.

Frequency and duration
A number of authors, including Rodgers (1987), have investigated this risk factor. Putz-Anderson (1988) stated that there is likely to be an increase in incidence of these disorders in jobs which have more that 1500–2000 repetitions per hour and/or a cycle time of 30 seconds, particularly if more than half is taken up by a single sequence of repeated actions. It is worth noting that a cycle time of 30 seconds is equivalent to about 900 production units per shift (Pheasant, 1991).

Posture
Posture can be classified as neutral, extreme (i.e. close to end of range), non-extreme but influenced by gravity, or non-extreme but influenced by geometry. In the case of the wrist, a number of studies have shown the effect of the non-neutral positions. Markison (1990) has been involved with musical instruments and their redesign to reduce the extreme postures, and the forces required to maintain finger positions at the keyboard against gravity were investigated by Rose (1991). Minimum key activation forces were specified as a result. A more recent study (Serina et al., 1999) showed that

wrist and forearm postures during typing were sustained at non-neutral angles; the mean wrist extension angle was $23.4 \pm 10.9°$ on the left and $19.9 \pm 8.6°$ on the right, and the mean wrist ulnar deviation was $14.7 \pm 10.1°$ on the left and $18.6 \pm 5.8°$ degrees on the right.

Hand tools
A number of factors that influence the task, including grip type, wrist posture, grip size, gloves and work behaviour, have been reported (Pheasant, 1986, 1991; Kuorinka and Forcier, 1995). Interactions occur such that grip strength varies with wrist position as well as handle size. Handle size was investigated by Pheasant and Scriven (1983), and they reported that maximum strength occurred with a handle 45 mm in diameter. Fraser (1980) listed certain basic requirements for the design of an efficient hand tool (Table 10.11).

TABLE 10.11
BASIC REQUIREMENTS FOR THE DESIGN OF AN EFFICIENT HAND TOOL (ADAPTED FROM FRASER, 1980)

It should effectively perform its intended function

It should be properly proportioned to the dimensions of the user

It should be appropriate to the strength and endurance of the user

It should minimize user fatigue

It should provide sensory feedback

Evaluation

A number of government bodies (HSE, 1990; NOHSC, 1990; OSH, 1991) have produced guides to prevent upper limb disorders, and the reader should refer to them. Furthermore, Kuorinka and Forcier (1995) have reviewed the evaluation of risk, but one specific tool warrants mention. McAtamney and Corlett (1992, 1993) reported a risk assessment tool for upper limb disorders. The tool, known as RULA (rapid upper limb assessment), although not specific to the wrist and hand, does include wrist and hand factors. Any evaluation should not forget the psychosocial aspects of musculoskeletal disorders, and Moon and Sauter (1996) have reported on this with regard to office work.

Summary

To summarize, key tips for the prevention of an upper limb disorder are:

1. Adopt a balanced joint position
2. Avoid static muscle work
3. Do not compress the nerves
4. Reverse the posture regularly
5. Exercise to stay fit
6. Apply ergonomic principles.

CONCLUSION

The management of occupational disorders of the hand provides the therapist with a clinical challenge. However, the greatest challenge for anyone working in the field of occupational health is the prevention of musculoskeletal disorders affecting the upper extremity, and in particular the hand.

REFERENCES

Barton, N. J., Hooper, G., Noble, J. and Steel, W. M. (1992). Occupational causes of disorders in the upper limb. *Br. Med. J.*, **304,** 309–11.

Boscheinen-Morrin, J., Davey, V. and Conolly, W. B. (1985). *The Hand. Fundamentals of Therapy.* Butterworths.

Boyling, J. D. (1994a). Ergonomics and the management of pain. In: *Pain Management by Physiotherapy* (P. E. Wells, V. Frampton and D. Bowsher, eds), pp. 29–38. Butterworth-Heinemann.

Boyling, J. D. (1994b). Prevention and treatment of upper limb disorders. In: *Physiotherapy in Occupational Health* (B. Richardson and A. Eastlake, eds), pp. 195–207, Butterworth-Heinemann.

Boyling, J. D. (1996). The 1996 Olive Sands Memorial Lecture: Work Related Upper Limb Disorders. *OCPPP In Touch*, **81,** 2–6.

Brennan, P. (1985). *RSI. Explorer's Guide Book.* Primavera Press.

Brown, M. C. and Dwyer, J. M. (1987). Repetition strain injury: an approach to treatment and prevention. In: *Readings in RSI* (M. Stevenson, ed.), pp. 80–90. New South Wales University Press.

Butler, D. (1991). *Mobilisation of the Nervous System.* Churchill Livingstone.

Cailliet, R. (1994). *Hand Pain and Impairment*, 4th edn. F. A. Davis Co.

Chao, E. Y., Opgrandi, F. and Axmere, M. (1976). Three-dimensional force analysis of the finger joints in selected isometric hand functions. *J. Biomech.*, **9,** 387–96.

Clark, G. L., Shaw Wilgis, E. F., Aiello, B. *et al.* (1993). *Hand Rehabilitation. A Practical Guide.* Churchill Livingstone.

Cohen, M. L., Arroyo, J. F., Champion, G. D. and Browne, C. D. (1992). In search of the pathogenesis of refractory cervicobrachial pain syndrome. *Med. J. Aust.*, **156,** 432–6.

Duff, S. V. (1997). Tendonitis, entrapment neuropathies, and related conditions. In: *Management of Cumulative Trauma Disorders* (M. J. Sanders, ed.), pp. 41–103. Butterworth-Heinemann.

Elvey, R. L. and Quinter, J. L. (1986). A clinical study of RSI. *Aust. Fam. Phys.*, **15(10),** 1314–22.

Ferguson, D. (1984). The 'new' industrial epidemic. *Med. J. Aust.* **March** 17, 318–19.

Fraser, T. M. (1980). Ergonomic principles in the design of hand tools. *Occupational Safety and Health Series No 44.* CIS 81–1226. International Labour Office.

Frieberg, A. and Levine, R (1989). Non-operative treatment of trigger fingers and thumbs. *J. Hand Surg.*, **14A,** 553.

Gemne, G., Pyykkoe, I. and others (1987). The Stockholm Workshop Scale for the classification of cold-induced Raynaud's phenomenon in the hand–arm vibration syndrome (revision of the Taylor–Pelmear Scale). *Scand. J. Work, Environ. Health*, **13(4),** 275–6.

Grant, R. J., Forrester, C. and Hides, J. (1995). Screen-based keyboard operation: the adverse effects on the neural system. *Aust. J. Physio.*, **41(2),** 99–107.

Grant, R. J., Jull, G. A. and Spencer, T. J. (1997). Active stabilisation for screen-based keyboard operators – a single case study. *Aust. J. Physio.*, **43(4),** 235–42.

Greening, J. and Lynn, B. (1997). Vibration sense in the upper limb in patients with repetitive strain injury and a group of at-risk office workers. *Int. Arch. Occup. Environ. Health*, **71(1),** 29–34.

Greening, J. and Lynn, B. (1998). Minor peripheral nerve injuries: an underestimated source of pain ? *Man. Ther.*, **3(4),** 187–94.

Hadler, N. M. (1993). *Occupational Musculoskeletal Disorders.* Raven Press.

Haj, A. A. and Wood, M. B. (1986). Stenosing tenosynovitis of the extensor carpi ulnaris. *J. Hand Surg.*, **14A,** 519.

Health and Safety Commission (1997). *Health and Safety Statistics 1996/7.* HSE Books.

Health and Safety Executive (1990). *Work-Related Upper Limb Disorders. A Guide to Prevention.* HS(G)60. HMSO.

Health and Safety Executive (1993). *Self-Reported Work-Related Illness. Results from a Trailer Questionnaire on the 1990 Labour Force Survey in England and Wales.* HSE Books.

Health and Safety Executive (1994a). *The Costs to the British Economy of Work Accidents and Work-Related Ill Health.* HSE Books.

Health and Safety Executive (1994b). *Hand–Arm Vibration.* HS(G)88. HMSO.

Health and Safety Executive (1998a). *Self-Reported Work-Related Illness. Results from a Household Survey.* HSE Books.

Health and Safety Executive (1998b). *Manual Handling. Manual Handling Operations Regulations 1992. Guidance On Regulations.* L23. HMSO.

Huskisson, E. C. (1992). *Repetitive Strain Injury. The Keyboard Disease.* Charterhouse Conference and Communications Limited.

Huskisson, E. C. and Dudley Hart, F. (1987). *Joint Disease: All the Arthropathies.* 4th edn. Wright.

Hutson, M. A. (1997). *Work-Related Upper Limb Disorders: Recognition and Management.* Butterworth-Heinemann.

Kahle, W., Leonhardt, H. and Platzer, W. (1992). *Color Atlas/Textbook of Human Anatomy, Locomotor System*, Vol. 1, Georg Thieme Verlag.

Kendall, F. P., McCreary, E. K. and Provance, P. G. (1993). *Muscles Testing and Function*, 4th edn. Williams & Wilkins.

Kraft, G. and Detels, P. (1972). Position of function of the wrist. *Arch. Phys. Med. Rehabil.*, **53**, 272–5.

Kuorinka, I. and Forcier, L (1995). *Work-Related Musculoskeletal Disorders (WMSDs): A Reference Book for Prevention.* Taylor & Francis.

Kuschner, S. H., Ebramzadeh, E., Johnson, D. *et al.* (1992). Tinel's sign and Phalen's test in carpal tunnel syndrome (original research). *Orthopedics*, **15**, 1297–1302.

Lamb, D.W. and Hooper, G. (1984). Benign tumour stenosing tenosynovitis. *Hand Conditions*, pp. 65, 99. Churchill Livingstone.

Louis, D. S. (1992). The carpal tunnel syndrome in the workplace. In: *Occupational Disorders of the Upper Extremity* (L. H. Millender, D. S. Louis and B. P. Simmons, eds). pp. 145–153. Churchill Livingstone.

Lowe, B. D. and Freivalds, A. (1999). Effect of carpal tunnel syndrome on grip force co-ordination on hand tools. *Ergonomics*, **42(4)**, 550–64.

Lucas, A. (1986). *Assessment and Treatment of Industrial Over-Use Syndrome (Upper Limb). A Clinical Manual for Physiotherapists.*

Macnicol, M. F. and Lamb, D.W. (1984). *Basic Care of the Injured Hand*, p. 68. Churchill Livingstone.

Markison, R. E. (1990). Treatment of musical hands: redesign of the interface. *Hand Clin.*, **6(3)**, 525–44.

Marks, M. R. and Gunther, S. F. (1989). Efficacy of cortisone injections in treatment of trigger fingers and thumbs. *J. Hand Surg.*, **14A**, 722.

McAtamney, L. and Corlett, E. N. (1992). *Reducing the Risks of Work-Related Upper Limb Disorders; A Guide and Methods.* Institute for Occupational Ergonomics, University of Nottingham.

McAtamney, L. and Corlett, E. N. (1993). RULA: a survey method for the investigation of work-related upper limb disorders. *Appl. Erg.*, **24(2)**, 91–9.

Millender, L. H., Louis, D. S. and Simmons, B. P. (1992). *Occupational Disorders of the Upper Extremity.* Churchill Livingstone.

Mital, A. (1999a). Non-fatal occupational injuries in the United States: Part I – overall trends and data summaries. *Intl. J. Indust. Erg.*, **25(2)**, 109–29.

Mital, A. (1999b). Non-fatal occupational injuries in the United States: Part III – injuries to the upper extremities. *Intl. J. Indust. Erg.* **25(2)**, 151–69.

Moon, S. D. and Sauter, S. L. (1996). *Beyond Biomechanics: Psychological Aspects of Musculoskeletal Disorders in Office Work.* Taylor & Francis.

Mottram, S. L. (1997). Dynamic stability of the scapula. *Man. Ther.*, **2(3)**, 123–31.

NOHSC (1990). *National Code of Practice for the Prevention and Management of Occupational Overuse Syndrome.* Australian Government Publishing Service.

OSH (1991). *Occupational Overuse Syndrome. Checklists for the Evaluation of Work.* Department of Labour, New Zealand.

Osol, A. (1973). *Blakiston's Pocket Medical Dictionary*, 3rd edn. McGraw-Hill Inc.

Pascarelli, E. and Quilter, D (1994). *Repetitive Strain Injury. A Computer User's Guide.* John Wiley & Sons Inc.

Pecina, M. M., Krmpotic-Nemanic, J. and Markiewitz, A. D. (1997). *Tunnel Syndromes*, 2nd edn. CRC Press.

Pelmear, P. L., Taylor, W. and others (1992). *Hand–Arm Vibration. A Comprehensive Guide for Occupational Health Professionals.* Van Nostrand Reinhold.

Phalen, G. S.(1966). The carpal tunnel syndrome. *J. Bone Joint Surg.*, **48A**, 211.

Pheasant, S. T. (1991). *Ergonomics, Work and Health.* Macmillan.

Pheasant S. T. (1994). Repetitive strain injury – towards a clarification of the points at issue. *J. Pers. Inj. Litigation*, **Sept,** 223–30.

Pheasant, S. T. and Scriven, J. G. (1983). Sex differences in strength – some implications for the design of hand tools. In: *Proceeding of the Ergonomics Society's Conference, 1983* (K. Coombes, ed.), pp. 303–15. Taylor & Francis.

Pheasant, S. T. (1986). *Bodyspace.* Taylor & Francis.

Putz-Anderson, V. (1988). *Cumulative Trauma Disorders. A Manual of Musculoskeletal Diseases of the Upper Limb.* Taylor & Francis.

Ramazzini, B. (1717). De Morbis Artificum Diatriba. In: *The Diseases of Workers* (W. Wright, ed., trans., 1940). University of Chicago Press.

Rempel, D. M., Harrison, R. J. and Barnhart, S. (1992). Work-related cumulative trauma disorders of the upper extremity. *JAMA*, **267(6)**, 838–42.

Rodgers, S. H. (1987). Recovery time needs for repetitive work. *Sem. Occup. Med.*, **2(1),** 19–24.

Rose, M. J. (1991). Keyboard operating posture and actuation force: implications for muscle overuse. *Appl. Erg.*, **22(3)**, 198–203.

Salter, M. I. (1987). *Hand Injuries. A Therapeutic Approach.* Churchill Livingstone.

Serina, E. R., Tal, R. and Rempel, D. (1999). Wrist and forearm postures and motions during typing. *Ergonomics*, **42(7)**, 938–51.

Simmons, B. P. and Koris, M. J. (1992). Occupational disorders of the hand and digits. In: *Occupational Disorders of the Upper Extremity* (L. H. Millender, D. S. Louis and B. P. Simmons, eds), pp. 105–15. Churchill Livingstone.

Terrono, A. L. and Millender, L. H. (1992). Evaluation and management of occupational wrist disorders. In: *Occupational Disorders of the Upper Extremity* (L. H. Millender, D. S. Louis and B. P. Simmons, eds), pp. 117–43. Churchill Livingstone.

Thomas, R. E., Butterfield, R. K., Hool, J. N. and Herrick, R. T. (1993). Effects of exercise on carpal tunnel syndrome symptoms. *Appl. Erg.*, **24(2)**, 101–8.

Tindall, A. (1993). *Tenosynovitis. A Case of Mistaken Identity.* Iron Trades Insurance Company Limited.

Vanderpool, D. W. (1968). Peripheral compression lesions of the ulnar nerve. *J. Bone Joint Surg.*, **50B**, 119.

11 The musician's hand

C. B. Wynn Parry

INTRODUCTION

Until quite recently, little attention was paid to musicians' physical problems – partly due to the natural instinct of players to keep their problems to themselves for fear of losing engagements, and partly because of doctors' ignorance of their causation and management.

The internationally famous pianist Gary Graffman 'went public' with his problem of dystonia in the hope of persuading the medical profession to take musicians' problems seriously and to warn his colleagues of the ineffectiveness of the therapies he had been prescribed (Graffman, 1986). An increasing number of reports were published indicating that musicians indeed suffered seriously from the exigencies of their art. In 1987, the International Conference of Symphony and Opera Musicians published the results of a survey carried out by questionnaire to over 4000 of its members. Some startling facts emerged.

Fifty-nine medical problems were noted, 34 of which related to the musculoskeletal system. Of the 2212 musicians who completed the questionnaires:

- 10 per cent were worried about their smoking habits
- 21 per cent were concerned about their alcohol intake
- 20 per cent were on some sort of drug for tension, anxiety or depression
- 84 per cent of the string players recorded at least one problem with pain in the shoulders, hands or fingers at some time
- 76 per cent of the total suffered symptoms severe enough to compromise their playing.

A series of articles revealing musculoskeletal problems in 485 musicians in eight orchestras found that 64 per cent were affected at some time or other. In 1996 questionnaires were sent to 55 orchestras world-wide, and 58 per cent of musicians complained of musculoskeletal problems.

The lay press regularly carries articles on tension in performance and in particular the problem of repetitive strain injury (RSI) in keyboard and string players.

In addition, there is in Britain a crisis in the arts; funding is at risk, sponsorship is more and more difficult to obtain, and musicians have to work increasingly hard to keep up a moderate standard of living.

It is a stressful life for orchestral musicians, with rehearsals, concerts, recordings, teaching and travel, and rushed, inadequate meals. They need to learn new repertoires, and contemporary composers make severe technical demands on players. Now too there is the rise of the authentic movement, so that many players have to alternate between very different techniques and styles of playing. String playing in particular is an artificial and unphysiological activity, with the players sitting on uncomfortable and poorly designed chairs, twisting the body for hours on end to read the score, keeping an eye on the conductor and listening to their colleagues in order to produce a technically difficult sound.

It is small wonder that the intellectual, emotional and physical stresses lead to tension and thus to muscular aches and pains. It is not only classical musicians who suffer. A recent survey of 100 rock musicians indicated a variety of stresses to which they are subjected, and these included high noise levels, lack of rehearsal time, bad playing conditions, loneliness on tour, exhaustion from travel, carrying heavy instruments, lack of sleep, and poor diet. These all lead to stress, tension and emotional and physical problems. However, it must be emphasized that musicians need not suffer significant or long-lasting problems.

If the technique is correct, the body fit and the mind calm, and if there is minimal general life stress, a lifetime in music need not be associated with any other than ephemeral problems. Despite some of the alarmist writings, not always confined to the lay press, there is no reason why prolonged music making should cause symptoms.

RSI is not inevitable, and the term in any event is a misnomer; it is not a strain, nor is it an injury. Musicians, unlike VDU operators or those involved in repetitive movements in industry, use their bodies more freely and their upper limbs in a much wider arc.

Young persons taking up a professional career need to be assured that they do not run a serious risk of injury or chronic strain provided they use their bodies sensibly. Much depends on enlightened teachers who understand the body's ergonomics and can prevent and correct poor technique and recommend the correct manner of playing for an individual's particular physique and temperament. This applies just as much to practice schedules and the manner of practice as to performance. Most problems arise during practice – players spend most of their professional life in practice, and it is here that early bad habits can become ingrained.

Lippman – one of the most experienced of music physicians – has stated (Lippman, 1991):

> There is no evidence that even intense and protracted playing in itself carries the risk of an overuse syndrome without a pre-existing injury or a chronic disease to disrupt normal play.

Treatment of so-called RSI by prolonged rest periods and the associated deconditioning or alienation in an otherwise healthy musician may be devastating, physically, psychologically and musically. The term 'overuse' obscures many possible causes of malfunction, which can be connected, that tend to lead the music physician/therapist astray. In practice, a second look will reveal that music playing beyond the point of fatigue and with disregard for pain and discomfort is *misuse*.

Overuse is a simplistic descriptive label that ignores various other possibly correctable causes of misfunction or malfunction in the playing of a musical instrument. The music physician is challenged to assess the physical, technical and behavioural bases of malfunction, the combination of which defines the trouble and leads to a diagnosis that can be a guide to remedial action. The majority of musicians who choose to spend a life with their instruments manage to emerge unscathed even after years of playing. This chapter is about what can go wrong, and how the multidisciplinary team can help to restore players to a normal performing life.

As will be seen later, many of the muscular aches and pains are due to muscle tension resulting from emotional stress and psychological factors. However plausible the players' explanations for their symptoms, such as overuse, may seem; the possibility of significant non-physical reasons should always be kept in mind.

The problems can be classified into four groups:

1. Problems induced directly by playing
2. Coincidental rheumatic disorders
3. Sequelae of injuries
4. Psychological/emotional problems.

The author's experience is based on 30 years in a musician's clinic in an orthopaedic hospital, a special musician's clinic in a general hospital, a clinic in a College of Music and, in the last 7 years, special clinics organized by the British Association for Performing Arts Medicine. Winspur and Wynn Parry (1997) reported on over 600 musicians seen at these clinics. Of these patients:

- 40 per cent had well-defined structural disorders, e.g. cervical spondylosis, osteoarthritis, ganglia, carpal tunnel syndrome etc.
- 40 per cent had symptoms that were adjudged to be caused by poor posture, poor technique, unsatisfactory lifestyle and bad practice methods
- 20 per cent were suffering from emotional or psychological stress, resulting in muscle tension, fatigue and consequent musculoskeletal symptoms.

These problems are discussed under the main headings of common rheumatic disorders, specific problems of technique, and emotional and psycho-logical problems. Problems following trauma need no special discussion, except to emphasize the importance of seeking a careful history of possible antecedent injury. It may well be that adequate rehabilitation was not instituted thereafter, and the sequence of restricted joint movement and reduced muscle power may be the cause of current symptoms. An intensive exercise programme may be all that is required.

COMMON RHEUMATIC DISORDERS

In assessing a musician, it is of course essential to make a thorough general examination – students can all too easily attribute fatigue and malaise to overwork before exams and before auditions, whilst the symptoms may in fact be due to general medical disorders such as anaemia, tuberculosis, thyroid disease, diabetes and so on. General examination of the musculoskeletal system may reveal scoliosis, kyphosis, early ankylosing spondylosis, shortening of the leg, or poor general physique, which will all predispose to aches and pains and may well need treatment. It must not be forgotten that depressive illnesses are not uncommon, may be precipitated by problems of a professional life, and require expert management.

Although this is a text on the hand, appreciation of problems of the neck, back and shoulder is vital. These may cause symptoms referred to the hand – for example, cervical spondylosis can cause pain in the hand and, conversely, pain in the wrist and fingers often leads to compensatory changes in the neck and spine that can in turn cause symptoms. Disorders of the C5 segment can refer pain to the trapezius, those of C6 to the biceps, those of C7 produce pain radiating to the dorsum of the forearm and wrist, and problems with C8 and T1 will refer pain to the fingers, particularly the little and ring fingers.

Poor posture of the neck and upper thoracic spine can cause both local pain and pain referred down the arms. In the author's experience problems of the upper thoracic spine are much commoner than realized, and any assessment of pain in the upper limb in musicians must take into account the mobility and posture of the thoracic spine as well as the cervical spine.

Thoracic outlet syndrome/cervical rib syndrome

The lower trunk of the brachial plexus may be compressed by a cervical rib or a band in the root of the neck. The classical symptoms are pain in the arm, particularly on the inner side of the forearm and the little and ring fingers, sometimes with paraesthesiae. This is made worse by holding and carrying heavy objects, particularly a musical instrument. The symptoms need to be distinguished from those of irritation of the ulnar nerve at the elbow, where the symptoms are predominately paraesthesiae in the ring and little fingers rather than pain. Sometimes there is a bruit that can be heard in the neck. There are various physical signs described that claim to be diagnostic – for example, Adson's sign is obliteration of the radial pulse on shrugging the shoulders and raising the arms above the head. However, it is generally agreed that these tests are unreliable, being reproducible in many normal subjects. In the author's experience, the only useful physical sign in the cervical rib syndrome is reproduction of the symptoms by pressure over the root of the neck on the affected side. In most patients the symptoms can be controlled by attention to posture, correct instrument technique, avoiding carrying heavy weights and carrying out a progressive programme of shoulder-raising exercises to strengthen the shoulder girdle muscles. If the patient does not respond to this regime and weakness and sensory loss develop, then clearly full investigation by a surgical team with the possibility of division of the band or removal of the cervical rib is essential.

Shoulder

One of the most common rheumatic problems in the shoulder is inflammation of the tendons making up the rotator cuff, particularly the supraspinatus tendon. The signs here are the characteristic painful arc (between 70° and 120°) when the patient abducts and elevates the arm as the inflamed tendon rubs against the acromion, and local tenderness. Sometimes symptoms of pain and paraesthesiae are felt down the arm and into the hand. Furthermore, in a surprising number of patients there is actual limitation of movement in the shoulder, particularly internal rotation, and this may be the presenting sign of an early frozen shoulder. It is vital to spot this early on and institute an intensive physiotherapy programme to restore full range of movement, particularly internal rotation, in order to try to prevent the development of the full-blown classic frozen shoulder and the appalling disability that this can cause for months or even years.

Some physiotherapists pay a lot of attention to the so-called neurotension tests, in which they demonstrate increased pain on the affected side when the arm is put into full abduction and external rotation. There are a number of publications from physiotherapists suggesting that this is relevant to musicians' problems. It is postulated that nerve roots become tethered in their sheaths, and the movement of playing an instrument causes stretching of these structures and pain. However, it is well known that nerves and nerve roots possess specialized ligaments that allow stretch of their length by at least 20 per cent. It seems more likely that these manoeuvres are demonstrating stiffness of joints, muscles and ligaments throughout the upper limb and neck, and correction of this shortening is clearly reasonable.

Elbow

Tennis elbow and golfer's elbow are often seen in instrumentalists. All instrumentalists and keyboard players are liable to strain of the extensor and flexor tendons, which is particularly common in percussion players. Prolonged maintenance of one position of the wrist with repetitive movements of the fingers is likely to strain the extensor and flexor origins. This emphasizes the importance of frequent breaks and isotonic exercises to counteract this effect. Although the treatment of choice is steroid injection, many musicians are loathe to accept such advice, having heard alarming stories of bad reactions to injections in their fellow artists. For these patients, conventional physiotherapy such as ultrasound, laser, progressive massage to release the scarring and even old-fashioned manipulation may well be successful. If these measures fail, the musician should be encouraged to submit to a steroid injection at the hands of an experienced doctor.

Hand

There are a number of common rheumatological problems affecting the hand that are of great importance in musicians.

De Quervain's syndrome
This is an inflammation of the extensor and abductor pollicis longus tendons, which become inflamed in their sheath through excessive repetitive use by playing, or by local damage through do-it-yourself activities around the home or garden. Characteristically, sharp ulnar deviation of the wrist with the forearm in the mid-position causes severe pain over the tendon just proximal to the wrist. Sometimes the tendon is inflamed and swollen in the sheath, but often there is nothing to be seen. Any form of resisted extension or abduction of the thumb or gripping movements causes exacerbation of the pain. In the early stages, ice, local support and rest are indicated. At a later stage ultrasound is particularly valuable, but if there is no response a local steroid injection repeated once or twice can be helpful. In recalcitrant cases, decompression of the tendon by surgical operation is necessary. This should only be performed by a skilled hand surgeon, as there is a real danger of damaging one of the branches of the superficial radial nerve, resulting in persistent causalgia.

Trigger finger
In trigger finger a nodule or localized thickening can be felt, usually in the flexor pollicis and flexor

superficialis at the site of entry of the tendons into the digital sheath. The nodular thickening should be easily palpable with the thumb over the volar surface of the metacarpophalangeal joint when the patient moves the digits backwards and forwards. Again, in the early stages ultrasound and massage can resolve the situation, but if this is not successful local steroid injection or surgical removal is necessary.

Flexor tenosynovitis

A classical true flexor tenosynovitis is characterized by a boggy swelling and a discrepancy between the full passive range of movement in the joint and limited active movement due to the swollen tendon. Playing is painful, and quickly becomes impossible. Tenosynovitis is far too frequently diagnosed when there are no physical signs other than mild tenderness in the muscle belly. It is very important not to confuse the upper limb pain syndrome, which will be described later, with true tenosynovitis. The latter is a real entity, with classical physical signs and symptoms, and can be treated in a specific manner with local physiotherapy, local and/or general anti-inflammatory drugs and steroid injections. There is a tendency to refer to all aches and pains in the hand as RSI or tenosynovitis. The condition of tenosynovitis is a clear-cut entity, whereas the upper limb pain syndrome with generalized aches and pains in different parts of the hand and forearm is another disorder altogether and requires a quite different approach.

True tenosynovitis follows an injury or repeated trauma, and is usually caused by extra-musical activities such as DIY in the home. However, occasionally poor technique or seriously excessive playing, particularly in guitarists where strong movements are required, may result in an inflamed tendon. Tenosynovitis is rare in string and keyboard players, as there is considerable free finger movement in execution.

Osteoarthritis of the carpometacarpal joint of the thumb

This is a not uncommon cause of pain in the older musician. Pain is felt at the base of the thumb and there is tenderness over the joint, which can be felt superficially. There may even be some wasting of the abductor pollicis brevis, and this can be confused with carpal tunnel syndrome. However, in an osteoarthritic joint there is no sensory loss, and electrical studies can easily distinguish between the two – although of course it is possible for both to coexist. X-rays will show the characteristic arthritic changes. In the early stages, local injection of steroid and self manual traction by the patient can be very helpful. The physiotherapist should teach the patient the technique of careful slow traction and holding the thumb in the extended position for 30 seconds, avoiding a jerky movement that can be harmful. At a later stage replacement of the joint or silastic interposition may be necessary, but this is clearly to be avoided for as long as possible.

Ganglia

Ganglia are not uncommon in and around the wrist joint, involving the extensor tendons. Usually these do not cause symptoms, and it is unwise to recommend removal of a ganglionic swelling simply for cosmetic reasons; it is impossible to be sure that the patient will not develop complications such as a keloid scar. However, very small ganglia that come and go and can sometimes be seen and felt on full flexion of the wrist can cause significant pain, and if persistent may require removal by an experienced surgeon.

Hypermobility

There is clear evidence that there is an increased incidence of hypermobility in musicians compared with the normal population. Whether this is because musicians select themselves due to their excessive mobility is not known, but it is a fact (Bird, 1988). Clearly flexibility of the fingers must be an advantage for string and keyboard players, and it is believed that Paganini owed his remarkable technical skills to his hypermobility. However, a price has to be paid in that the musician must develop increased strength in the intrinsic and extrinsic hand muscles in order to cope with the excessive movement. Lack of this power results in aches and pains in the hand and forearm.

The full hypermobility syndrome comprises the ability for the thumb to touch or approximate to the radius, 90° passive movement of the MCP joints with the wrist hyperextended, 10° or more of hyperextension of the elbow, and hypermobility of the spine, knees and ankle. In practice, the full syndrome affecting all the joints mentioned is rarely seen. However, it is not at all uncommon to find musicians with symptoms of aches and pains in the hand and wrist with hypermobile MCP joints and thumb joints.

Dropping of the bow can result if there is hypermobility of the third metacarpal joint on the right. Recurrent dislocations of the IP joints can cause digital nerve lesions, and marked hypermobility of MCP joints can produce difficulties in the pianist's strike. Easy fatiguability of muscles with aching in the wrists and fingers are the main symptoms. It is vital to test for hypermobility in all musicians reporting problems of pain in the upper limb. This may be the only finding. Attention to building up both extrinsic and intrinsic power with progressive resistance exercises can speedily resolve the problem. These can of course be carried on at home after being taught by a hand therapist.

In general, within a few weeks of such a programme patients lose their symptoms and can play
difficult passages that had previously caused problems, with ease.

Carpal tunnel syndrome

This is a common syndrome, particularly in middle-
aged females. The majority of cases are idiopathic
and are not caused by specific playing problems.
However, excessive hyperextension of the wrist in
pianists and excessive flexion of the wrists in string
players can predispose to this syndrome, and in
some cases may indeed cause it.

It has also been described in guitarists, who have a
particular tendency to hyperflex the wrist. The
symptoms are well known – paraesthesiae and pain
in the median distribution (sometimes the whole of
the hand), particularly at night, relieved by rubbing
the hands and shaking them about. At a later stage
weakness and wasting of the abductor pollicis brevis
(APB) can occur, but the diagnosis should be made
well before these signs appear. There is commonly a
positive Tinel's sign at the wrist, and there may be
some weakness of the intrinsic hand muscles
supplied by the median nerve. There can be
coexisting flexor tenosynovitis, so that there is a
doughy swelling at the wrist and difficulty in
bending the fingers. Electrical investigations will
reveal the extent to which the median nerve is
compromised, and the objective readings that these
tests can provide will determine whether surgery is
required. A motor conduction delay of more than 7
milliseconds from wrist to APB and reduction by
more than 50 per cent of the sensory action potential
compared with the normal side will normally lead to
the recommendation for surgery. In the early stages a
night splint (see Chapter 12) and sometimes a
steroid injection will resolve the symptoms. The
majority of cases are self-limiting, and surgery is
only required in a small proportion of patients.
Clearly musicians are very anxious to avoid surgery
if possible; they do not like to have a scar and are
naturally afraid of surgical procedures. If symptoms
persist, then careful attention to a musician's
technique with advice from an experienced player
may be all that is required to relieve and prevent the
symptoms. However, musicians are just as likely to
suffer from a common condition as the general
population, and their playing technique may not be
relevant. Surgical decompression may be necessary
to avoid progressive symptoms, permanent weakness of muscles and the loss of sensitivity of the
fingertips that is so vital to musicians.

Careful and regular reviews with appropriate
electrical tests are mandatory.

Dupuytren's contracture

This condition can interfere with performance,
particularly if it has proceeded to the stage of
limitation of flexion of the fingers. In the very early
stages where there is simply a thickening and no
deformity, no surgery is required. However,
patients need to be seen at regular intervals of at
least every 6 months in order to spot any early
development of deformity, and thus allow surgery
to be introduced to prevent progressive deformity
at a stage when surgery is relatively easy. The
longer it is left the more deformity occurs, and the
more difficult it is to obtain a satisfactory result
surgically. There is no place for physiotherapy or
stretch splinting in this condition, although it
makes sense to suggest to the patient that rubbing
in some cream will keep the skin as supple as
possible.

Herberden's nodes

These are the outward sign of osteoarthritis of the
terminal interphalangeal joints. They can become
inflamed and require anti-inflammatory treatment,
both local and general. There is no indication for
surgical treatment unless the node becomes recur-
rently infected and interferes with playing. It is
usually a familial condition, and patients can be
reassured that they are not developing a progressive arthritis and that the condition is usually
self-limiting.

Wrist

Chronic pain in the wrist is notoriously difficult to
diagnose and treat. Sprains can produce a chronic
painful wrist, causing difficulty in playing and
practice. This may be due to damage to the
triangular fibrocartilage, and requires arthroscopy
or arthrography for diagnosis and surgical treatment. It is usually associated with clicking and pain
over the ulnar side of the wrist. Persistent pain in
the wrist joint should always lead to specialist
referral.

Upper limb pain syndrome

One of the commonest presentations of musculoskeletal symptoms seen by the author in clinics is
the so-called upper limb pain syndrome (ULPS).

The patient complains of generalized aches in the
palms, dorsum of the hand and volar aspect of the
wrists, later spreading to the flexor and extensor
muscles of the forearm. In severe cases, pain and
aching is felt in the upper arms and neck, and even
in the thoracic and lumbar spine. The presentation
is reminiscent of the clinical picture seen in many
VDU operators, mistakenly known as RSI.

At first the symptoms are felt after practice or
performance and are located predominantly in the
hands and wrists. Later the symptoms spread to the
forearm and are felt at the end of a session, then
actually during a session, and ultimately immediately the performer starts playing. In the most
severe cases, performance for more than 5 minutes

becomes impossible and the simple activities of daily life become difficult. Patients find they cannot open jars, cut up food, sew, drive or garden.

The outstanding feature of this condition is the paucity of signs. Apart from mild muscle tenderness, there are no objective signs – no swelling, no crepitus, no limitation of movement, no sensory loss and no true weakness, although the patient may be reluctant to proffer a strong contraction in the expectation of pain.

The marked discrepancy between the often dramatic symptoms and their effect and the physical findings is the key factor in diagnosing ULPS. The condition is due to muscle fatigue and not to tendonitis or nerve compression. It is vital not to confuse the two – the management of the two disorders is entirely different.

The ULPS usually follows a period of increased practice and playing under stress, whether building up to exams, learning a new repertoire quickly, or an unaccustomed intensity of playing, such as summer courses for music students. If the patient persists in playing, the fatigue increases and a vicious circle is established of pain – anxiety – tension – excessive muscular effort – more pain, anxiety, etc.

A central pain state in the central nervous system at spinal level and even higher develops, and inhibitory pathways are alerted to stop further motor neuronal discharges in an attempt to limit pain. This transference of the disorder from neuromuscular to spinal level explains why severe limitation of functional activities develops despite little in the way of physical signs. Patients readily accept the explanation that the nerve centres are acting to prevent further activity but that the body over-reacts.

A careful history is essential to establish the antecedent factors – excessive playing, faulty technique, change of instrument or teacher, or emotional stress and tension.

It must be clear from the lack of physical signs, in particular the absence of the signs of tendonitis, that the remedy does not lie in local measures but in attention to the factors that precipitated the disorder. Thus, replanning of practice and performance schedules, attention to technique, and exploration of psychological and emotional factors is essential. Often help from the appropriate professional teacher, psychologist, and counsellors is necessary.

Immediate management must be by rest until the acute aches and pains have settled, but prolonged rest is counterproductive – skills are easily lost, confidence ebbs, and patients deprived of music making easily become depressed. Therefore, as soon as symptoms are settling patients are encouraged to play for 5 minutes at a time twice daily, gradually and slowly increasing their playing and keeping a careful record of the time played and the nature and onset of symptoms. They should be exhorted to 'make friends with their instrument again' and play for sheer pleasure, with no thought of exams or concerts. This must be accompanied by a profound study of their technique, posture, attitude, practice schedules, home and work attitudes, emotional state and ambitions. Patients may well require the services of a counsellor to help them over an emotional crisis, a musician who is experienced in the ergonomic approach to their instrument, instruction in relaxation and posture, and an overhaul of their lifestyle. Most important is insistence on frequent breaks during practice, with relaxation and general exercises.

The author deplores the practice of sentencing musicians to prolonged rest (it has been known for months or even years of no playing to be recommended), with the limb placed in a sling and used for no activities whatsoever. This attitude misunderstands the pathophysiology of the condition. Rehabilitation after a short period of initial rest is essential. Patients have been seen in whom prolonged rest has not only totally destroyed their confidence and chance of a career, but also led to disuse atrophy, stiff joints and even dystrophy. It is illogical to treat normal muscles with rest when it is the neural system that is at fault.

Provided that this condition is recognized for what it is – and not for what it is not, i.e. local musculoskeletal pathology – the multifaceted approach is almost always successful provided too long has not elapsed since symptoms began.

Complex regional pain syndrome

Complex regional pain syndrome is a rare condition characterized in the acute stage by severe pain, heat and swelling of the hand, often with allodynia and hyperpathia and osteoporosis of the hand bones. In the later stages, swelling subsides and a cold, weak hand results, frequently with restricted movements of the MCP, PIP and wrist joints and severe functional impairment. It follows quite trivial injuries such as a minor fracture or strain, and appears to be due to sympathetic overdrive centrally triggered by local tissue damage (Roberts, 1986). The most successful approach to treatment is by sympathetic blockade, either locally by guanethidine infusions or by serial stellate blocks. This almost always relieves pain sufficiently for the therapist to start an intensive rehabilitation programme to restore movement to stiff joints and power to weak muscles. In severe cases, this may necessitate several plasters and stretches, splintage, TENS, desensitization procedures and treatment of concomitant stiffness of elbow and shoulder (Wynn Parry, 1991). It is not uncommon to see minor degrees of osteoporosis in the bones of the wrist after prolonged disuse of the hand in the ULPS, but this is not to be regarded as full-blown complex regional pain syndrome and the radical measures described above are not needed. Some units appear to over-diagnose this condition, and patients are subjected to prolonged and unnecessary treatment that is both uncomfortable and expensive.

SPECIFIC PROBLEMS OF TECHNIQUE

A careful assessment of the patient's playing conditions and technique must be undertaken in all cases of musculoskeletal problems in musicians where there is not a clear-cut traumatic cause. There are some well-recognized problems that can arise as a result of faulty technique. The commonest is the violinist who pushes the shoulder forward instead of keeping it back in line with the trunk, which produces pain in the neck and the upper arm. Violinists who have long necks may find that the standard violin chin rest is too shallow and they have to hunch their neck towards the shoulder, causing neck and shoulder pain. A violinist and Alexander teacher, W. Benham, has devised a special custom-built rest for violinists with long necks; this can easily be attached to the violin and will speedily resolve symptoms (Benham, 1991). One of the problems of a violinist bringing the left shoulder forward to support the instrument is that not only will it cause neck and shoulder pain but it will also hinder free forearm rotation, and thus the musician will have difficulty in reaching the G or C strings. The bowing arm can present its own problems – incorrect posture of the spine, or any physical tension, can cause pain in the bowing arm. It is most important to use the whole arm in string playing and not just the forearm, which can limit freedom of movement.

If a cellist has a correct stance, it should always be possible to put a fist between the neck of the cello and the chest. If the cello is held too close, there will be tension in the neck and shoulder. The whole arm should be used for bowing, rather than just the elbow or wrist; poor bowing technique is a potent cause of shoulder pain, and can lead to a true tendinitis. Many of the cellists' problems are related to an unrelaxed posture, for sitting crouched over the cello with the muscles of the neck and upper trunk tense will undoubtedly produce pain.

Joan Dixon, the doyenne of ergonomic problems with cellists, stated that there would be no 'RSI' if movements were balanced and free and without tension. No group of muscle should ever be held in tension for more than a very short time, and there should be a constant flow with alternating relaxation and contraction. If the forearm is kept tense, then pain will develop. If the thumb grip is too tight, pain will develop along the extensor aspect of the thumb up to the elbow. Pressing the fingers too hard will produce pain in the forearm muscles and the elbow. Many cellists use maximum force all the time rather than only when it is necessary, and this

is a potent cause of cumulative symptoms. After the shoulders have been raised they should be relaxed again; some cellists use the shoulders in an emotional way and tend to keep them raised for far too long. Humeral rotation should be used as much as possible rather than radioulnar rotation, as this gives a freer and stronger movement. Throughout her teaching Dixon stressed that music is movement in sound, and most musculoskeletal problems develop through lack of proper relaxation and use of too much energy for the movement required.

One of the features that constantly emerges from interdisciplinary meetings between artists, teachers and doctors is that teachers on the whole are not trained in the ergonomics of instrument playing and do not understand the way the locomotor system works. Often they impose a rigid training technique on their pupils without taking into account the individual's physique and temperament. A great deal of harm has been done by teachers insisting on a specific type of approach to the instrument regardless of the musician's physique, temperament and desires. The teachers who are particularly involved in assessing pupils' ergonomic problems are adamant that teachers as a whole must take a great deal more interest in this field. A lot of the problems that musicians, particularly students, present are preventable by a correct approach to the instrument, both physically and emotionally. Most of the music colleges now employ an Alexander teacher, and where any musician coming to the author's clinic has any sort of postural problems or muscle tension it is practice to recommend a course of Alexander lessons.

Guitarists are very prone to aches and pains in the neck and shoulders from the uncomfortable and abnormal position in which they play. John Williams, the world famous guitarist, pays special attention in his student teaching programmes to regular exercises and relaxation between practice sessions. He is also a great exponent of the Alexander technique. He emphasizes that all teachers have noticed that musicians, particularly students, who have recurrent problems with their locomotor system are likely to develop bad habits during practice. Many people feel impelled to play daily for many hours on end to achieve a high standard of performance. This may well be unnecessary, but if a lot of practice is required it should be broken up into short sessions of 20–30 minutes each, followed by complete relaxation and a general exercise regime (even if for only a few minutes) before starting again.

Pianists suffer the same problems as string players, with aching in the wrists, fingers and forearm muscles if their approach towards the instrument is too tense. The arms should be held balanced and slightly away from the body, with the elbow in line with the fifth finger, allowing execution of all technical passages, especially rapid movements from one end of the keyboard to the other. Many problems in pianists are due to hyperextension of the wrist, fingers and thumb, which causes wrist sprain and chronic pain in the extensor compartment of the forearm.

Woodwind players, particularly clarinettists and flautists, have problems because of the way in which their instrument is held. The flautist has a most unnatural position, with severe hyperextension of the wrist and little finger and an extended position of the thumb. Clarinettists often develop pain in the thumb as a result of supporting their instrument, and various forms of sling can be recommended.

Many of the patients attending the author's clinic have developed symptoms as a result of changing their technique or their instrument. A slight alteration in the breadth of a lute or guitar can lead to stress on the wrist and forearm. For many years the musician has coded his or her nervous system in a particular way, and even a slight change in the mechanics will lead to the necessity for recoding centrally, a potent cause of stress and locomotor symptoms. Careful enquiries should always be made into the circumstances into which the symptoms first started. Common causes that are only revealed by a careful history include a change in technique, instrument, practice schedules or teacher, or a change in the style in which the music is played – e.g. with authentic instruments or eighteenth-century keyboard fingering techniques. Emotional stress inevitably leads to a tense approach to the instrument. This means that muscles are under tension rather than freely relaxed, and this can be an important cause of symptoms. Thus not only technical problems need to be addressed, but also careful enquiry should be made regarding the patient's lifestyle at that time. Was there some problem at home? Have there been problems with the teacher? Has the patient recently had an unhappy love affair? The latter may even be with some other member of the orchestra, and is not uncommon these days with frequent travel abroad as a group. Where students are concerned, the co-operation of the teacher is all-important. Only the teacher will be able to state whether the student is likely to make the grade or whether the persistence of symptoms is a subconscious way of the patient finding an honourable means of not continuing with a career. Unfortunately, teachers may be so obsessed with their pupil's success that they cannot see the problem. Moreover they are not trained in the ergonomic aspect of playing an instrument, and may not notice that the poor technique is due to poor posture, particularly if the teacher follows a rigid style of instrument playing.

At this clinic, there is access to a small, select group of experts for each instrument who are prepared to look at a student's performance and can spot not only technical errors but errors of posture and general approach to the instrument. However, there are not enough dedicated and knowledgeable teachers for these huge demands – the ultimate answer must be better training of teachers to understand the technical, physical and emotional problems of musicians.

EMOTIONAL AND PSYCHOLOGICAL PROBLEMS

The realization that tension in performance is a potent cause of musculoskeletal symptoms leads to consideration of the player's general approach to the instrument and an understanding of his or her lifestyle and emotional state. There are some key periods in a musician's life when things can go wrong.

First, in the final year at school, admission to music college will depend on successfully passing exams. Students have to increase their tempo of work, and there may also be the question of whether they are emotionally and technically up to the grades required. At this stage a student may break down with musculoskeletal symptoms, and it is important to appreciate the real basis of the symptoms. No useful purpose is served by persisting with the myth that the student has RSI and requires therapy and rest, when in fact the problems are emotional, technical, or quite simply a lack of requisite ability.

The second period is during the first year at college, when students have carried all before them in school but now find at college that they among hundreds of people all equally good and all competing. Breakdowns are not uncommon at this stage. There are two particular problems of which the therapist involved with music students should be aware:

1. Students who are desperate to impress uncaring and hostile parents who resent the money spent on their musical education and have supplemented it under some duress; these students may work far too hard and be too emotionally and physically tense to give of their best.
2. Students with parents who are excessively caring and ambitious, who see in their child the possibility of a successful musical career that was denied to them. These students will again be overanxious to impress and please, and this may lead to over-practising and an over tense approach and the development of symptoms as already explained.

Children are also very sensitive to the atmosphere created by family problems – it is always important to explore carefully the interfamily relationships and if necessary to discuss these in depth with the parents and any other relevant person, particularly the general practitioner. There have been a number of instances of young students whose aches and pains did not seem to relate to any specific disorder or to any abnormal playing technique, but whose symptoms were revealed to be due to tension at home. These circumstances may require a multi-disciplinary team of psychologists, therapists, counsellors and doctors.

The third period is at the stage of final exams, before musicians are let loose on the public and their career starts. Of necessity they will have a great deal of work to put in, and if the practice regime and technique are faulty and the emotional state fraught this may well cause breakdown.

The fourth period is in mid-career. There is often a mid-life crisis in musicians who can see younger competitors coming up and threatening their career. Each generation of keyboard and string players seem to be technically more brilliant than the last, and there is a very real fear among artists even of great international repute that they will be ousted by the younger generation. It is at this stage that counselling, with a careful look not only at their technique but also at the whole physical and mental approach to playing, is vital. Many players feel that they must accept every engagement and that if they do not somebody else will take their place, or they will be ousted from their position at the top. It is very important to explain to musicians that they must guard their resources and look after their minds and bodies; that there is a point of no return when taking on too many engagements produces general and local fatigue, a fall off in performance, a vicious circle of muscular aches and pains, and a serious impairment of their career. It is astonishing how often players of international reputation fear for their future. It is not uncommon to hear them say that they are only as good as their last performance and that at their next concert there will be a disaster or they will forget the notes, or they will be unable to play. Reassurance is constantly required, and again the holistic approach is vital. Such players find it a great help to have some form of physical and mental discipline, such as yoga, relaxation, the Feldenkrais method or the Alexander technique. Orthodox physiotherapy and medicine alone may not be adequate to deal with their problems.

Fundamental to the whole of music medicine is prevention, and here the installation of good disciplines early in practice and performance are vital. A general approach is essential for all musicians. They should have adequate time for recreation and should have some sort of sport – obviously not one that involves body contact, but one that uses their body freely such as swimming and walking. It is unnatural to be hunched over a piano, cello or violin all day, and there must be a relaxation period to stretch muscles and move joints and to improve general cardiovascular efficiency. Some sort of body control technique is extremely helpful, whether the Alexander technique, Feldenkrais method, yoga or similar disciplines. Musicians must have adequate holidays and complete rest from their instrument. They should if possible have a guru, particularly when they become well known and increasing pressure is put on them to take on ever more engagements of increasing technical difficulty. They must have a teacher to whom they can go from time to time who understands ergonomics and basic technical problems. They must pay careful attention to their seating (11 per cent of cellists and 21 per cent of double bass players have low back pain). They must make sure they have an adequate diet, which is often difficult with rushed meals between rehearsals and travelling. The necessity of a warm up before playing and a cool down after playing is more often honoured in the breach than in the observance. They must have correct practice techniques and divide up their time sensibly – if necessary they should have specific exercise programmes if they have any weakness of muscles (e.g. hypermobility or chronic back pain). Finally, they should have an understanding agent who will relieve pressure in times of stress and not insist that they fulfil engagements when they are clearly physically or emotionally unfit.

DYSTONIA

Dystonia is a nightmare for players. It usually affects players in mid-career when they have been playing for 20 years or more, and starts with the inability to move a particular finger at the speed required. This gradually gets worse so that the finger may become disobedient and the player has to leave it out of the pattern and compensate by putting more stress on the neighbouring fingers, which will in turn develop the same problem. Either the patient develops cramp so that the finger will simply not move, or the finger is disobedient and moves in an uncontrolled and unwanted manner. Gradually the condition appears at an earlier stage of the practice or the performance, and it may end up with inability to play at all.

The physical symptoms are of aching of the forearm and wrist. The common manifestation in pianists is the inability to extend the ring finger, and in violinists the inability to extend the little finger. Wind players have problems with their embouchure, so that they find it increasingly difficult to blow high notes or execute particularly difficult passages. Other functions are entirely normal. Thus a pianist who is quite unable to extend the ring and little fingers is perfectly able to carry out activities at home and in the office. Similarly, a wind player who cannot blow certain notes can whistle and sing and has no difficulty with chewing. There is now no doubt that this is an organic condition and is a fatigue phenomenon of the central connections, akin to writer's cramp, where the co-ordination of complex voluntary movements takes place, presumably in the basal ganglia. The more the patient tries to conquer the problem by practising the difficult passages that bring on the weakness, the more the condition is compounded. If treated in the early stages a complete cure can be promised, but if the patient has been having problems for months or years it may be difficult or impossible to regain the highest standard of playing. It is imperative to make a full neurological examination with appropriate special investigations to make sure that there is not a rare underlying structural lesion such as a brain tumour. If these investigations are negative, the approach must then be a short period of rest from the instrument until any physical signs such as inflammation of tendons or marked muscle tenderness have subsided, with relief of pain by physiotherapy and analgesic or anti-inflammatory drugs. As soon as the symptoms have settled, the patient must begin at the beginning and start building up practice sessions with very simple technical exercises gradually increasing in complexity. The author has found the Feldenkrais approach the most successful, and this has enabled a number of international keyboard players with dystonia to return, completely cured, to their instruments. The aim of this regime is to help the patient to understand and feel the movements of the body, starting with the simplest movements and gradually building up to the most complex. Clearly careful attention to any problems of technique or change of instrument or lifestyle is very important. These may be potent factors and attention to them may substantially relieve symptoms, but some form of re-education discipline is essential if the patient is to regain a satisfactory performance standard. Chamagne (1983) has stressed the importance of correct scapular control, and has noted how there is often a profound disturbance of control of muscles around the shoulder. Kember (1995) has also insisted on the value of close attention to thoracic mobility and muscular control around the shoulder, combined with attention to correct posture and technique. Some neurologists treat the condition of writer's cramp by paralysing the neuromuscular junction with botulinum toxin. However, the literature suggests that it is impossible to achieve correction of the dystonic state without causing weakness of muscles, and this of course is to be avoided at all costs in musicians.

Physiotherapists can be of great help in advising the patient on general and specific fitness for the instrument. Moreover, physiotherapists should be aware of dystonia, particularly if a patient is referred without a clear diagnosis for physiotherapy and the therapist suspects that the dystonic state has been missed. Continuing a progressive exercise programme without attention to the fundamental cause of this fatigue state can only compound the issue.

SUMMARY

In the management of upper limb problems in musicians:

1. A holistic approach is required, with an understanding of the patient's lifestyle, emotional state and psychological approach, the technical skills required for the instrument, the patient's general physique, and any underlying abnormalities that may predispose to locomotor symptoms. Thus the approach will involve an assessment of any underlying abnormalities such as scoliosis, kyphosis, poor posture, cervical spondylosis, osteoarthritis of the spine etc.
2. Any general disorders that masquerade as general malaise or fatigue (e.g. anaemia, diabetes, blood dyscrasia or post-viral fatigue syndrome) must be eliminated.
3. A careful look should be taken for obvious pathology such as tenosynovitis, carpal tunnel syndrome, rotator cuff lesions and ganglia.
4. An assessment must be made regarding the extent to which the symptoms are due to poor practice and performance technique or inadequate training for the instrument, both physically and technically, and how much is due to the true underlying structural disorder. Both may well coexist. All the conventional physiotherapy techniques for relieving pain, improving muscle function, restoring mobility, attention to posture and general lifestyle are relevant, but must be seen against a background of a full understanding of the musician's technical, emotional and psychological problems.

Only by a clear understanding of these will players have the confidence in their therapist to follow the regime. Therapists should see performers in action when possible, and always ask them to bring their instrument (if feasible) to the clinic to demonstrate the particular problems as they arise. In cases where the instrument cannot come to the consulting room or the therapy department, any opportunity should be taken to see patients in action in their home or studio; it may then be possible to spot a particular problem which is only evident in that environment. The more therapists involve themselves with the players' playing, the more confidence they will instil in those players and the more rewarding it will be for all parties concerned.

ADDENDUM

In the past few years an association of doctors and therapists interested in the medical problems of musicians has been formed, The British Association of Performing Arts Medicine. Regular meetings, seminars and workshops are held to discuss such problems. Videos have been made demonstrating examination of the upper limb with special reference to musicians' musculoskeletal ailments, and of good and bad technique in string players. In addition, a network of specially trained general practitioners has been set up such that each major orchestra has its own medical advisor to help with any physical, emotional and psychological problems facing the players.

A quarterly journal, *Medical Problems of Performing Artists*, is published in the USA, and the *Textbook of Performing Arts Medicine* by Satalof *et al.* (1991) has recently been published there.

Arts psychologists work closely with the medical team, and are of great value in the management of stage fright, performance anxiety and emotional problems affecting performance. In addition, a network of ergonomically minded instrumentalists who have made a special study of technical faults leading to muscular symptoms are available for advice.

REFERENCES

Benham, W. (1991). Emus and violins – alternative chin rest for long-necked violinists. *Strad.*, **102**, 406–9.

Bird, H. (1988). Body flexibility in dancers and musicians. *ISSTIP J.*, **5**, 5–11.

Chamagne, P. (1983). Approches kinestherapigne des crampes fonctionelles dites proffessionelles. *Semestres de l'Hopital de Paris*, **59**, 3080–86.

Graffman, G. (1986). Doctor can you lend an ear? *Med. Probl. Perf. Art.*, **1**, 3–6.

Kember, J. (1995). You and your guitar. Parts 1–7. *Classical Guitar*, **14**, 3–8, 12.

Lippman, H. I. (1991). A fresh look at the overuse syndrome in musical performers. Is overuse overused? *Med. Probl. Perf. Art.*, **6**, 57–60.

Roberts, W. J. (1986). A hypothesis on the physiological basis for causalgia and related pains. *Pain*, **24**, 297–312.

Sataloff, R. T., Brandfonbener, A. G. and Lederman, R. J. (1991). *Textbook of Performing Arts Medicine*. Raven Press.

Winspur, I. and Wynn Parry, C. B. (1997). The musician's hand. *Br. J. Hand Surg.*, **22B**, 433–40.

Wynn Parry, C. B. (1991). Painful peripheral nerves. In: *Management of Pain in the Hand and Wrist* (C. B. Wynn Parry, ed.). Churchill Livingstone.

FURTHER READING

Amadio, P. C. and Russor, G. M. (1990). Evaluation and treatment of hand and wrist disorders in musicians. *Hand Clin.*, **6(3)**, 405–16.

Fischbin, M. and Middlestart, S. E. (1988). Medical problems among the ICSOM musicians – overview of a national survey. *Med. Probl. Perf. Art.*, **3**, 1–8.

Fry, H. J. H. (1986). Incidence of overuse syndrome in the symphony orchestra. *Med. Probl. Perf. Art.*, **1**, 1–5.

Merriman, L. (1986). A focal movement disorder of the hand in six pianists. *Med. Probl. Perf. Art.*, **1**, 17–19.

Rosenthal, R. (1987). The Alexander technique. What it is and how it works with three musicians. *Med. Probl. Perf. Art.*, **2**, 53–7.

Spike, M. (1989). The Feldenkrais method. An interview with Arat Baniel. *Med. Probl. Perf. Art.*, **4**, 159–62.

Tubiana, R. and Amadio, P. (2000). *Medical Problems of the Instrumental Musiciam*. Martin Dunitz.

Winspur, I. and Wynn Parry, C. B. (1998). *The Musician's Hand*. Martin Dunitz.

Occupational Cramp (Focal Dystonia) (1991). *Med. Probl. Perf. Art.* (Special issue), **6**.

12 Splinting the hand

Lynn Cheshire

Splinting is well documented in a large number of publications on hand rehabilitation and, as this chapter is a limited selection of types and choices of splinting rather than a complete treatise, the reader is encouraged to pursue the references and suggested literature. The splinting described here is intended as an integral part and never as the sole element of the hand patient's care and rehabilitation. The hand therapist must always avoid being coerced by pressures into becoming solely a splint technician, as it is the integrated and balanced provision of all elements of hand therapy that result in proper outcomes for the patient.

Rheumatoid arthritis is dealt with in Chapter 16, and brachial plexus lesions and burns are covered in Chapters 8 and 9 respectively.

Suppliers of materials and equipment are listed in Appendix A.

PATIENT POSITIONING, CONTROL AND CARE IN UPPER LIMB SPLINTING

The way in which therapists position both themselves and patients has a profound effect on the efficiency, ergonomics, comfort and control of the whole procedure of splinting. Correctly managed, pain, stress, tension, and fatigue can all be minimized and a suitable psychological and physical ambience created in which the patient and therapist can focus properly on all aspects of the treatment.

Positioning of the patient

The patient is seated comfortably, taking into account any disability or limitations other than in the hand that is being treated. The affected arm rests on a table beside rather than in front of the patient, so that the elbow and forearm are fully supported, with the elbow flexed and the shoulder relaxed and supported in adduction – i.e. as when sitting in a well-proportioned armchair.

If the shoulder is stiff or painful, the table can be moved diagonally to support it in internal rotation. If oedema is present, a pillow or two will support the forearm in elevation, and a foam pad will protect a bony or painful elbow. The degree of forearm rotation, depending on safe positioning, wound aspect and comfort, is checked. Mid-pronation/supination of the forearm provides the optimum for splinting, allowing unstrained positioning of the wrist and hand, although there are important exceptions to this (e.g. rheumatoid arthritis).

Positioning of the therapist

The therapist is seated comfortably facing the patient and in front of the hand that is to be treated. This gives the therapist good manual control of the patient's limb, and allows varied positioning of the patient's hand for assessment or splinting. It also minimizes stress and discomfort for both therapist and patient (Figure 12.1) and provides good eye contact, which is essential in order to:

- establish rapport and gain the patient's fullest attention
- listen and attend alertly to what the patient is saying
- observe the patient's movements, expression, body language and, most importantly, any discomfort or pain.

Positioning during splinting

The patient's hand can be supported on a purpose-made hand block or wedge to maintain the desired position. This encourages relaxation and is particularly suitable for a weak or painful limb, and when forming the splint on only one aspect of the hand. When a splint must be fitted around the hand, it is more effective if the patient's elbow is on the table and the hand is held upwards. This stabilizes the shoulder and elbow and allows the therapist two-hand control for simultaneous positioning of the patient's limb and moulding of the splint.

PRINCIPLES OF SPLINTING

- Understand the optimum safe positions for post-trauma and post-surgical immobilization for nerve repair, flexor tendon repair, extensor

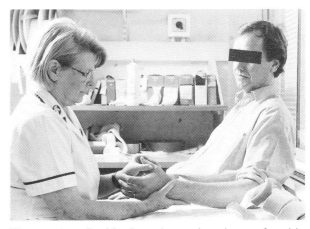

Figure 12.1 Positioning: the patient is comfortable and relaxed while the therapist controls the affected hand and arm with maximum ease and minimum strain. Eye contact and observation of patient discomfort and emotional expression are all within the direct field of vision.

tendon repair, and all other specific conditions, with particular reference to the positioning of the collateral ligaments of the MCP and IP joints of the fingers to prevent their contracture. (Descriptions are given in the relevant sections of this chapter.)

- Understand the optimum functional positioning for non-acute intermittent splintage and the rationale for this (p. 239).
- Ensure that any splint is positioning the joints in both a therapeutic optimum as well as a normal plane: e.g. the tips of the fingers in flexion converge on the scaphoid; the metacarpals are at an angled plane to the forearm; the arches of the palm are maintained.
- Splint only those joints that require control. Do not, for instance, immobilize or hyperextend the DIP joint in a Capener splint that is only intended to extend the PIP joint.
- With regard to pain, ensure that adequate pain control is effective during splinting procedures unless this compromises patient safety. The mental distraction of pain also reduces the efficacy of patient education, assessment, and collaboration in the procedure of splinting.
- Where a painful procedure is essential to treatment, for example joint mobilization or passive range testing, the patient should be adequately educated and prepared and then given real control of the therapist's actions. This should include the ability to give clear instructions to stop the therapist at any time, and never being put under undue psychological pressure to exceed personal tolerance limits. (See also Chapter 3.)
- Health and Safety issues must all be incorporated in hand therapy practice and organization of the splinting room and service (Dival, 1997).
- Apply sound mechanical principles (Brand and Hollister, 1993; Brand, 1995a, Dival and Wilton, 1997; van Lede and van Veldhoven, 1998). The effects and measurement of force on human tissue and on the hand are complex subjects still requiring much research, but an increasing amount of written work is now available.
- Apply force at a right angle (90°) to the relevant bone, not at 80° or 100°, as this will cause shearing stress to the soft tissues and greatly reduce mechanical efficiency.
- Consider the effects of the law of interaction, i.e. that every action has an equal reaction. What effect does an applied force have on tight tissues, and will it remain constant? (Dival and Wilton, 1997; van Lede and van Veldhoven 1998). For instance, the amount of force may change within a few minutes following application of the splint, due to adaptation of the tissues. Therefore it can be more effective to have an easily adjustable mechanism, e.g. a strap that can be tightened by the patient.

- Make an appropriate and effective choice of static or dynamic splinting to mobilize a joint. Certain general rules have been found to apply (Colditz, 1995a; Fess, 1995):
  a. At the acute/inflammatory/acutely painful stage of healing, use static or serial static splinting. At the proliferative stage of healing, use serial static, static progressive or dynamic splinting. At the chronic stage of healing, use serial static or static progressive splinting.
  b. Apply gentle, slow traction and not fast, forced traction which will result in additional tissue damage and scarring.
  c. Apply splintage for sufficient periods of time to maximize 'total end range time' (TERT; Flowers and Michlovitz, 1988; Flowers and La Stayo, 1994); that is, the amount of time that the joint is maintained at the end of its range to stimulate tissue growth and therefore to adapt in length (Brand and Thompson, 1992). Some authors give this as a total of approximately 12–14 hours per day, but definitive time/duration-related evidence has yet to be shown (Prosser, 1995).
  d. Continue splintage until scar and tissue formation ceases to be contractile.
  e. If a joint has a 'soft end feel' (when at maximum passive stretch the joint feels as if it will move further) use dynamic splinting, and if a 'hard end feel' (where at maximum passive stretch the joint feels unyielding) use static progressive splinting which allows prolonged wear.
- Whenever possible, measure the amount of force applied using springs, elastic traction or other tensile material, and keep it within accepted safe limits (Brand and Hollister, 1993; van Lede and van Veldhoven, 1998; Dival, 1997), though evidence of effective forces and application is debated.
- Use the natural pressure-bearing areas of the hand (the finger pulps and palmar pads) to bear splint pressure, and also the muscle bellies.
- Avoid constriction by dressings, taping or straps, especially when there is the risk of increased oedema or infection. The digits are particularly vulnerable to such strangulation, so consider spiral, stretch and diagonal fastenings.
- Maintain elevation of the hand for 3–7 days post-surgery or post-trauma, and longer if indicated by infection, inflammation or oedema. Provide a suitable arm sling (see Figure 5.2) to maintain elevation and accommodate the patient's splint. Triangular slings are frequently unsuitable, as they pull the shoulder and neck forward into a poor, cramped posture. Wide foam strapping such as Velfoam or Betapile makes a more therapeutic sling. If folded into a loop at either end and secured with Velcro, the sling can be worn diagonally across the patient's back to give comfort and proper posture. The

Boscombe Sling (Promedics Ltd) is an excellent commercial version provided that it is fitted across the patient's back and not around the neck.

- Always check for any areas of numbness or hyposensitivity to ensure that a splint does not cause unforeseen skin damage. The patient may have an overlooked or undiagnosed sensory nerve deficit or an old injury that has previously posed little risk.

- Provide advice on prevention of cold intolerance. This is always a risk following hand trauma and hand surgery, particularly if nerve damage is present, and it is increased by the presence of a splint that prevents the normal use of a glove. Prevention is the optimum treatment for cold intolerance, as other methods have a poor success rate. Suggest the use of long baggy sleeves to keep the hand warm, or a mitten made from old tracksuit trousers. Sports shops may supply 'hand bags' used in low-temperature sports, or these can be made from fleece fabric to fit over a splint and fasten with a drawstring or Velcro.

- Prevent undue sweating and skin maceration in a splint by lining it with absorbent fabric or applying tubular cotton gauze. Alternatively, use an open-mesh thermoplastic such as X-lite to allow cooling. Thermoplastics with smaller perforations may provide little or no ventilation if the splint fits snugly and there is no movement, and therefore no conduction, of air across the skin.

- Allergic reactions to splinting materials are rare, but if they occur prompt action must be taken to change the material or lining and improve hygiene. Most reactions are attributable to sweat rash, so measures to reduce warmth and sweating are appropriate.

- Written instructions must be given to the patient. Trauma and surgery are exceptionally stressful events, and the patient may have been given advice and verbal instructions by several staff in varying terminology. Recalling every detail will be impossible, and stress is a known reducer of memory; therefore the patient needs *written* notes on the care of the hand and the use of the splint. Consider the implications of illiteracy (which is often concealed) and foreign language translation. Instructions should include the intervals and duration of splint wear, cleansing, adverse indications, and the recommended course of action should pain or inflammation increase. Complex, difficult to fit splints may require a diagram of the desired positioning. Contact details of the therapist are also essential.

- Ensure that comfort, cosmesis, and patient preference for materials and colour are addressed. Patient satisfaction and compliance may hinge on these factors and dictate the success of treatment.

- Allow sufficient practice time to develop style, technique and expertise in the art and science of splinting, particularly the acquisition of current skills.

WRIST/HAND SPLINTS

Static splints

Paddle-type thermoplastic splints are the most commonly used static wrist/hand splints. They are usually fitted to the volar aspect, but a dorsal forearm component with a volar finger support is a useful option. The thumb support should be excluded when superfluous.

Paddle splints are essential for:

1. Safe positioning in the acute stage of trauma, post-operatively, and in acute infection and inflammation. The POSI (position of safe immobilization) is used to prevent the contractures that can rapidly occur in the acute inflammatory stage, namely extension contracture at the finger MCP joints, flexion contracture at the IP joints, and adduction of the thumb (Boscheinenen-Morrin *et al.*, 1992). POSI is:
   - wrist at 30° extension (in some units only a few degrees of extension, or neutral, is preferred)
   - MCPs in 70–90° flexion
   - IPs in extension
   - thumb in abduction but lying lateral to the index finger, i.e. similar to the lateral pinch position.
   NB: This POSI position is *not* the safe position for many surgical procedures and conditions, such as tendon repairs. The specific protocols of the hand surgery team must be carefully followed.

2. Positioning for intermittent splinting (i.e. resting, night, or non-acute splinting that will be interrupted by mobilization, exercise or function):
   - wrist at 20–30° extension with slight ulnar deviation
   - MCPs in 45° flexion
   - PIPs and DIPs at 30° and 10° respectively
   - thumb in palmar abduction.
   NB: Variations on this position are important in certain conditions, particularly rheumatoid arthritis (see p. 276).

3. Serial and stretch splinting. A paddle splint may be needed to act on several joints to gain the desired range or to gain adequate leverage or distribution of skin pressure to act on one joint alone, for example to extend the wrist.

Interesting and useful models for extension gain are the Thomas static progressive wrist extension splint (Thomas, 1996) and the Palmer's flexor stretch orthosis (Palmer, 1991), which acts on the long flexors of the fingers (Figure 12.2).

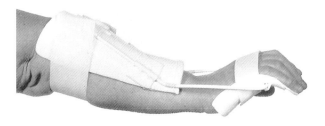

Figure 12.2 Palmer's flexor stretch orthosis (static). The rigid wire frame is shaped in maximum extension of the wrist. When applied to the hand the splint levers the wrist into the extended position, acting on the long flexors. Extension is increased by angulation of the wire at a point just proximal to the ulnar styloid (photograph reproduced by kind permission of Philip Palmer).

Dynamic splints

Most dynamic wrist/hand splints have outriggers, and are known as dynamic high- or low-profile splints. There are numerous designs, and regrettably many are extremely cumbersome, not very low in profile and inefficient. Every effort should be made to study the available literature and materials to find cosmetically acceptable and effective designs (Figure 12.3). These splints have dynamic elastic or spring components to give individual control of one or more fingers. They usually act on the MCP or PIP joints and are used to:

- control the range of motion of individual digits
- provide controlled resisted or assisted motion or exercise
- protect a joint or soft tissues in addition to controlling motion.

(See also dynamic splinting for rheumatoid arthritis, p. 304, and peripheral nerve palsy, pp. 251 and 255.)

WRIST SPLINTS

The positioning of the wrist is the 'pre-set' to the positioning and function of the whole hand. Due to tenodesis action (the reciprocal movements of the wrist and fingers due to the balance of tension of the extensors and flexors), stability of the wrist is essential to the control of hand function, and efficient grasp and pinch are not possible in the absence of wrist extension. Even in the totally paralysed upper limb, passive extension of the wrist produces some flexion of the digits, while flexion of the wrist gives extension and 'opening' of the hand. Therefore, splinting of the wrist can be the fundamental key to function of the hand.

Where normal range of motion in the wrist is an unrealistic goal, 12° of extension will allow some power grip, whereas 20° of extension is adequate for a large proportion of function. Thirty to forty degrees is normal for power grip.

Static wrist splints

These can be classified as soft or rigid splints.

Soft splints

There is a wide range of ready-made wrist splints in a choice of materials and linings. Neoprene (Figure 12.4) is a first choice, as the edges can be trimmed with scissors to fit properly round the thumb and MCP joints. Its appearance is neat and acceptable as it is similar to sports braces and is machine washable. Elastic fabric may be preferred for extra support or a closer fit, but unfortunately this material requires edge binding, which tends to dig

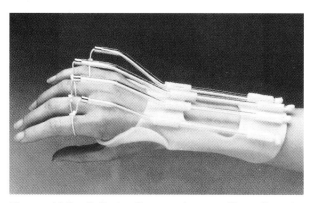

Figure 12.3 Orfitube System low-profile splint. An example of modern materials that provide ease of fabrication with a 'hi-tech' finish. This model would need the addition of suitable finger slings (photo courtesy of North Coast Medical Inc., www.ncmedical.com).

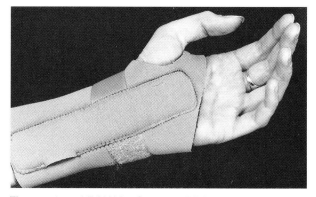

Figure 12.4 VM Wrist Support (VM Marketing Ltd) – a Neoprene soft splint with metal insert to position the wrist. The cotton terry towel lining relieves sweating and synthetic fabric allergy. Different lengths and strapping options are available.

into the skin around the thenar area or to force the index MCP joint into ulnar deviation. Any tight edge binding is also unsuitable for sensory deficits.

Some wrist supports incorporate a cotton lining suitable for reducing sweat rash and for patients allergic to synthetic fabrics. A choice of fabric and colour is a compliance plus, while optional fastenings are important for firm fitting with one hand.

Rigid splints

These can be moulded to the volar, dorsal, ulnar or radial aspects of the wrist, or circumferentially where total support is needed. The volar type is most commonly used.

The design is determined by the following factors:

- allowing full movement of the thumb and MCP joints
- full, limited, or partial support to the thumb
- strong or minimal support at the wrist (rigidity and length of splint)
- avoidance of painful, bony areas or wounds
- suitability for function, especially for employment conditions
- cosmesis.

Indications

1. Carpal tunnel syndrome. In conservative treatment of this condition, a splint may be used to maintain the wrist in the neutral position to reduce pressure in the carpal canal (Falkenstein and Weiss-Lennard, 1999). It is used at night when symptoms are most frequently experienced, but may also be used during the day if symptoms are severe or exacerbated by function. Following surgery, a splint may be used to support the wrist until inflammation has subsided.
2. Wrist extensor weakness. A splint is used to act as an extensor assist, preventing a non-functional flexed position and over-stretching of the extensors. It is also used to stabilize the wrist and facilitate hand function.
3. The 'intrinsic minus' (claw) hand. A splint is used to reinstate the normal functional position of the hand using a tenodesis action – by bringing the wrist into extension, the MCP joints are drawn into flexion and the thumb into some abduction.
4. Painful or unstable wrist. A splint is used to provide support for function, employment and leisure activities.

Fabrication

When making the splint:

- maintain the wrist in the optimum position of extension and slight ulnar deviation unless contraindicated

- maintain the palmar arches
- ensure there is no unintended blocking of range of movement of the thumb or MCP joints
- consider the types of strapping and fastening for ease of patient use
- consider using diagonal straps for better hold.

(See also splinting for rheumatoid arthritis, p. 299.)

Dynamic wrist splints

These are mainly used for radial nerve lesions to support a dropped wrist, but may also be used as a dynamic assist where the extensors are weak rather than paralysed. (See p. 255.)

FINGER SPLINTS

Finger splints can be broadly classified as protective or mobilizing. Both may be static or dynamic and are often of similar design. Indications are given under the different splints described. Mobilizing splints, particularly for the PIP joints, need careful selection to be effective, and guidelines are given under Principles (p. 237).

If oedema is present Coban wrap or a Lycra finger-sleeve can be worn between the skin and the splint, and for scarring, tenderness, skin fragility or hypoaesthesia a gel-lined Digitube (Silipos) can be worn under the splint to soften the scar or protect the skin.

Dynamic finger extension splints

There are many different designs of these splints. They are known generally as Capener splints and are made of spring wire, usually incorporating a coil at either side of the IP joint. Variations of Capener splints include the Cambridge, Odstock and Simpson splints. Most models are designed for use on the PIP joint, while others combine PIP and DIP joint control. The latter models must be carefully fitted to prevent an imbalance of force that may result in hyperextension of the less resistant DIP joint. They can be custom- or ready-made, and some suppliers will make them to order in the desired strength and size.

Measurement of effective force (from 100–300 g) and length of moment arm are recommended by many authors, including Brand and Thompson (1992), and there is much discussion of the practicalities, treatment results (Colditz, 1995a; Prosser 1995) and, importantly, the tolerance of the patient's skin to amount of splint force and pressure.

Custom making requires the skill to produce accurate work to a high standard of comfort, mechanical efficiency and cosmesis, although ready-made coil spring wire is obtainable (Orfit Joint Jack Coil Spring, in 0.7 mm wire). It is often more cost-effective and cosmetically acceptable to use ready-made splints. A variety of types and sizes can be stocked to give an appropriate choice of resistance and shape, especially for swollen and painful fingers. Different designs can be tried on the patient to find the most efficient and comfortable splint, and minimal time is needed for adjustment of the leverage, padding and strapping.

The patient must be taught to apply and remove the splint properly and, when appropriate, to adjust the resistance so the leverage can be increased or reduced. A graduated regimen for wearing the splint may initially be necessary, increasing over the first few days until the patient can tolerate the skin pressure required. An advantage of dynamic splinting is that the patient can actively flex against the splint to reduce any joint stiffness caused by prolonged splinting.

Some ready-made options

1. The Steeper finger extensor (Steeper RSL; Figure 12.5). This has all-white spring wire and plastic parts with a very neat clean appearance, and is supplied in several sizes. It requires simple adjustment to shape around the finger webs, and padding on the distal bar; it is easy to fit and adjust and no strap is needed. It has exceptionally efficient leverage and can be fitted in two different ways to give either average or extra strong resistance, and also has the unusual feature of a rigid proximal phalanx bar that prevents the spring coils from impinging on the PIP joint.
2. The Simpson Splint (Promedics Ltd; Figure 12.6) is a Capener-type splint, with a short distal cuff specifically designed to leave the DIP joint free. The standard model is rarely of adequate resistance, so the 'extra-strong' model should be stocked.

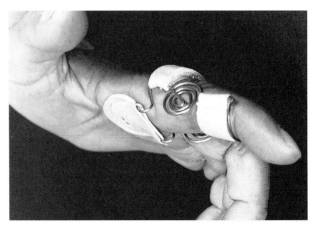

Figure 12.6 Simpson Capener (Promedics Ltd) – a dynamic PIP extensor designed with a short distal cuff to leave the DIP joint free.

3. The LMB Spring Coil Extension Assist (North Coast Medical Inc.) leaves the DIP joint free and has user-friendly moulded foam pads. It is particularly suitable when pressure must be applied over scars or fragile skin. **NB**: LMB manufacture several designs of splints on similar principles.
4. The Spring Mallet Splint (Promedics Ltd) is designed for mallet finger deformity. This strong spring wire splint can also be useful to give almost static extension of the PIP joint, or of the PIP and DIP joints combined. It can be used in reverse on the volar aspect or dorsally for a variety of IP joint problems, and is worth having in the splint store.

Unfortunately, with many of the ready-made Capeners the standard strength model is often too weak to provide adequate resistance. Some suppliers provide stronger versions and unusual sizes. On some models tightening the strap may cause unacceptable pressure from the wire, particularly on either side of a swollen joint, and replacing the strap with a rigid band of thermoplastic can be the solution.

Custom-made finger splints

Reinforced Lycra finger-sleeves Reinforced Lycra finger-sleeves are used for flexion contracture of the interphalangeal joints, especially in acute injury and in the presence of oedema. They have been used for many years as compression therapy to reduce oedema and to control scarring. It was observed that wearing a finger-sleeve on a single digit interrupts the normal cascade of flexion of the fingers at rest, with the inference that the finger-sleeve is assisting extension of the digit. It was a natural progression to add an extra layer of Lycra over the dorsum of the finger-sleeve to increase this

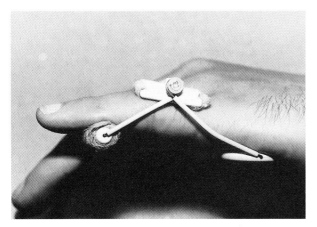

Figure 12.5 Steeper finger extensor (Single Digital Extension Splint, Steeper RSL) for dynamic PIP joint extension.

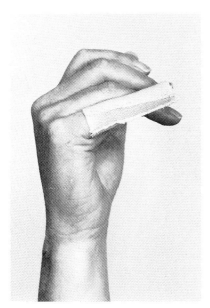

Figure 12.7 Dorsally reinforced Lycra finger-sleeve.

effect while still allowing relatively unhindered movement (Figure 12.7).

In the presence of oedema, according to McGrouther (1990) and Brand (1995b), tissue fluid spreads into the dorsal skin, which is more distensible than the inelastic volar skin. This flexes the proximal interphalangeal joint. If there are volar scars they will have contractile elements, which will contribute to flexion contracture. Brand (1995b) advocates gentle constant tension to give scars the message to lengthen. If the tissues keep receiving the same message for days at a time, the cellular activity of absorbing collagen and relaying it will lead to sustained lengthening. The Lycra finger-sleeve can be worn constantly, fulfilling these criteria (Kennedy *et al.*, 2000).

The finger-sleeve is constructed by drawing around the finger, with the pen perpendicular to the finger. The pattern is enlarged to allow for the depth of the finger, and is then cut out double on the fold line of the Lycra (Powernet Lycra), together with a strip of Lycra of equal width to the finger tracing. This strip is sewn into place and the longitudinal seam of the finger-sleeve is sewn using a zig-zag stitch (Figure 12.7).

Low-profile/outrigger splints These may be more practicable when more than two or more fingers need splinting simultaneously, and extra-wide finger loops can also be incorporated to control both PIP and DIP joints simultaneously. Because of their bulk they are not suitable for use in most employment or for household tasks.

Extensor splints for paralysis See Peripheral nerve lesions, pp. 254–7.

Static finger extension splints

Full hand/wrist splint
A full hand/wrist splint extending from the forearm may give the best control if all four fingers are involved, and will be correct if extension is being limited by the long flexors. If not, a simple volar splint extending from the wrist crease to the fingertips will have adequate leverage. If a thermoplastic with good drape is used, close moulding can ensure that individual fingers are each held in maximum extension.

Finger gutter
A small gutter splint or palm-based splint is suitable to extend an individual finger, and is altered progressively to gain extension. By forming a U-shaped bridge in the centre, purchase can be increased when the strap is tightened.

Plaster of Paris serial splinting
This is suitable for all stages of healing, and particularly for joints that are inflamed, painful or difficult to move. Mild contractures are better treated with a simple gutter splint. Serial splinting is also indicated for joints that are contracted or stiff in more than 45° of flexion, when dynamic splinting is mechanically ineffective. The splints can be of cylindrical or figure-of-eight construction, the latter allowing exposure of the dorsum of the joint, and are usually applied in the position of maximum active extension or slight passive traction. The plaster is removed and remade every few days. Bell-Krotoski (1995) recommends renewal of the plaster every day or every other day, and continued use while improvement is evident.

Joint Jack
This is a commercially produced metal splint with felt padding. It can be applied to the finger and the thumb joints. It may be the only splint with adequate leverage for some contractures, as it can exert an exceptionally precise force due to its unique design and its minutely adjustable screw mechanism (Figure 12.8).

NB: The Joint Jack is powerful enough to sublux a joint, and should not be used on an insensate digit or a patient who might be over-motivated.

The Joint Jack is bent to conform to the finger to be treated, leaving space for the stiff joint to be corrected. It is then strapped firmly to the finger with a foam or compressed wool pad under the strap. The adjusting screw is turned gradually and gently until some pressure is evident, and after 1–2 minutes a further turn of the screw can be made if the joint position has changed. This can be repeated until the pressure is adequate. The method of application and adjustment must then be carefully rehearsed with the patient.

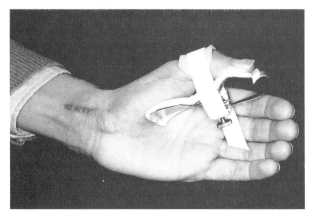

Figure 12.8 Joint Jack – a powerful extensor splint for a digital joint. It is minutely adjustable by turning the screw, and can be used on fingers or thumb (photo with permission of the Joint Jack Co.).

Buddy splinting

This is one of the simplest methods of assisting range of motion of a finger joint. The affected finger is strapped or splinted to an adjacent finger by various methods. Adhesive tape is speedy and firm but is not suitable for more than a few days use, when a removable strap or splint is best. Velcro works well, leather is more durable, synthetic leather resists wet and sweating, thin thermoplastic gives firmer control, and Lycra fabric will also control oedema. To achieve the best purchase, the material is joined on both volar and dorsal surfaces. A double finger-stall can be made on the same principles. The fingertip should be left free for tactile function.

THUMB SPLINTS

The thumb contributes about 50 per cent of the function of the hand, and this should be taken into account when splinting any part of the hand. If thumb opposition and abduction are limited in any way, the role and movement patterns of the fingers and hypothenar area are greatly affected. The thumb is their essential opposing force and their partner in the action of pinch.

An adducted thumb can only produce a cramped or lateral pinch, which forces the fingers to claw and the palm to flatten. Once a patient can pinch effectively, the hand becomes useful and can then be instrumental in its own rehabilitation.

Thumb stabilizer (thumb post)

This splint controls the CMC and MCP joints of the thumb, usually in the pinch position (Figures 12.9, 12.10). It is also used to maintain the arches of the metacarpals and palm to reduce any flattening of the hand when claw-hand posture is present.

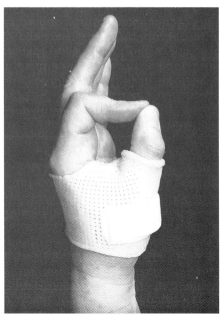

Figure 12.9 Thumb stabilizer, fabricated in Turbocast soft-surface thermoplastic.

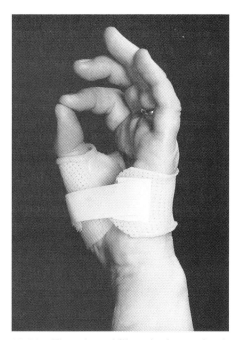

Figure 12.10 Thumb stabilizer (palmar view).

Indications and options:

1. Osteoarthritis, pain or inflammation of the CMC joint. The splint is used to reduce the mechanical stresses on this joint, particularly during function, or to alter the position used for pinch so that the painful joint posture is avoided. The patient may habitually pinch in the same position, resulting in a small area of worn cartilage in

the CMC joint. If this is the case, by splinting in a 'new' position, undamaged cartilage can be utilized and the pain avoided.

2. Rupture or damage of a collateral ligament of the MCP joint. Any lateral subluxation of the joint is corrected and maintained by the splint. This allows the ligament to heal and contract to its normal length over a period of at least 6 weeks.

3. Median nerve palsy (see Peripheral nerve lesions, p. 252).

4. Scar contracture. Silicone moulding compound (Otoform) is moulded to the scar, and the splint is then moulded over the silicone. Silicone gel sheet can be used in the same way.

5. Stiffness or contracture. The splint should be applied immediately after mobilizations, then remoulded every few days to maximize progress.

Correct positioning of the whole hand and wrist during the fitting of this splint is essential for effectiveness and comfort. The wrist must be in extension, the palm cupped, the fingers in some flexion, and the thumb and index finger in pinch. The softened splint (Figure 12.11) is wrapped around the dorsum of the hand, drawing the thumb into opposition. The central lip of the splint is then stretched closely over the thumb web into the palm and moulded against the thenar eminence. As the thermoplastic sets, the hand is cupped and the thumb held in palmar abduction and pinch. The edges of the splint are carefully shaped and lipped for comfort and to allow unrestricted range of the wrist, thumb IP joint and finger MCP joints.

There is a wide choice of thumb stabilizing splints providing varying degrees of control of one or all joints. Types of 'soft' splint are described below.

Soft thumb stabilizer/thumb support
Using a similar pattern to the rigid thumb stabilizer (above), this splint is made of Neoprene, synthetic suede, leather or Lycra (pressure garment material). The custom-made Neoprene MCP support and CMC support are described in detail below. Several versions are available commercially under such names as Wrist/Thumb Wrap, Thumb Support, etc.
Indications include:

1. Where the thumb needs to be gently progressed to the pinch position.
2. When gradual reduction in support is needed, e.g. later stage motor recovery in nerve palsy.
3. Where the skin is tender or fragile.
4. With an elastic strap, to give semi-dynamic opposition of the thumb.
5. With a moulded thermoplastic C-piece over the thumb web, to maintain abduction (Fig.12.12).
6. With both C-piece and elastic strap, for a nerve palsy.
7. With a stiff reinforcement on the dorsum of the thumb, to protect the MCP joint or to reduce mechanical stress during movement.

Neoprene thumb MCP support (custom-made)
A standard pattern is used (Figure 12.13) and up-sized or down-sized to fit. It can support to the proximal wrist crease, or be extended along the forearm to give additional wrist support. It is cut

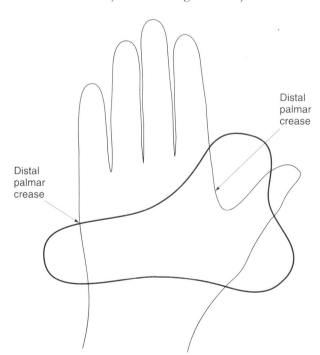

Figure 12.11   Pattern for thumb stabilizer.

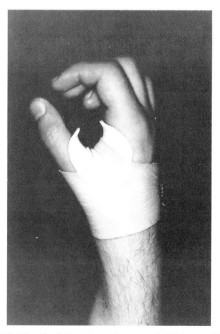

Figure 12.12   Soft leather thumb stabilizer with thermoplastic C-piece to maintain abduction.

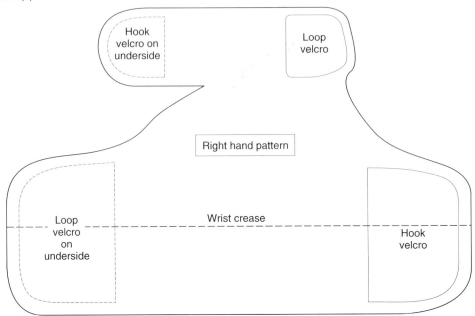

Figure 12.13 Pattern for Neoprene thumb MCP support.

out of 3 mm (1/8 inch) Neoprene, with the pattern orientated so that the longitudinal borders coincide with the selvedges of the Neoprene. Velcro is added where indicated (Figure 12.14).

Neoprene thumb CMC support (custom-made) A standard pattern is used (Figure 12.15) as for the thumb MCP support, and is cut out in the same way. The radial and palmar darts are cut out and sewn butt-edged with a wide, close zig-zag seam, and the Velcro added (Figure 12.16).

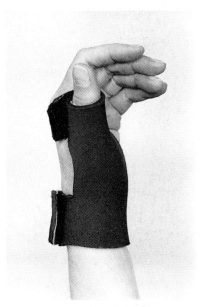

Figure 12.14 Neoprene thumb MCP support.

Thumb web spreader (C-splint)
Nearly all conditions of the thumb cause some loss of span of the first web space, and a thumb web spreader splint is therefore used. This static splint (Figure 12.17) is best made in a thicker thermoplastic to ensure rigidity. It should conform well, and is moulded very closely while the thumb web is stretched into abduction of the CMC joint. Care must be taken to prevent forcing the thumb MCP into radial deviation or the index MCP into ulnar deviation.

Best results are achieved if the splint is moulded with the thumb CMC in palmar abduction and extension and is worn every night. Some additional periods of wear during the day may be needed for a severe contracture, particularly if hypertrophic scarring is present. The splint is remoulded frequently to ensure progress. Diligent use can produce dramatic results within a fortnight.

Firm strapping is essential to secure this splint. A figure-of-eight strap encircling the thumb web and the wrist works well. Velfoam strapping is good where skin protection is needed, and elastic Velcro gives optimum conformity and comfort, holding the splint well down into the thumb web.

Options include:

1. An extra wide splint to spread and reduce pressure, or to apply pressure to scar tissue (Figure 12.17)
2. Silicone moulding compound or gel under the splint to treat contracted or dry scars
3. Extending the splint to the fingertips or just to the IP joints.

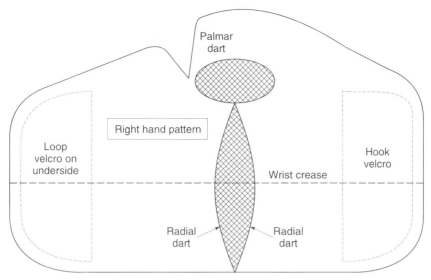

Figure 12.15   Pattern for Neoprene thumb CMC support.

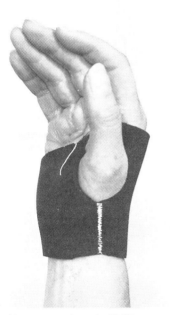

Figure 12.16   Neoprene thumb CMC support.

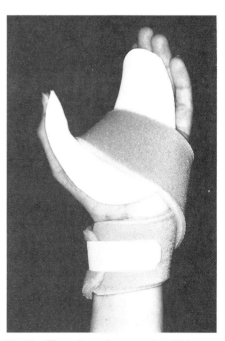

Figure 12.17   Thumb web spreader. This extra-wide version can be used for web scar control with a silicone insert, or to distribute pressure on fragile or painful skin.

Thumb spica

This splint controls the wrist and thumb together (Figure 12.18). It is most commonly used for De Quervain's tenosynovitis (of abductor pollicis longus and extensor pollicis brevis), and is therefore moulded on the radial aspect of the hand and forearm. The IP joint of the thumb is usually left free to prevent stiffness and maintain function, but may also be splinted for a short period while inflammation is severe. It can also be used for

damage to the MCP joint or its collateral ligaments when a shorter splint is ineffective, and for pain or swelling of both the wrist and thumb.

For De Quervain's, the positioning should be 25° extension and slight radial deviation of the wrist, slight flexion of the first MCP joint, and mid-palmar abduction at the first CMC joint.

For MCP collateral ligament healing, there should be slight flexion at this joint and correction of any lateral deviation.

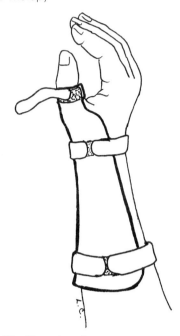

Figure 12.18 Thumb spica.

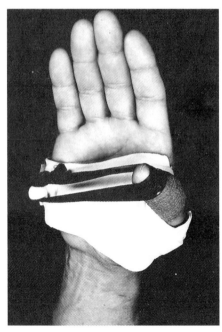

Figure 12.19 Thumb IP flexion stretch splint with Theraband thumb loop (also showing Coban wrap on thumb to reduce oedema).

Other thumb problems and splinting solutions

Joint stiffness

Capener-type splints are not suited to the thumb, and most therapists find it best to use other types of dynamic or static splinting. Traction can be applied in flexion or extension by arranging pulley points on a static base splint. The splint stabilizes the thumb proximal to the stiff joint, and traction is applied by an elastic or static cord attached to a thumb loop. Fine rubber ribbon (Theraband) is particularly good for thumb traction, as it conforms well and clings in place on the skin or fingernail (Figure 12.19).

It is possible to apply traction to either the IP or MCP or to both simultaneously by a suitable arrangement of pulleys (Colditz, 1995c; Wilton, 1997a).

Extreme joint stiffness

A Joint Jack splint can be used in the same way as serial splinting. The change in joint positioning is achieved in seconds simply by turning the adjustment screw (Figure 12.8). The Joint Jack must be used with care, as it is possible to sublux a joint by over-zealous adjustment.

'Physio thumb'

Pain or hyperextension of the IP or MCP joints caused by mechanical stresses from giving mobilizations is a common occupational hazard for physiotherapists, particularly those who treat back pain. Preventive splinting is the wise course of

action, and should be used as soon as discomfort is noticed. There is a choice of support:

1. Adhesive taping (strapping). This will give some support whilst still allowing a certain amount of movement of the affected joint.
2. A small closely-fitting tube splint made in semi-rigid thermoplastic (the tubular construction prevents movement). A very close fit is essential to avoid any play in the affected joint. To prevent the splint from pinching the skin during the application of mobilizations, its distal edge is moulded against the thumbnail as a counterforce but the thumb tip pulp is left free to allow contact and sensation. A little hand lotion eases removal.
3. A thumb stabilizer, using any of the design options. This gives greater support than the thumb tube.

FLEXOR TENDON REPAIRS

Splinting and hand therapy must be provided in harmony for the successful outcome of flexor tendon repairs. Effective post-operative regimens centre on patient compliance, which is the result of correct management by the hand team (see Chapter 3).

Immediate post-operative splinting

The Kleinert splinting system greatly advanced the results of flexor tendon surgery by using controlled,

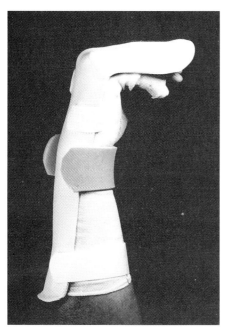

Figure 12.20 Protective splint for repair of flexor tendons of the fingers. Positioning may vary according to the protocol of the hand surgery team.

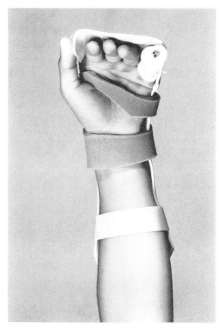

Figure 12.21 Protective splint for flexor tendon repair (volar view).

regular excursion exercise to prevent the formation of adhesions and preserve tendon glide. It involved a dorsal protective splint and the use of elastic traction on the affected digits. Excursion of the repaired tendons was exercised by active extension against the elastic, followed by passive flexion on return to the resting position. Most hand units now practice early passive or early active exercise regimens in which the elastic traction is no longer used, although this has been reintroduced in some units for patients who are at unusual risk of re-rupture.

Basic protective splint

A basic protective splint (Figures 12.20 and 12.21) is still essential to most of these regimens, and is usually made in thermoplastic in approximately the following positions:

- wrist in neutral or slight flexion; if the wound is at wrist level, 30–40° of flexion is sometimes preferred
- MCPs in 70–90° of flexion; if the wrist is splinted in flexion, a less acute position of 45° of MCP flexion may be used
- IPs at 0°, allowing full extension of these joints within the splint.

Note that the latter point regards the position of the splint. The IP joints themselves are held in relaxed flexion, as the fingers are not usually strapped against the splint but left free. All four fingers are included in the splint in the above position,

regardless of whether one or all fingers are affected. This is to discourage functional use of the hand and particularly any strong flexion, which might cause re-rupture.

Repair of flexor tendons of the thumb

For repair of the flexor tendons of the thumb, the splint is made in the following position:

- wrist in neutral or 25° of flexion, plus slight ulnar deviation, thus there is the minimum tension on the thumb flexors; if finger flexor repairs are also present, wrist flexion must be at 40°
- CMC in some palmar abduction
- MCP in 30° of flexion
- IP in extension.

The splint should tuck neatly into the thumb web to prevent the splint from slipping and to maintain some abduction. Most importantly, the splint must allow unhindered flexion and extension of the thumb during the exercise regimen.

Nerve and flexor tendon repairs combined

Where lesions of the median, ulnar or digital nerves also have occurred, the splint is fitted in additional flexion to ensure that there is no tension on the nerve repair.

With or without a nerve repair, it is always wise to check for any areas of sensory deficit before fitting the splint so that an undetected or old nerve lesion is not subject to skin damage in the splint.

Splint comfort

A narrow piece of foam lining along the centre of the splint reduces pressure on the bony prominences of the ulnar styloid and MCP heads, and prevents slipping of the splint. Tubular cotton stockinette may be fitted to reduce sweating.

Strapping should be comfortable and firm but not tight, and must allow full flexion of the fingers and thumb. Velfoam, Betapile and other foam-layer straps are best, especially post-operatively where oedema and painful wounds are present. They are trimmed to conform to the contours of the wrist and in particular to the palm to allow flexion at the MCPs.

Approximately 3 weeks after surgery, any extreme angulation of the splint may be reduced a little to increase comfort, subject to agreement with the surgeon.

Discontinuing the splint

Full-time wear of the splint is usually discontinued at 6 weeks post-surgery. Sleeping, travel on public transport, crowd participation and social occasions involving alcohol require continued wear of the splint for at least a further 2 weeks. For children the optimum time will be longer to prevent accidental damage.

Stiffness of the IP joints following flexor tendon repair is a common complication, especially if the wound is distal to the palm. Solutions include:

- buddy splinting – strapping to an adjacent unaffected finger
- a static gutter finger splint – suitable in early stage of healing
- a dynamic Capener-type splint – care must be taken that the finger is not flexed strongly against the spring before tendon healing is adequately established.

Once the dorsal protective splint is discarded any wrist and finger deficits can be treated more aggressively, including appropriate splinting (e.g. a dynamic outrigger with elastic traction or a combination of dynamic and static wrist/hand splints). Individual finger deficits may require a splint chosen from those described under Finger splints (p. 241).

EXTENSOR TENDON REPAIRS

Both therapist and patient must be aware of the potential problems of rupture and adhesions that can occur in poorly managed extensor tendon repairs. It may be particularly difficult for the patient to appreciate the seriousness of an injury with what is often a very small wound, and little pain or swelling.

The exact site and zone of the wound and of the repair must be ascertained before the immediate post-operative plaster slab and bandaging are removed. The injured wrist and hand must be kept in extension throughout the splinting process, so it is preferable to use a shaped splinting block or wedge for support, not forgetting the thumb if this is also involved.

Static protective splinting, which is combined with early passive or active mobilization regimens (except for Zones 1 to 4), is described here. Many hand surgery units prefer the use of dynamic splinting, using outriggers and elastic, in specific mobilization regimens. The duration of splinting also varies from unit to unit.

Zone 7

If the wrist extensor tendons only are involved, use a palmar splint extending from the upper forearm to the transverse palmar crease, with the wrist in 45° extension and the MCP and fingers left free. If the finger extensors are involved, splint as for Zones 5 and 6.

Zones 5 and 6

If using a volar wrist and hand splint, the MCP joints must be included but the IP joints can be left free. If there is any danger that the splint might slip into the wrong position or might be replaced incorrectly after cleansing or dressings, it is best to ensure safety with a full-length splint that includes the IP joints. Positioning is:

- wrist in 45° of extension
- MCPs in 25° of flexion
- IPs at 10–30° of flexion.

The duration of splinting is 4–6 weeks.

Zones 3 and 4

To prevent the Boutonnière deformity that may result at this level of tendon repair, the PIP joint is splinted in full extension and the DIP joint is left free to encourage active flexion. If the PIP joint cannot be passively moved into full extension on day 1 of treatment, then it must be serially splinted to gain extension. This is vital to the prevention of long-term deformity and loss of function of both the DIP and PIP joints.

Any finger splint that maintains full extension is suitable, including:

- a plaster of Paris cylinder
- a thermoplastic gutter to the dorsal or volar surface with, if necessary, a foam wedge to obtain full extension
- a double thermoplastic gutter to sandwich the finger.

Duration of splinting is for 6 weeks continuously, with 4 or more further weeks of night splinting if loss of range is present.

Zones 1 and 2

This produces the typical mallet deformity. To provide the best possible chance of successful approximation and healing of the avulsed tendon, usually with its fragment of bone from the distal phalanx, a mallet splint should be fitted as soon as possible. This holds the DIP joint in 10–20° of hyperextension, and should leave the PIP joint free.

Mallet splints are commonly available in a variety of ready-made types and sizes, or can be custom-made from thermoplastic or foam-lined aluminium strip (Zimmer splint). If is it difficult to obtain hyperextension of the DIP joint, a firm foam wedge can be inserted between the finger pulp and splint or taping. Adhesive taping secures the splint effectively, and this is placed just distal to the PIP joint to allow free movement of this joint.

There are a number of common problems that occur, any of which take the DIP joint into flexion and disrupt or destroy any healing achieved:

● the splint becomes loose as the swelling subsides
● the patient or an inexperienced staff member removes the splint for cleansing and does not maintain uninterrupted extension of the joint
● the strapping on the splint is dislodged
● the splint is discontinued before the optimum of 6–8 weeks.

A custom-made splint may be necessary to prevent the problems described. For successful treatment it is imperative that the patient is correctly educated about the diagnosis, care and contraindications. Regular follow-up of the patient is needed to check that the splint is effective and for reinforcement of patient education.

Thumb: extensor pollicis longus repair

A volar splint extending from mid-forearm to thumb tip is fitted in the 'hitch-hiker' position, with:

● wrist in 30°extension, with slight radial deviation
● CMC in extension
● MCP in extension
● IP in full extension.

The splint should fit comfortably to the palm and into the thumb web, but allow full function of the fingers.

Patients usually learn to use the 'thumb' of this splint as an opposition post to provide crude pinch. This should be encouraged, as this basic function provides exercise for the whole limb.

Thumb and finger extensor repairs combined

This requires a paddle-type wrist/hand splint with all the digits supported in extension in the positions given here and as above for finger extensors. The duration of splinting is 6 weeks.

Once the protective splint is discontinued, there may be varying degrees of loss of range and function. At this stage dynamic splints are the most effective, but they must only be used when it is safe to apply tension to the tendon repair. Gentle traction may be needed for at least the first 2 weeks, and this should be agreed with the surgeon.

Splinting goals at this stage are:

● to increase active and passive range of the finger joints
● to apply stretch to reduce adaptive shortening of an immobilized muscle
● to reduce any tendon excursion deficit.

A suitable splint can be selected from the section on Finger splints (p. 241).

PERIPHERAL NERVE LESIONS

The fundamental aims of early stage splinting are:

● to protect surgical repair of the nerve
● to protect a fragile damaged nerve when surgical repair is not required
● to reduce tension on a repaired or fragile nerve to maximize the speed and quality of healing
● to prevent complications of immobilization, i.e. stiffness and contractures
● to facilitate recovery and return of function.

Types of nerve lesion (Tubiana *et al.*, 1996) and indications for splinting

1. Neurapraxia (first degree, Sunderland's classification). There is usually spontaneous recovery within weeks. Splinting is required to prevent over-stretching of the nerve and paralysed muscles, and may also be considered, when safe, for function and to minimize interruption of the patient's employment.
2. Axonotmesis (second and third degree). Recovery may take many months. Protective splinting is needed to protect a frail nerve and prevent further injury. Functional splinting should be provided to normalize hand function and to prevent contractures and complications, and unless contraindicated the patient should return to work and normal activity.
3. Axonotmesis (fourth degree) and neurotmesis (fifth degree). Surgical repair is necessary for recovery, and this must be maintained by protective splinting to prevent tension, distraction or rupture of the repaired nerve. After 3–4 weeks, the repair will have sufficient tensile strength and the protective splint can be discarded. It should then be replaced by functional splinting as described for each type of nerve palsy.

Assessment

Full motor and sensory assessments are made (see pp. 28 and 42). The majority of these tests are carried out by the hand therapists, but this should be a team task involving surgeons and electromyography.

These assessments are fundamental to the splinting plan, as they accurately detail the patient's sensory and motor deficits. The motor deficits will determine which movements the splint will need to control or substitute, and the sensory deficits are monitored carefully to ensure that any splint contact does not cause skin damage. Vasomotor deficits are included in the patient's education and treatment.

If there is weakness of a movement, as opposed to complete paralysis, then the assessment must determine the need for splinting to assist motion rather than to substitute it.

A useful tool when checking which motor deficits are present is a table of the nerve supply of the upper limb. A suitable one appears in Lister (1993).

Protective splinting

This maintains the nerve in a safe position by protecting it from rupture at the site of the repair, and from poor or slow healing due to adverse tension of the nerve.

Median nerve lesions

High lesions require static elbow splintage and positioning of the paralysed areas of the hand. Lesions in the distal forearm require static wrist and hand splintage, and those in the palm require splintage of the wrist and affected digits – in other words, control of any joint movement that would cause adverse tension on the nerve.

Positioning is as follows:

- elbow in 90° flexion
- radio-ulnar joints in the mid-position
- wrist in the neutral position
- MCPs in 45° flexion
- PIPs in 30° flexion
- IPs in 10° flexion
- thumb CMC in some abduction and opposition (functional resting position)
- thumb MCP and IP in 20–30° flexion.

Ulnar nerve lesions

For a high lesion in the elbow region or upper forearm, the elbow is splinted. For a lesion in the distal forearm, wrist or hand, only the wrist and affected digits are splinted.

Positioning is as follows:

- elbow in 30–60° flexion
- wrist in the neutral position or slight extension
- MCPs in 45° flexion

- PIPs in 30° flexion and DIPs in 10° flexion
- thumb in the neutral position

NB: If the nerve repair has been difficult and has been sutured under tension, then the splint positioning may be more flexed, particularly at the joints adjacent to the repair site. This should be agreed with the surgeon.

Radial nerve lesions

These are often high lesions at the radial groove of the humerus or in the region of the elbow. The elbow is therefore held statically to protect the repair, and the wrist is also splinted to prevent contractures and overstretching of the paralysed extensors:

- elbow in 90° flexion
- wrist in 30° extension.

A static night resting splint to position the wrist and hand is usually needed.

Functional splinting

After nerve repair, or nerve 'immobilization' where surgery is inappropriate, functional splinting can be commenced as soon as it is safe for the protective splint to be discarded. Dynamic functional splints are unsuitable for night wear, so the patient is also fitted with a static resting splint, this being particularly important in radial nerve palsy to prevent over-stretching of the wrist extensors.

The objectives of functional splinting are to:

- 'normalize' function of the hand by providing a splint that largely substitutes for the actions of the paralysed muscles
- prevent disuse contractures by facilitating a near-normal range of motion
- prevent denervated muscles from remaining in an over-stretched position (Colditz, 1995d)
- maintain the power and action of unaffected muscles by eliminating trick movements and allowing function
- facilitate recovery by acting as a muscle substitute in the early stages and as a muscle assist in the recovery stage.

If possible, functional splints should fit closely to the limb so they do not impede the use of the hand. This is especially important for such activities as putting the hand in a pocket, tucking in a shirt or pulling on a sleeve when dressing, and when travelling, driving, caring for infants and children, and working in confined spaces or on machinery.

History and design Before the designs for nerve palsy splints described by Bunnell in the USA, including the Oppenheimer splint (Boyes, 1964), and Wynn Parry and Barr in the UK (Wynn Parry, 1973), cumbersome outriggers with elastic pulleys were used. The newer, neater splints promoted by these pioneers were made mainly of spring wire, and were designed to conform closely to the hand and arm and give a full range of movement at all joints. Because of their contiguity with the hand they were much more functional than the outrigger splints and could be worn for a much wider variety of activities, especially in the work environment. Some of the radial nerve palsy splints were almost undetectable when worn under the sleeve of normal clothing, and even allowed the wearer to put the hand in a pocket.

It is regrettable that many hand therapists now seem unaware of these splint designs, do not understand their advantages and are not familiar with their publication (Wynn Parry, 1973; Barr, 1975). It is the author's opinion that many of these designs remain 'state-of-the-art' and should be more widely used, employing modern materials when suitable.

Median nerve palsy

The objectives are to:

- provide opposition and abduction of the thumb for functional pinch and grasp
- prevent contractures
- facilitate recovery.

Options include:

1. A static thumb stabilizer or opponens splint (Figure 12.9) – many designs are available. The splint force should be applied to the dorsal aspect of the first metacarpal just proximal to the MCP joint to achieve opposition, and to the ulnar aspect to achieve palmar abduction. It is usually necessary to stabilize the thumb MCP joint in the splint but leave the IP joint free. Semi-rigid thermoplastic usually gives optimum comfort for the static thumb stabilizer. Stability is provided by the strap, which also allows some adjustment of the degree of opposition and can be easily altered by the patient for differing activities.
2. Dynamic thumb opposition splints – various designs are available; simple models that do not involve outriggers are the most effective and are best accepted by the patient (Figure 12.22).
3. A static thumb web spreader (C-splint; Figure 12.17) may be needed in addition to the above splints to stretch or prevent thenar web contracture.

Patients may need to try several types of splint to find their preferred model, and may like to have more than one type, for work and leisure for instance, particularly if recovery is prolonged.

NB: Anaesthetic areas must be constantly monitored for splint pressure and skin damage.

(See also Thumb splints, p. 244.)

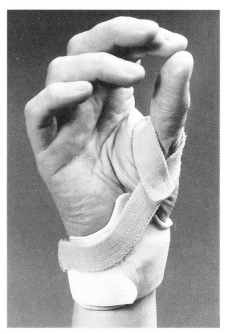

Figure 12.22 A simple dynamic thumb opposition splint with a static thermoplastic base. The elastic Velcro strap (stretch loop Velcro) draws the thumb into opposition. It can be adjusted by refastening on its hook Velcro attachment, which is distal to the wrist crease to prevent pulling the wrist into flexion. To give opposition, and not MCP flexion, the thumb loop must sit proximal to the MCP joint.

Ulnar nerve palsy

The objectives are to:

- prevent MCP hyperextension
- facilitate IP extension
- prevent clawing deformity and contractures.

Options include:

1. A dynamic ulnar nerve palsy splint, 'Chessington' type (after the design originating from the Royal Air Force Medical Rehabilitation Unit at Chessington and published by Wynn Parry, 1973). This provides very precise fit and accurate spring resistance. The spring-wire and coil construction incorporates pressure pads made from thermoplastic, or sheet aluminium covered with leather (Figure 12.23). An accurate pattern can be made directly on the patient by using a length of soldering wire (soft solder wire approximately 1.3 mm in diameter). This is easily formed and allows quick alterations, including the direction and position of the spring coils, before the splint is made up in the spring wire (steel spring wire/piano wire, approximately 1.0–1.3 mm, depending on the size and strength of the patient's hand). A simpler version of this splint has thermoplastic parts joined by a spring coil wire (Figures 12.24 and 12.25).

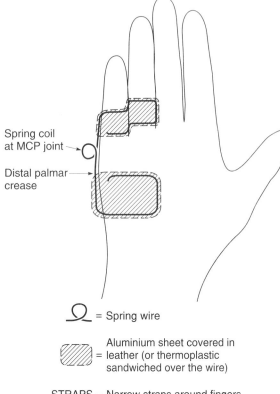

Spring coil at MCP joint

Distal palmar crease

$\mathcal{Q}$ = Spring wire

= Aluminium sheet covered in leather (or thermoplastic sandwiched over the wire)

STRAPS – Narrow straps around fingers and around metacarpals

Figure 12.23 Pattern for dynamic ulnar nerve palsy splint ('Chessington' type; after Wynn Parry, 1973).

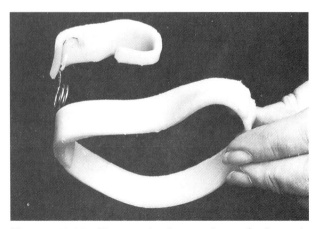

Figure 12.25 Thermoplastic version of dynamic ulnar nerve palsy splint, showing construction.

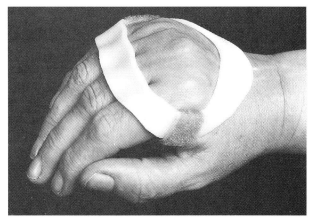

Figure 12.26 Static ulnar nerve palsy splint/MCP extension block, with Velcro palmar strap.

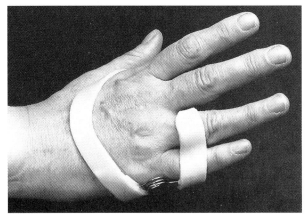

Figure 12.24 Thermoplastic version of the dynamic ulnar nerve palsy splint. This can be fabricated with a custom-made coil or with an Orfit knuckle bender coil spring (Orfit Industries).

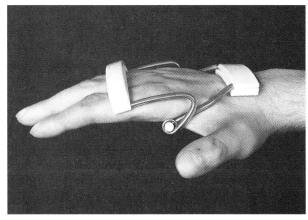

Figure 12.27 Dynamic Steeper knuckle duster splint (Steeper RSL) for ulnar nerve palsy. Suitable for the stronger hand and for heavy work conditions, where it can be worn over an industrial glove.

2. A static MCP block (Figure 12.26). This splint blocks extension of the MCP joints by setting the splint in 30–45° MCP flexion, which corrects clawing whilst allowing active flexion of the MCP joints. Unfortunately, because the splint does not move with the hand it can be difficult to achieve a perfect fit.

3. A Steeper knuckle duster (Figure 12.27). This is a ready-made dynamic splint with strong spring construction and foam-padded bars. It is easily adjustable, durable and particularly suitable for work, as it is usable at higher temperatures than are possible with regular thermoplastics (e.g. in hot water). It is well-suited to the powerful hand, as it has high resistance.

4. For loss of little finger abduction due to paralysis of the third palmar interosseous muscle, a small Velcro strap is added round the base of this finger to keep it in alignment with the ring finger.

5. An MCP flexion stretch splint (Figure 12.28) applies stretch by elastic traction to the ring and little finger MCP joints, or to all four fingers. It can be used in conjunction with any of the above splints to reduce extension contracture, which can occur in ulnar nerve palsy if mobilization has been neglected.

Combined median and ulnar nerve palsy

It is not easy to achieve a satisfactory splint that is both comfortable and effective. When correctly

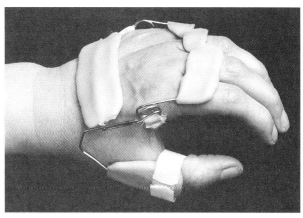

Figure 12.29 Dynamic spring wire splint for combined median/ulnar nerve palsy (after Wynn Parry, 1973).

fitted, the model described by Wynn Parry (1973) fulfils all the criteria (Figure 12.29), and it is efficient, contiguous to the hand, and durable. A splint made on the same principles enabled one of the author's patients to return to work as a laboratory technician. The patient had found it impossible to hold a pipette and glass containers, but by using the splint she could manage nearly all manual tasks and was able to return to work, where she continued to use the splint for over 6 months until the nerves recovered.

This splint is made in spring wire (piano wire), 1.25 mm in diameter for a lighter splint (for a small woman) and up to 1.6 mm in diameter for a heavier splint (for a large man). An accurate pattern (Figure 12.30) can be made directly on the patient's hand using soft soldering wire as described for the ulnar palsy splint, Chessington type. The three pressure pads on the metacarpals, fingers and thumb are of thermoplastic, which is sandwiched round the wire. For greater durability the pads can be fabricated from thin aluminium sheet, covered with fine leather. Drinks cans make a convenient aluminium sheet substitute. When fitted on the patient, narrow Velcro straps are attached across the palm and round the thumb, and the angulation of the wire is adjusted to give the required resistance and comfort.

Spring wire coils can be made with round-nosed pliers, but the use of a spring wire coil jig (Smith and Nephew) will greatly assist in producing an acceptable level of accuracy and cosmesis.

Radial nerve palsy

Radial nerve palsy is characterized by 'wrist drop', and the inability to open the hand and fingers prior to grasping an object. There is typically loss of extension at the wrist, the finger MCP joints and the thumb, although only a wrist extension deficit may

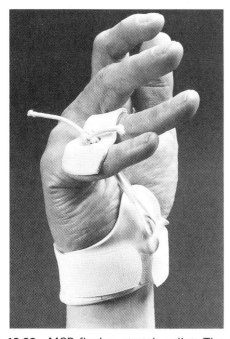

Figure 12.28 MCP flexion stretch splint. The elastic cord traction is adjusted simply by retying on the finger bar. To prevent the elastic pinching the finger web, it is covered with soft plastic tubing.

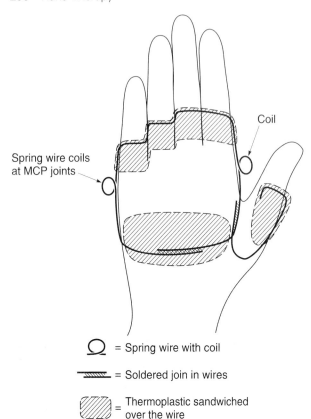

Spring wire coils
at MCP joints

Coil

$\bigcirc$ = Spring wire with coil

$\overline{}$ = Soldered join in wires

⬜ = Thermoplastic sandwiched over the wire

STRAPS – Narrow velcro straps across distal palmar crease and proximal phalanges

Figure 12.30 Pattern for combined ulnar/median nerve palsy splint (after Wynn Parry, 1973).

be present depending on the level of the lesion and on the stage of recovery. The type and design of splint is determined by assessment of the motor deficits and the suitability of the splint to minimize these deficits.

When splinting for loss of wrist extension alone, a static wrist extension splint may be the first choice for establishing a stable functional position of the wrist. A soft Neoprene splint will be suitable for an elderly or confused patient, or one who is at risk of pressure and skin damage from a more complex splint, and the more active patient will usually prefer a custom-moulded thermoplastic splint that firmly stabilizes the wrist during function.

Dynamic wrist extension splints can offer immediate 'normalization' of function. They fulfil the important aims of functional splinting listed above, and in so doing become rehabilitation tools in themselves.

In radial nerve palsy where there is wrist drop, it is particularly important to prevent overstretching of the denervated extensor muscles (Colditz, 1995d, 1987).

Choosing a radial nerve palsy splint

Radial nerve palsy splinting is a complex subject, and hand therapists frequently have difficulty in the selection of a suitable design. The author is most grateful to Dominique Thomas, who has kindly contributed the following text and illustrations on this complex subject.

Lively splints: the ultimate low-profile Since ancient times, therapists have tried to compensate for functional impairment resulting from radial palsy by splinting. By 1919 there were already 21 designs listed by Athanasio (cited by Nadeau, 1983), and since then many more models have been added. This profusion of designs leads to the presumption that the ideal splint does not exist.

Radial palsy splinting principles are well established:

1. Substitution of wrist extension during reach and wrist stabilization during pinch and grasp
2. Substitution of metacarpophalangeal extension
3. Eventual substitution of thumb extension.

A splint that fulfils all these functions, as proposed by Sutter, is complex, difficult to make and can be cumbersome. Many therapists therefore opt for simple wrist stabilization. Wrist stabilization by static splintage allows resisted grasp, but does not greatly improve reach and precision pinch.

Thus there are two approaches:

1. Wrist stabilization only
2. Substitution of wrist, MCP and thumb extension, plus wrist stabilization.

Six splint designs can be placed in the second group; the completely flexible 'Sutter' splint, the Oppenheimer, the Bryan Thomas, the Granger, the Chapel Hill, and the Radial Bis variation of the Chapel Hill design. However, the cumbersome Bryan Thomas, which is less used nowadays, will be excluded from the following descriptions.

The complete mobility 'Sutter' splint (Figure 12.31) was described by Sutter in the 1950s. This lively splint allows independent finger and wrist flexion and extension. Finger and wrist suspension cuffs are made from leather so that contact between the palmar skin and any object is virtually unimpaired. The wrist is not fully stabilized during heavily resisted activity. This beautifully physiological splint presents several disadvantages; manufacture is time-consuming and requires skills that most therapists do not possess.

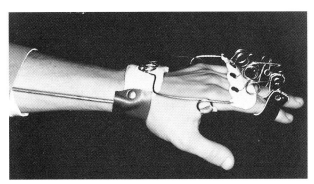

Figure 12.31 The Sutter complete mobility hand splint.

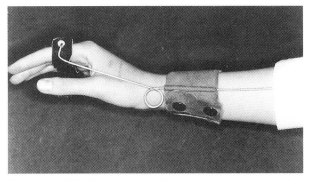

Figure 12.32 The revised Oppenheimer radial palsy splint. The fingers 'hang' from the dorsal bar.

The Oppenheimer splint is a classic lively splint. It has several disadvantages:

• the palmar bar in the original model is positioned on the palmar surface of the proximal phalanges, and gives only global, not independent, extension of the wrist and digits
• during prehension the bar creates an obstacle between the fingers and the seized object
• the bar prevents normal function of the transverse metacarpal arches
• finger flexion pushes the splint in a proximal direction
• it does not allow independent flexion of the wrist and fingers
• friction of the skin can occur from the lateral coils and the dorsal bar at the wrist
• fabrication of the coils in heavy-gauge spring wire, even with a proper jig, requires strength and skill.

The revised Oppenheimer (Figures 12.32 and 12.33) solves all the above disadvantages except for wire-bending, independence and wrist stabilization during heavy resistance. This splint becomes a realistic option when:

• the palmar bar is bent into a dorsal position above the proximal phalanges, and the digits are then suspended from the dorsal bar by leather slings
• the wire and the coils are separated from the wrist by a leather band glued onto a circular leather wrist cuff; the leather cuff, besides being comfortable, prevents the splint from slipping.

The Granger splint (Figure 12.34) was described by Crochetiere *et al.* in 1975. This elegant splint is identical to the revised Oppenheimer, except that the wire frame is static, not lively. It is made from plain (not spring) wire, and has

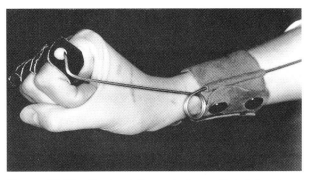

Figure 12.33 Revised Oppenheimer. Detail to show how the metal frame and coils are kept at a distance from the wrist by the leather cuff, and how grasp is controlled by this splint.

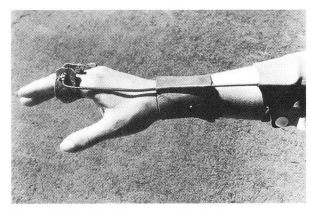

Figure 12.34 The Granger splint design.

no built-in coils. The Granger splint has been slightly modified by Romain *et al.* (1997) and Wilton (1997b). Finger extension results from releasing flexor muscle contraction. The weight of the hand then causes the finger slings to swivel under the dorsal bar, bringing the MCPs and wrist into extension. Because this splint design does not allow wrist flexion, the wrist is stabilized during heavily resisted activities.

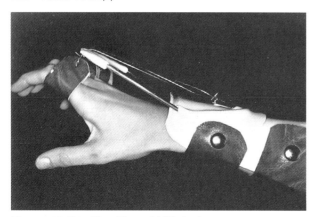

Figure 12.35 The Chapel Hill design.

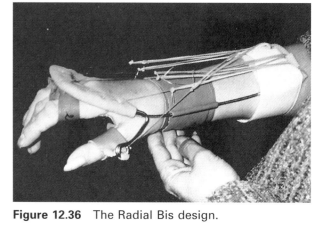

Figure 12.36 The Radial Bis design.

The Chapel Hill design (Figure 12.35) was described by Hollis in 1978, and differs from the Granger splint in that the finger cuffs are not attached directly to the dorsal bar but to adjustable static traction lines that pass over it. This bar is fixed to a thermoplastic forearm piece which, when not properly fitted, slips distally during finger flexion and the friction damages the dorsum of the wrist/forearm. It is easier to adjust than the Granger splint, but is more cumbersome for function. It does not allow independent movement of the wrist and fingers, and because it does not allow wrist flexion the wrist is stabilized during heavily resisted activity.

The Radial Bis design (Figure 12.36) was described by Thomas in 1990, and its static wire frame is identical to Granger's. The wrist is protected from frame contact by a leather cuff.

The individual finger and wrist traction is achieved by leather slings placed under the proximal phalanges at the level of the proximal finger creases and a separate sling at the distal palmar crease. A dynamic traction line that passes over the dorsal bar pulls each sling into extension, making individual digit and wrist extension and flexion possible.

To provide wrist stability during heavily resisted activities, wrist flexion excursion is limited by placing a stop on the wrist traction lines. This splint enables activities requiring precise individual finger movements.

Posterior interosseous nerve palsy In this particular form of radial palsy, as well as in certain patterns of reinnervation, wrist extension is preserved or returns before finger extension. A hand-based lively splint made out of piano (spring) wire, enabling individual

finger and thumb and thumb extension and flexion, appears to be the most user-friendly, efficient and reliable design.

Which design of radial palsy splint is best? There is no unequivocal or simple solution to radial nerve palsy splinting. Application depends on two factors; the patient's needs and the therapist's skill/available technical assistance.

A manual labourer who needs mass extension and flexion of the digits and wrist stabilization might be the right candidate or at least a reasonable indication for a Granger type of splint. A person whose activity requires mass finger/wrist flexion and extension and less wrist stabilization will be better fitted with a revised Oppenheimer splint, while someone who requires fine, skilled, individual finger function will prefer the Radial Bis design as demonstrated by Thomas in 1992.

A therapist who cannot master wire and coil bending will be more at ease with making a Chapel Hill splint, whilst a more skilled practitioner will be able to make the more user-friendly revised Oppenheimer or Radial Bis designs.

Recovery stage splinting of peripheral nerve palsies Dynamic splintage must not prevent any reinnervated, recovering muscle from regaining its power. Because the splint has been designed to substitute muscle action, it will, at the recovery stage, be preventing its full use. The resistance of the splint can be reduced by remaking the splint in narrower gauge wire, or the original splint can be worn for gradually decreasing periods of time.

RETURN TO EMPLOYMENT

If the patient can safely return to work or to lighter employment, this greatly reduces the adverse effects of injury and loss of function. Any splint must be adapted to this end; washable or coated thermoplastic, high-durability materials, non-rusting (stainless) steel wire and aluminium sheet covered in leather are all appropriate if they restore independence.

PATIENT EDUCATION AND COMPLIANCE

As nerve palsies often require long and tedious treatment of many months' duration, the patient must be carefully educated to appreciate the necessity and benefits of splinting and all aspects of coping with a nerve lesion. Many patients need choice in their splinting requirements and different splints for different activities; for example, a 'dirty', tough splint for work and a 'clean', cosmetic splint for home and leisure.

Patient education must be reinforced by support. This means regular and open appointments and access to the therapist, especially during the difficult 'plateau' periods. Treatment should not be terminated if the patient prefers not to wear a splint. Non-use of a splint should not necessarily be seen as non-compliance, and the patient should not be persecuted for preferring to be free from such encumbrance (does the therapist always wear gloves for washing dishes?). Treatment sessions should continue, or perhaps be increased, to ensure proper client-centred care and to give psychological support to a patient who may be finding recovery or disability difficult to cope with (see Chapter 3, p. 66)

BRACHIAL PLEXUS LESIONS

Splintage for brachial plexus lesions is highly specialized and should, when possible, be undertaken by the hand therapist as part of a dedicated treatment team that includes bioengineers and orthotists in a specialist unit (see Chapter 8).

DUPUYTREN'S DISEASE

Splinting has been found to have little effect on Dupuytren's contractures themselves, though there is evidence to show that it can retard concomitant contractures in surrounding soft tissues and joints. Extension splints are almost always used post-operatively.

The aims of post-operative splinting are to:

- maintain or regain extension of the hand by ensuring that all healing and scar tissues are kept at maximum length
- prevent any contracture of scar tissue, particularly into a flexed position
- correct or maintain the surgical release of any joint contractures
- reduce hypertrophic scarring.

The post-operative thermoplastic splint is fitted to the volar surface of the hand to include the palm and the fingers, and extends from the wrist crease to the fingertips. It may include all four fingers and the thumb, or one digit alone, provided that splint rigidity is not compromised. Care must be taken that all areas subject to scar tissue formation, both in the skin and deeper within the palm, are included and held in sufficient extension. Therefore, the extent of the fasciectomy or fasciotomy must dictate the extent of the splint, as this may well be greater than the evident area of the surface wound. A distressing outcome is a palmar contracture that has been allowed by too small a splint.

In some hand surgery units dorsal splinting is used, particularly for open wound (open palm) techniques.

Immediate post-operative regimen

One to seven days post-operatively, the bulky outer dressings are removed unless they are needed to absorb bleeding. Sterile dressings are kept in place or renewed. A volar thermoplastic splint (Figure 12.37) is moulded closely to the palm and fingers, and as the splint hardens the maximum passive extension is held. The splint edges are trimmed or

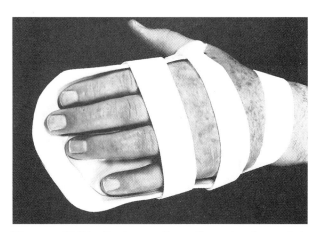

Figure 12.37 Post-operative Dupuytren's splint, moulded to the palm with fingers in maximum extension.

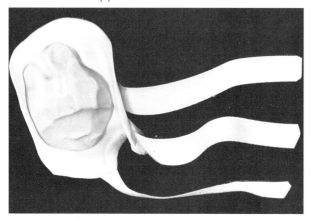

Figure 12.38 Post-operative Dupuytren's splint showing moulded Otoform silicone lining for scar therapy.

lipped to allow free movement of unaffected areas, especially of the thumb and wrist. Firm strapping is essential to hold the positioning, and a pressure strap lined with semi-rigid foam can be fitted across the proximal phalanges to keep the IP joints extended.

For the first 3–7 days the splint is worn continuously day and night, with frequent removal for mobilization exercises. Thereafter it is worn at night only for 4–6 months. The duration of splinting is dictated by the scar tissue – that is, the length of time needed for the scar to become mature and non-contractile.

At 4 months post-surgery the splint is discontinued for 2 nights, and if no further flexion occurs the splint can be discarded. Any tendency to contracture requires continued splint use.

If IP joint flexion contractures cannot be fully controlled by this splint combined with mobilization, then individual dynamic and/or static splinting must be used during the day and should commence as soon as the wound is healed.

Contracture or thickening of scar tissue following Dupuytren's surgery is a common occurrence, and it is therefore wise to apply silicone as soon as the wounds have fully closed. Either silicone moulding compound (Otoform) or silicone gel can be used. Moulding compound may be preferable to gel, as it gives complete contact to any pitted areas of the scar; it is also considerably cheaper (about £2/US$3.50 per application in 1999) and very durable. It is moulded to the patient's skin to fully cover the scar area. The splint is fitted over the silicone (Figure 12.38), and pressure is applied to ensure close contact and to expel any air bubbles until the silicone is set. The silicone can be anchored to the splint by punching holes in the plastic so the soft silicone can form 'rivets'. The silicone also is used until the scar has matured.

FRACTURES

Plaster of Paris or other cast methods are commonly preferred, but thermoplastics are needed if:

- normal or partial range of movement at adjacent joints is needed whilst also stabilizing the fracture site
- a lighter, more durable, splint is needed
- the splint is to be removed for exercise, or only used for night or protective wear
- skeletal pins need to be accommodated or covered
- extension block splinting is chosen for an intra-articular fracture
- specialized traction or controlled range and resistance devices are needed, e.g. distraction or active traction splinting for intra-articular fractures.

If thermoplastic splinting is used immediately post-operatively it is best applied to the volar aspect of the hand for stability and comfort, but dorsal splinting may be necessary to allow exercise. As swelling subsides, it is important to remould the splint to ensure an accurate fit. A combination of splints may be used to reduce IP stiffness (e.g. a dynamic Capener day splint and a static night splint).

Distraction, dynamic traction, or active traction splinting is often the preferred choice for fractures within (or close to) a digital joint. Traction is applied to the fracture in such a way that movement at the involved joint can occur simultaneously with the traction. Thus bony union and joint range do not compromise each other and, most importantly, healing of cartilage is enhanced in the presence of sufficient synovial fluid activity, which is in turn dependent on joint movement (Schenck, 1994, 1997). This is achieved either by an arctuate outrigger splint (Schenck, 1994), or preferably by a less cumbersome dynamic traction splint (Dennys et al., 1992) or active traction splint (Murray and McIntyre, 1995). Other types of splinting on similar principles include the Suzuki frame (Suzuki et al., 1994), which is not fixed to a hand or forearm-based splint and is therefore particularly acceptable to the patient.

A skeletal pin is inserted distal to the fracture and elastic traction is applied to this on both sides of the finger. The design of the splint allows traction to be maintained as the finger joint is moved into flexion or extension. The splint is applied within hours post-fracture, and is worn continuously for approximately 4 weeks. Some patients find this type of splinting too difficult to tolerate either physically or psychologically, although others are intrigued and enthusiastic. Multidisciplinary support and education and frequent appointments are essential to success and to avoidance of complications.

REFERENCES

Barr, N. R. (1975). *The Hand. Principles and Techniques of Simple Splintmaking in Rehabilitation.* Butterworths.

Bell-Krotoski, J. A. (1995). Plaster cylinder casting for contractures of the interphalangeal joints. In: *Rehabilitation of the Hand*, 3rd edn (J. M. Hunter, E. J. Mackin and A. D. Callahan, eds), pp. 1609–16. C. V. Mosby.

Boscheinen-Morrin, J., Davey, V. and Conolly, W. B. (1992). Introduction. In: *The Hand. Fundamentals of Therapy.* 2nd edn, pp. 3–5. Butterworth-Heinemann.

Boyes, J. H. (1964). *Bunnell's Surgery of the Hand*, 4th edn, p. 173. J. B. Lippincott.

Brand. P. W. and Thompson, D. E. (1992). Mechanical resistance. In: *Clinical Mechanics of the Hand*, 2nd edn (P. W. Brand and A. Hollister, eds), pp. 92–128. Mosby.

Brand, P. W. and Hollister, A. (1993). *Clinical Mechanics of the Hand.* 2nd edn. Mosby.

Brand, P. W. (1995a). The forces of dynamic splinting: ten questions before applying a dynamic splint to the hand. In: *Rehabilitation of the Hand*, 3rd edn (J. M. Hunter, E. J. Mackin and A. D. Callahan, eds), pp. 1581–7. C. V. Mosby.

Brand, P. W. (1995b). Mechanical factors in joint stiffness and tissue growth. *J. Hand Ther.*, 8, 91–3.

Colditz, J. C. (1987). Splinting for radial nerve palsy. *J. Hand Ther.*, 1, 18–23.

Colditz, J. C. (1995a). Therapist's management of the stiff hand. In: *Rehabilitation of the Hand*, 3rd edn (J. M. Hunter, E. J. Mackin and A. D. Callahan, eds), pp. 1141–59. C. V. Mosby.

Colditz, J. C. (1995b). Spring-wire extension splinting of the proximal interphalangeal joint. In: *Rehabilitation of the Hand*, 3rd edn (J. M. Hunter, E. J. Mackin and A. D. Callahan, eds), pp. 1617–29. C. V. Mosby.

Colditz, J. C. (1995c). Anatomic considerations for splinting the thumb. In: *Rehabilitation of the Hand*, 3rd edn (J. M. Hunter, E. J. Mackin and A. D. Callahan, eds), pp. 1161–72. C. V. Mosby.

Colditz, J. C. (1995d). Splinting the hand with a peripheral nerve injury. In: *Rehabilitation of the Hand*, 3rd edn (J. M. Hunter, E. J. Mackin and A. D. Callahan, eds), pp. 679–92. C. V. Mosby.

Crochetiere, W., Goldstein, S., Granger, C. V. and Ireland, J. (1975). The 'Granger' orthosis for radial nerve palsy. *Orthot. Prosthet.*, 29, 27–31.

Dennys, L. J., Hurst, N. H. and Cox, J. (1992). Management of proximal interphalangeal joint fractures using a new dynamic traction splint and early active movement. *J. Hand Ther.*, 1, 16–23.

Dival, T. A. (1997). Resources, materials and methods. In: *Hand Splinting. Principles of Design and Fabrication* (J. C. Wilton, ed.), pp. 43–4. W. B. Saunders.

Dival, T. A. and Wilton, J. C. (1997). Biomechanical principles of design, fabrication and application. In: *Hand Splinting. Principles of Design and Fabrication* (J. C. Wilton, ed.), pp. 22–42. W. B. Saunders.

Falkenstein, N. and Weiss-Lennard, S. (1999). Cumulative trauma. In: *Hand Rehabilitation. A Quick Reference Guide and Review*, pp. 224–5. C. V. Mosby.

Fess, E. E. (1995). Principles and methods of splinting for mobilization of joints. In: *Rehabilitation of the Hand*, 3rd edn (J. M. Hunter, E. J. Mackin and A. D. Callahan, eds), pp. 1589–98. C. V. Mosby.

Flowers, K. R. and Michlovitz, S. L. (1988). Assessment and management of loss of motion in orthopaedic dysfunction. *Postgraduate Advances in Physical Therapy II–VIII.* American Physical Therapy Association.

Flowers, K. R. and La Stayo, P. (1994). Effect of total end range time on improving passive range of motion. *J. Hand Ther.*, 7, 150–57.

Hollis, I. (1978). Innovative splinting ideas. In: *Rehabilitation of the Hand*, 1st edn (J. M. Hunter, J. H. Schneider, E. J. Mackin, J. A. Bell, eds), p. 641. C. V. Mosby.

Kennedy, S. M., Peck, F. H. and Stone, J. T. H. (2000). The treatment of interphalangeal joint flexion contractures with reinforced Lycra finger-sleeves. *J. Hand Ther.*, 13(1), 52–5.

Lister, G. (1993). In: *The Hand: Diagnosis and Indications Reconstruction*, 3rd edn, pp. 238–9. Churchill Livingstone.

McGrouther, D. A. (1990). Factors influencing recovery. In: *Principles of Hand Surgery* (F. D. Burke, D. A. McGrouther and P. J. Churchill, eds), pp. 18–19.

Murray, K. A. and McIntyre, F. H. (1995). Active traction splinting for proximal interphalangeal joint injuries. *Ann. Plast. Surg.*, 35(1), 15–18.

Nadeau, G. (1983). Ortheses et paralysie radiale. *Rev. Readapt. Fonct. Prof. Soc.*, 10, 8–11.

Palmer, P. (1991). Introducing a new design of orthosis for applying serial stretch to the volar aspect of the hand and wrist. *Br. J. Hand Ther.*, 1(3), 7–8.

Prosser, R. (1995). Splinting in the management of proximal interphalangeal joint flexion contracture. *Aust. J. Physiother.*, 41(1), 53–7. (This article was also published in 1996 in *J. Hand Ther.*, 9, 387–86.)

Romain, M., Durand, P.-A., Rouget, E. and Pellegrin, R. (1997). Orthese de tenodese dans la paralysie radiale. Presented at the XXXIII Meeting of the French Society for Surgery of the Hand, Paris, 11 December, 1997.

Schenck, R. R. (1994). The dynamic traction method. Combining movement and traction for intra-articular fractures of the phalanges. *Hand Clin.*, 10(2), 187–97.

Schenck, R. R. (1997). Advances in reconstruction of digital joints. *Clin. Plast. Surg.*, 24(1), 175–88.

Suzuki, Y., Matsunaga, T., Sato, S. and Yokoi, T. (1994). The pins and rubber traction system for treatment of comminuted intra-articular fractures and fracture-dislocations in the hand. *J. Hand Surg.*, 19B(1), 98–107.

Thomas, D. (1990). L'Attelle Radiale Bis. *Ann. Kinesither.*, 17(5), 271–4.

Thomas, D. (1992). Etude comparative de deux attelles de paralysies radiales. *Ann. Kinesither.*, 19(3), 148–51.

Thomas, D. (1996). Physiotherapy and rehabilitation of upper extremity reflex sympathetic dystrophy. *Baillière's Clin. Orthopaed.*, 1(2), 339–58.

Tubiana, R., Thomine, J.-M. and Mackin, E. (1996). *Examination of the Hand and Wrist*, 2nd edn, pp. 364–5. Martin Dunitz.

Van Lede, P. and van Veldhoven, G. (1998). *Therapeutic Hand Splints. A Rational Approach.* Provan bvba.

Wilton, J. C. (1997a). Splinting to address the thumb. In: *Hand Splinting. Principles of Design and Fabrication* (J. C. Wilton, ed.), pp. 159–60. W. B. Saunders.

Wilton, J. C. (1997b). Splinting to address the wrist and hand. In: *Hand Splinting. Principles of Design and Fabrication* (J. C. Wilton, ed.), pp. 106–9. W. B. Saunders.

Wynn Parry, C. B. (1973). Peripheral nerve injuries. In: *Rehabilitation of the Hand*, 3rd edn, pp. 90–101. Butterworths.

FURTHER READING

Bain, G. I. and Janak, A. M. (1998).The proximal interphalangeal joint: surgical and mobilisation options. *Br. J. Hand Ther.*, **3(4),** 13–18.

Capener, N. (1956) The hand in surgery. *J. Bone Joint Surg.*, **38B(1),** 28–151.

Capener, N. (1967). Lively splints. *Physiotherapy*, **53,** 371.

Malick, M. H. (1972). *Manual on Static Hand Splinting.* Harmarville Rehabilitation Center, Pittsburgh.

Malick, M. H. (1974). *Manual on Dynamic Hand Splinting with Thermoplastic Materials.* Harmarville Rehabilitation Center, Pittsburgh.

Malick, H. M. and Carr, A. C. (1982). *Manual on Management of the Burn Patient.* Harmarville Rehabilitation Center, Pittsburgh.

CD ROM

Colditz, J. C. and McGrouther, D. A. (1998). *The Interactive Hand.* Therapy Edition. Primal Pictures Ltd., 4th floor, 16–18 Ramillies Street, London W1V 1DL.

Section 2

13 Rheumatoid arthritis and its effects on the hand

Ann Birch and Lynda Gwilliam

THE DISEASE

Although hand structures are frequently affected by the rheumatic diseases, these effects cannot be viewed in isolation. The therapist who undertakes treatment of the hand must therefore not only have detailed knowledge of the anatomy of this structure and how rheumatic disease can affect it, but also a proper understanding of the systemic manifestations of the disease, and must take into account the multitude of problems, physical, psychological and social, that the sufferer may be experiencing.

Rheumatoid arthritis is the commonest of the connective tissue disorders, and is really an inflammatory synovitis rather than an arthritis. This is a chronic, inflammatory, systemic disease that affects synovial joints, but is often associated with extra-articular features. Swanson (1990) states that:

> the most widely accepted theory of the pathogenesis of Rheumatoid Arthritis is that of an immunological response taking place in the synovial tissues . . . this inflammatory synovium forms a pannus, a granulomatous mass, which grows over the surface of the cartilage, into and around the tendons and into the ligament attachments. If unchecked, this invasion results in loosening of ligaments, destruction of joint surfaces and disability of tendons to function, all of which are typical of the advanced rheumatoid process. Every derangement or deformity of the musculoskeletal system seen in rheumatoid arthritis is the result either primarily or secondarily of this synovial invasion.

However, the disease is not confined to joints. During its course, many features may occur that affect extra-articular tissues and organs. The patient with severe disease is often unwell, with weight loss, lassitude and sometimes low-grade pyrexia; involvement of the lungs, heart, spleen, blood vessels, eyes and other soft tissue structures is not uncommon, especially in those patients who have a strongly positive rheumatoid factor.

Rheumatology is an important medical, surgical and therapeutic speciality, if only because rheumatic diseases afflict many individuals, frequently in the prime of life, and thus it imposes a considerable financial and social burden on the community and an enormous amount of personal suffering on the individual. Although patients with rheumatoid arthritis account for only 5–10 per cent of all patients with rheumatic disease, the severity and progressive nature of the disease ensures that they demand a disproportionate share of health care services. Since most rheumatic diseases are of a chronic nature and often involve many joints and extra-articular organs, the importance of a team approach in their management is obvious. The rheumatologist provides the continuity in management, but the team should also include a specialist nurse, an occupational therapist and a physiotherapist, a social worker, a clinical psychologist and an orthopaedic surgeon who has a special interest in rheumatoid arthritis. At different times these team members will become involved in the patient's management and rehabilitation to a greater or lesser extent. This multidisciplinary approach should be maintained through regular clinical meetings, ward rounds, combined medical and surgical clinics, and case conferences for those patients who present particular difficulties of management or rehabilitation.

Prevalence

Rheumatoid arthritis affects about 5 per cent of British women and 2 per cent of British men, the peak incidence for disease onset being from 35–55 years in women and 40–60 years in men. The reason for its predilection for women is not known. There is a genetic influence in the development of the disease in that it is more prevalent in first degree relatives, but the hereditary load is small.

Onset

The onset of this disease may be slowly progressive over several months, or it may be very acute. The patient may be able to date the onset from an infection or traumatic incident, or from childbirth. These may well be precipitating factors, or they may simply focus the attention on pre-existing disease.

The patient with *insidious onset* rheumatoid arthritis may present with:

- loss of appetite and weight
- anaemia
- pain in one or more joints
- stiffness – particularly in the mornings or following periods of inactivity.

As the disease progresses more and more joints become involved, with inflammation, pain, swelling and loss of function that may appear out of proportion to joint involvement. The small joints of the hand, particularly the metacarpophalangeal joints (MCP) and the wrist joints, are frequently involved, as are the tendon mechanisms. It is unusual for the proximal interphalangeal joints (PIP) to be a primary target of synovial invasion in sero-positive rheumatoid arthritis; this is usually more characteristic of psoriatic arthritis, sero-negative juvenile arthritis and gout.

The patient with *acute onset* disease may present with multiple joint involvement from the very beginning, with swollen, acutely inflamed joints leading very rapidly to loss of function. The constitutional symptoms may also be present.

Clinical course

The disease can be arbitrarily divided into three phases; acute, sub-acute and chronic.

1. In the acute phase there is acute pain and swelling with 'hot joints', and the patient often feels unwell.
2. In the sub-acute phase there is chronic synovitis and deformities are developing. The patient suffers acute 'flare-ups' from time to time.
3. In the chronic phase the disease activity is 'burnt-out' and there are fixed deformities.

TREATMENT

Since there is no cure for this disease, treatment is directed towards minimizing the effects on a given individual. The evaluation and treatment must be an ongoing process due to the changing and progressive nature of the disease. The diagnosis of rheumatoid arthritis brings with it an inevitable decrease in function as a result of pain, joint and tendon involvement and systemic manifestations. The ultimate goal of all treatments is to minimize functional impairment for as long as possible. To this end, treatment can be divided into medical, therapeutic, and surgical.

Medical management

This takes the form of rest and medication.

Rest

Rest often forms an initial part of the treatment, particularly if joints are acutely inflamed. Characteristically, the inflamed joint is painful and this pain is increased by movement, so resting the joint is frequently a useful measure as it produces symptomatic relief. The patient will often adopt a position that predisposes to deformity in which to rest the inflamed joint; great care must therefore be taken during periods of complete or partial bed rest to avoid these deforming positions. Often bed rest is best administered in the hospital environment, where it can be regulated in keep-

ing with the local and systemic manifestations of the disease.

Medication

The two major considerations in the drug therapy of most rheumatic diseases are the relief of pain and the reduction of inflammation. The drugs used range from simple analgesics and non-steroidal anti-inflammatory drugs known as *first line*, which have a local effect on inflammation, through to the suppressing agents known as *second line*, such as gold, cytotoxins, antimalarials and immunosuppressants. Steroids still remain a very effective way of reducing active inflammation, and are commonly given intra-articularly for an acutely inflamed joint, and used systematically in severe disease. In the future there may be new treatments, some of which are currently under investigation. One such treatment is immunotherapy. Immunotherapy is a means of treating patients using targeted antibodies against components of the immunological system.

Therapeutic management

The therapist has a major role in achieving the overall goal of treatment for the patient with rheumatoid arthritis.

Treatment is aimed at:

1. Relieving pain
2. Maintaining/increasing joint mobility
3. Maintaining/increasing muscle strength and endurance
4. Prevention of deformity
5. Assisting with the emotional adjustment to disability
6. Educating the patient about the condition
7. Maintaining/increasing functional abilities
8. Supporting the patient in the community.

Surgical management

Before undertaking the care of a patient with a systemic disease such as rheumatoid arthritis, the surgeon should liaise closely with the rheumatologist and anaesthetist. This will ensure the best care for the patient, who frequently requires continued medical management and can pose an anaesthetic risk.

The goals of surgery are:

1. To relieve pain
2. To improve function
3. To prevent further deterioration.

The mere existence of deformity is not for many patients an indication for surgery. Many individuals with severe deformities continue to function at a level acceptable to them and experience no pain.

Indications for surgery

The indications for surgery include:

1. *Pain*
   - as a result of inflammation in joints and tendon mechanisms, which have not responded to adequate medical/therapeutic management
   - as a result of mechanical problems in and around the joints, i.e. secondary degenerative changes/instability etc.
2. *Loss of function.* All patients with rheumatoid arthritis have loss of function, which results from pain, stiffness, instability and/or deformity. For the patient with multiple joint problems it is crucial to identify which of the main affected joints is contributing most to the functional deficit and why.
3. *Prevention of deterioration*
   - the destructive effects of persistent synovitis are all too easy to see in the majority of patients, and synovectomy as a surgical procedure is indicated when the medical/therapeutic management fails to halt the cycle of synovitis > destruction > instability > deformity > synovitis
   - once there is an established instability or subluxation the deformity is progressive and time/effort related, stabilization procedures such as radio-lunate arthrodesis are specifically aimed at halting this progressive deterioration.

A more subtle effect of surgery is the joint protection programme, which is enforced during the postoperative phase when the motivation to 'look after' the 'new' hand is most powerful.

Procedures frequently performed include:

1. Synovectomy of joints and tendon mechanisms
2. Soft tissue reconstructions
3. Joint arthroplasties
4. Joint arthrodeses.

EFFECTS ON THE HAND

The hand as an organ is capable of both great strength and precise manipulation. Joints, tendons and nerves are dependent on each other's integrity to achieve this level of complex activity. The effects of rheumatoid arthritis can be seen very clearly in the hand, affecting as it does joints, tendons and peripheral nerves. Destruction of a joint and/or invasion of tendon/nerve substance by proliferative synovitis can have a devastating effect on the ability of the hand to carry out its multiplicity of functions.

Joint deformities

The development of specific deformities in the wrist and hand is a very complex process. Since the joints are so intimately related in both structure and function, destruction and deformity in one will inevitably have a 'knock-on' effect on the others. This influence is most likely to be from proximal to distal. The shoulder and elbow are frequently damaged by the disease and the pain, and restriction in movement resulting from this will compound the effects of any hand deformities. Also, if one hand is more affected, the less disabled hand will be subject to additional function and mechanical stresses.

The wrist

For certain patients deformity can be almost exclusively confined to the wrist and distal radio-ulnar joints, with the hand joints being left largely unaffected. In these patients the problem at the wrist joint is most likely to be erosion of the joint surfaces, producing fusion or fibrosis in both the radiocarpal and intercarpal joints. This tends, of course, to lead to stiffness and pain, and in this way it inhibits hand function even though hand deformity may be minimal. Although this may be a disabling condition, it remains confined to the wrist joint and does not lead to secondary deformities in the hand. In other patients the whole carpus shifts in an ulnar direction on the radius, which can happen without much destruction at the intercarpal joints. This deformity will lead to radial deviation of the metacarpus, thus encouraging ulnar deviation of the fingers in order to compensate and maintain the relationship between wrist and hand.

A third common scenario is one where the volar radiocarpal ligament is disrupted, resulting in volar subluxation of the hand on the forearm. Functionally this is a very disabling deformity as the resulting instability robs the hand of its power. This deformity predisposes to extensor tendon rupture. In very severe wrist destruction it is possible for the wrist to completely dislocate in an ulnar direction, leaving the hand virtually at right angles to the forearm.

The distal radio-ulnar joint

The distal radio-ulnar joint (DRUJ) plays a vital part in hand function, allowing the forearm to rotate and the hand to be placed in the variety of positions that are needed for sophisticated function.

There are two main ways in which it is affected:

1. The collapse of the DRUJ ligaments allows dislocation of the ulnar head dorsally.
2. The extensor carpi ulnaris (ECU) may slide in a palmar direction, allowing the hand to supinate on the forearm and thus exaggerating the prominence of the ulnar head.

The resulting tension on the extensors to the ring and little fingers, coupled with destructive synovitis, puts these tendons at risk of rupture.

Metacarpophalangeal joints
The combination of movements possible at these joints, i.e. flexion, extension, radial and ulnar deviation and rotation, coupled with the complexity of the muscular system surrounding them, makes them vulnerable to deformity when ligamentous structures are weakened by rheumatoid disease.

Volar subluxation The powerful pull of the strong flexor muscles, when transmitted across the MCP joints in order to give strength to the grip, will result in volar subluxation of these joints since the periarticular structures have been weakened by synovitis. This in turn causes the effective lengthening of the long flexors of the fingers, which diminishes their power. Since the extensor mechanism is also weakened by synovitis, this subluxation can proceed to full dislocation, making it impossible to open the hand. This results in a fixed flexion deformity, which often proves more disabling than the more widely recognized ulnar deviation.

Ulnar deviation The factors producing ulnar deviation are numerous. The normal anatomy predisposes the MCP joints to move in an ulnar direction when a strong grip is applied. Under normal circumstances the radial collateral ligaments act as a check to excessive movement, but when these become weakened by the disease process the forces cause excessive mobility. The weakening of the attachments of the extensor expansion allow the extensor tendons to be dislocated into the groove on the ulnar side of each metacarpal head. This in turn leads to more force being applied in an ulnar direction. Laxity of the pulleys supporting the flexor tendons has a corresponding effect, allowing the flexor tendons to pull in an ulnar direction. Once the deformity is established, every use of the hand serves to reinforce and worsen it. In the worst cases the volar subluxation and ulnar deviation deformities coexist, leading to gross loss of function.

The proximal interphalangeal joints
There are two collapse deformities of the finger that are initiated at the PIP joints; the *swan-neck* deformity and the *boutonni'ere* deformity. The one that inhibits function the most, if it is allowed to progress and become fixed, is the swan-neck deformity.

Swan-neck deformity Swanson (1990) gives a very full and comprehensive description of this deformity:

This deformity is usually caused in rheumatoid arthritis, by synovitis of the flexor tendon sheaths, which results in restriction of interphalangeal joint flexion. Flexor power becomes concentrated in the MCP joint and in this position intrinsic muscle pull on the central tendon is facilitated, resulting in unbalancing of forces to the extensor aspect of the joint. Hyperextension of the middle phalanx on the proximal phalanx occurs . . ... As the hyperextension deformity is increased, the transverse fibres of the retinacular ligament are stretched out, allowing the lateral tendons to sublux dorsally, which further magnifies the deforming power through its extensor pull, now located above the centre of the axis of rotation of the joint. The oblique retinacular ligaments are stretched, a relative lengthening of the lateral tendons occurs, and the DIP joint becomes flexed by the pull of the flexor profundus tendon.

Because of the effect of the flexor tendons now exerted at the MCP joints, a pre-existing swan-neck deformity can exacerbate volar subluxation at the MCP joints, and *vice versa*.

The combination of these two deformities renders the hand almost useless, as the patient is neither able to open the hand fully nor to make a fist.

Boutonnière deformity The boutonnière deformity is the opposite collapse deformity at the PIP joint, resulting in flexion of the PIP joint and hyperextension of the DIP joint. The central tendon is lengthened by bulging synovium, and the lateral bands tend to slide forwards in front of the the axis of the joint and are no longer able to contribute to the extension of the PIP joint. Any attempt at active extension results in hyperextension at the DIP joint.

Not all of the patients who have involvement of the PIP joint develop collapse deformities; synovitis and bony erosion can lead to either stiffness or ligamentous instability, which is confined to the PIP joint.

Distal interphalangeal joints
The DIP joint is of course affected in the collapse deformities of the PIP joint as described above. Individual deformity of the DIP joint is not very common in sero-positive rheumatoid arthritis, although it is sometimes seen. However, it is more commonly affected in sero-negative arthritis, juvenile arthritis, psoriatic arthritis and gout, where the erosive changes make the joint very unstable. Destruction of the distal attachment of the extensor tendon can also occur, leading to a mallet finger deformity. With time, a neglected mallet finger deformity always results in a swan-neck deformity. This is the reverse process of that described by Swanson above.

The thumb
The thumb contributes between 40 per cent and 50 per cent of hand function because of its ability to

oppose to the other fingers. It is a three-joint unit, and deformity at one joint very often leads to problems at the adjacent joint or joints. For the thumb to function adequately, there are certain qualities that must be present:

1. *Absence of pain.* Pain inhibits any power activities.
2. *Sensation.* To carry out fine manipulative tasks, sensation in the thumb is vital. The threat to sensation is carpal tunnel syndrome, and this must be treated as a priority if permanent loss of sensation is to be avoided.
3. *Stability.* The disease process can lead to distension of joints and invasion of ligaments by synovium. This will ultimately lead to joint destruction and instability.
4. *Control.* The thumb is controlled by four long tendons and the intrinsic thenar muscle. Control can be lost either by rupture of the tendons or by loss of nerve supply. The long tendons are the extensor pollicis longus, extensor pollicis brevis, abductor pollicis longus and flexor pollicis longus. The abductor pollicis longus is rarely affected by the disease, but the other three are frequently involved and their absence obviously leads to imbalanced movement of the thumb. The thenar muscles are supplied in the main by the median nerve, and are therefore at risk of weakness or paralysis in severe carpal tunnel syndrome.
5. *Adequate length.* In a certain type of arthritis, the so called 'arthritis mutilans', bone is reabsorbed and the digits are considerably shortened. This is particularly disabling in the case of the thumb, because it becomes too short to oppose to the other fingers.
6. *Mobility.* In order to oppose the thumb to the fingers, and abduct and extend it to pick up objects, there must be adequate movement in the three thumb joints. Function can be more or less maintained if either the MCP joint or the PIP joint is stiff, but lack of movement at the CMC joint always leads to loss of function.

As previously stated the thumb functions as a unit, which means that deformity in one of the three joints in some way affects the other two. There are two well-recognized patterns of deformity; boutonni'ere and swan-neck.

Boutonnière deformity The first is the so-called 'boutonnière deformity'. Although similar in appearance to the finger deformity of the same name, the mechanism is slightly different. The primary cause is synovitis of the MCP joint causing stretching of the extensor mechanism. The attachment of the extensor pollicis longus (EPL) is lengthened, and thus the ability to extend the MCP joint is diminished. The EPL and extensor insertions of the intrinsic muscles extend the distal joint,

eventually leading to hyperextension at this joint. If not corrected the destruction of the joint surfaces follows and the tissues become contracted, making the deformity fixed.

Swan-neck deformity The second of the combined deformities of the thumb is the so-called 'swan-neck deformity'. Once again it has a different mechanism from the deformity of the same name in the finger, and is usually initiated by synovitis of the CMC joint of the thumb. This leads to stretching of the joint capsule and subluxation of the base of the metacarpal on the trapezium. Abduction becomes painful and there is abduction spasm, which eventually leads to abductor contracture. The lack of movement at the metacarpal causes excess movement of the proximal phalanx at the MCP joint into extension in order to get the thumb out of the palm of the hand. This causes stretching of the volar plate and the MCP joint becomes hyperextended. These deformities, once established, are progressive and time/effort-related.

Tendon pathology

Extensor tendons
Preservation of extensor tendon function is a high therapeutic and surgical priority, since rupture results in substantial functional deficit.

Digital extensors Inability to extend the fingers can occasionally cause a diagnostic problem. It may be the result of the extensor tendons dislocating and 'slipping' in an ulnar direction off the metacarpal heads and losing the leverage necessary to extend the fingers. This happens when the MCP joints are involved in the disease process, but the combination of ruptured extensor tendons and ulnar drift is in fact uncommon.

Involvement of the extensor tendons in the disease process is often at the level of the wrist joint or on the back of the hand, and is frequently associated with wrist joint disease and deformity (Sterling, 1995). In particular, it is the supination of the carpus and involvement of the ulnar head that give rise to attrition rupture of the extensor tendons, whilst space-occupying synovitis on the dorsum of the wrist and hand will result in ischaemic rupture of the extensor tendons. Tendon ruptures are often progressive and frequently follow a set pattern – e.g. the extensor digiti minimi tendon is the first to rupture, followed by the common extensors to the little, ring and middle fingers. The common extensor to the index finger is often spared, as is also the extensor indices (Ryu, 1998). This is the most frequent pattern of rupture, but very occasionally the tendons to the ring and middle fingers rupture whilst the tendons to the index and little fingers remain intact.

Rupture of the digital extensor tendons results in the inability to actively extend the metacarpophalangeal joint, making it difficult to open the hand to grasp large objects or to let go after gripping.

Extensors of the thumb The commonest problem affecting the extensor tendons of the thumb in rheumatoid disease is rupture of the extensor pollicis longus. This tendon often ruptures early in the disease, during an inflammatory phase and before articular erosion has occurred. Frequently the cause of this is attrition of the tendon on Lister's tubercle on the dorsum of the radius; where it crosses this point the tendon is vulnerable because of the change in direction in its line of pull.

Rupture of the extensor pollicis longus results in the inability to actively extend the first metacarpal dorsal to the plane of the hand, although quite often the patient can still actively extend the interphalangeal joint of the thumb through the action of the intrinsic muscle. This is a subtle deformity, frequently hidden amongst complex thumb deformities, and is often overlooked until patients report that their hand is 'clumsy' and a careful examination is performed.

Flexor tendons

Involvement of the digital flexor tendons in the disease process can result in severe functional loss in the hand as a consequence of:

1. *Pain.* Active movement of the digits, particularly during periods of inflammation, causes pain, which inhibits full range of movement and power.
2. *Loss of tendon excursion.* This results from
   - synovial hypertrophy
   - tendon nodules, which will impede the movement of the tendon through the sheath and frequently result in the tendon becoming locked in either flexion or extension
   - tendon adhesions, resulting from repeated episodes of synovitis, forming between the tendon and the tendon sheath, and between flexor digitorum profundus (FDS) and flexor digitorum superficialis (FDS).
3. *Joint stiffness.* Since the tendons are incapable of full excursion, the interphalangeal joints become stiff because they are not maximizing the full range of movement possible in these joints. This is further compounded by the degenerative effects of the disease on the joints themselves.
4. *Tendon rupture.* Unresolved and untreated flexor tenosynovitis causes ischaemia of the tendons and ultimately results in rupture; there can be either single or multiple ruptures.
5. *Rupture in continuity.* Frequently tendon rupture in the rheumatoid hand is incomplete, and the tendons attempt to heal themselves. This healing causes lengthening of the tendon and so weakens the action of the flexor muscles, resulting in loss of power in the hand. Approximately 50 per cent of patients with the diagnosis of rheumatoid arthritis experience flexor tendon involvement of either a remittent or chronic nature (Wynn Parry, 1993).

During an *acute* episode of flexor tenosynovitis there is often pain in the palm of the hand, particularly at the level of the A1 pulley. This pain is made worse when digital flexion and grip are attempted. The effects of synovitis may be visible and palpable along the length of the tendon, and there may be a characteristic sound when finger flexion is initiated. Active range of movement at the interphalangeal joints may be limited because of the pain and swelling associated with synovitis, but passive range, in the absence of articular changes in the joint, is usually full. It is not unusual for the patient to report a significant reduction in hand function, with even self-care activities being difficult to perform.

During the *sub-acute* phase of the disease the effects of flexor tenosynovitis are not as obvious. As a result of loss of differential glide between the FDS and FDP, and also reduced excursion of the tendons within their sheath, there is usually a greater passive range of movement at the interphalangeal joints than there is active range (Stanley, 1992). There will almost certainly be a decrease in the functional capacity of the hand, particularly in those activities that involve grip and power. Pain may still be a feature, but it is not a significant one in the absence of acute flexor tenosynovitis. The integrity of the flexor tendons is essential to the normal biomechanics of the hand. When they are damaged by disease their action is changed, and they thus contribute to the development of two of the most disabling hand deformities; swan-neck deformity of the PIP joints and subluxation of the MCP joints.

The effects of *chronic* flexor tenosynovitis are not easily detectable, hidden as they often are amongst articular problems and deformities. Pain is rarely a feature and synovitis is difficult to detect, but the long-term legacy of tendon adhesions – loss of differential glide between the tendons, poor range of movement in the interphalangeal joint, possible tendon ruptures and greatly reduced hand function – can be found if sought.

Extra-articular manifestations of rheumatoid arthritis in the hand

Not all of the of the manifestations of rheumatic disease in the hand are confined to articular structures; some are extra-articular. Sturge (1984) summarized these as:

1. *Rheumatoid nodules.* The presence of nodules is important since they are of prognostic significance, often indicating sero-positive RA and

severe erosive disease. Their presence on the dorsal aspect of the hand gives rise to concerns about the appearance of the hand rather than loss of function or pain. However, on the volar surface of the hand nodules will result in discomfort and interfere with function, particularly if they are situated on the radial border of the index finger or pulp of the thumb.

2. *Vasculitis.* Ulceration and gangrene as a result of vasculitis are fortunately uncommon in the digits, but the more common nailfold and distal pulp space microinfarcts are seen in the digits with sero-positive RA. In themselves they cause few functional problems, but they can indicate that wound healing following injury or surgery may be problematic, and their presence is an indicator that any pressure or friction from a splint will be poorly tolerated by the skin.

3. *Raynaud's phenomenon.* This is more frequently seen in connective tissue diseases, particularly in systemic lupus and scleroderma. In severe cases the patient may develop peripheral ulceration resulting in amputation of a digit, but more commonly Raynaud's causes varying degrees of pain and loss of function, particularly in the winter months.

4. *Peripheral nerve involvement.* The sensory and motor loss associated with peripheral nerve involvement can have a marked affect on hand function, and it may also give rise to deformities as a result of muscle imbalance. The effects of peripheral nerve compression syndromes are frequently seen in the rheumatoid hand, notably from the ulnar nerve at the elbow or the median nerve in the carpal tunnel; it is not uncommon for the cervical spine to be the source of peripheral neuropathy. Cervical myelopathy associated with atlanto-axial or subaxial instability will result in what is often initially an unexplainable deterioration in hand function through loss of motor function and sensation. The nerve involvement may, however, be non-compressive in origin, as the nerve itself can be infiltrated by the disease process.

5. *Muscle wasting.* When joints are stiff and painful, their associated muscle groups will suffer from disuse atrophy. This may be the primary cause of loss of muscle bulk, but it can be compounded by the muscle wasting associated with motor branch nerve compression. There is also an inflammatory process that causes muscle fibre degeneration, this gives a clinical picture of reduced power and marked muscle wasting in the hand.

REFERENCES

Ryu, J., Saito, S., Honda, T. *et al.* (1998). Risk factors and prophylactic tenosynovectomy for extensor tendon ruptures in the rheumatoid hand. *J. Hand Surg.,* **23B(5)**, 658–61.

Stanley, J. K. (1992). Conservative survery in the management of rheumatoid disease of the hand and wrist. *J. Hand Surg.,* **17B**, 339–42.

Sterling, C. and Feldon, P. (1995) Extensor tendon ruptures in rheumatoid arthritis. *Hand Clinics,* **11(3)**. 449–59.

Swanson, A. B. (1990). Pathomechanics of deformities in hand and wrist. In: *Rehabilitation of the Hand* (J. M. Hunter, E. J. Mackin and A. D. Callahan, eds), pp. 891–902. C. V. Mosby.

Sturge, R. A. (1984). The remote effects of rheumatic diseases on the hand, and their management. In: *Clinics in Rheumatic Diseases,* (C. B. Wynn Parry, ed.) Vol. 10(3). pp. 479–77. W. B. Saunders.

Wynn Parry, C. B. and Stanley, J. K. (1993). Synovectomy of the hand. *Br. J. of Rheum.* **32**, 1089–95.

14 Conservative treatment of rheumatoid arthritis

Lynda Gwilliam

INTRODUCTION

Since rheumatoid arthritis is a lifelong, chronic, systemic disease, affecting multiple joints and organs, the evaluation and treatment of its effects must be an ongoing process that takes account not only of physical factors but also the social and psychological consequences of the disease. It is essential that sufferers have the benefit of a multi-disciplinary team approach (Ahlmen, 1988) directed towards the management of the disease, and that they are encouraged and empowered to have input into the decision-making processes that determine individual treatments (Roche and Klestov, 1995). Donovan (1991) has shown that involvement of the patient in their care enables short- and long-term treatment plans relevant to individual needs and personal beliefs to be formulated; this in turn improves compliance to the treatment plans suggested as well as outcomes.

Although hand structures are frequently affected, hand involvement cannot be viewed in isolation. Therapists who undertake the treatment of the rheumatoid hand must have a detailed knowledge of the anatomy of the hand and the effects of the disease on it, in addition to a proper understanding of the rheumatic disease. They must be able to take account of the multitude of disabling effects that coexist for the sufferer.

The changing nature and varied course of this disease dictates that the therapeutic emphasis will be different according to the stage of the disease and the patient's needs.

Acute phase

The early stages are often characterized by periods of acute disease activity, where medical management in the form of medication and rest is indicated to bring the disease under control. Avoiding positions of deformity and the development of contractures during bed rest is vital, as is support for inflamed joints. The hands, particularly the meta-carpophalangeal (MCP) joints and the wrists, are often affected early in the disease, and the provision of hand/wrist rest splints during this period is common practice (Chapter 16). It is essential that during this early phase the therapist endeavours to establish a communication network with the patient and build rapport. This is an appropriate time to explain the multidisciplinary team approach to the management of rheumatoid arthritis. It is vital, even at this very early stage, to encourage the patient into this partnership, to give them the opportunity to discuss and learn about how the disease affects them and what they, and the therapeutic team, can do about it. Education close to the time of onset or diagnosis has been shown to be beneficial in preventing anxiety and increasing compliance (Tucker and Kirwan, 1991). There is much to be said for early admission to hospital (Vliet Vieland *et al.*, 1996). Alternatively, providing the patient with immediate and easy access to the therapeutic team on an outpatient basis is appropriate so that participation in education programmes and the opportunity to discuss fears, emotions and difficulties can be initiated. Early intervention is currently seen as the key to preventing disability and enabling patients to manage their disease more effectively themselves (Emery, 1994). The therapeutic team should not take control of the patient's illness and life. There is evidence to suggest that disability progression is more influenced by psychological factors than by physical, and that many symptoms of the advanced stages of the disease are the result of insufficient 'digestion' of the problems posed earlier (Brattstrom, 1987).

Sub-acute phase

For the patient with established disease, medication and rest will have brought it under control so that they have infrequent 'flare-ups' of disease activity. It is during this phase that specific hand deformities are developing (see Chapter 13). Patients are usually by this stage familiar with their medication regime, and have contact with the various members of the therapeutic team. For many this is still a period of emotional turmoil; they have grave concerns for the future and fear dependence on others for their everyday needs. Depression is a well-recognized psychological disturbance in chronic illness, and rheumatoid arthritis is no exception. Depression can significantly increase disability, since sufferers feel they have no control over what is happening to them or that they lack the emotional reserves to cope with the situation (Wells *et al.*, 1989). This feeling of helplessness is frequently compounded by the very real and often profound effects that chronic illness has on the social and economic lifestyles of individuals and their families. It is during this phase that the therapeutic team aims to assist individuals to accept that they have a chronic disease and help them minimize its effects, be they physical or psychological, by the timely introduction of information, treatment and support.

Chronic phase

In late stage disease, many patients will have multiple fixed deformities (see Chapter 13) and greatly diminished capacity in terms of social activity and function. The way in which individuals deal with this varies enormously, and this in turn has a marked effect on their functional capabilities and the level of therapeutic input they require (Taal et al., 1996). Some patients deny that they have difficulties and try to do everything for themselves no matter what the consequences, whilst others exaggerate their problems and depend on others. Both of these extreme reactions pose problems for the therapist; it is impossible to help patients who do not recognize that they would benefit from assistance, and equally difficult to help those who magnify their disabilities and deny their abilities. Thankfully most patients steer the middle course and, through appropriate interventions, maintain some degree of independence.

It is evident that the amount and type of therapeutic input each patient requires varies throughout the course of the disease. Therapy will only be of value if patients understand the benefits of it and are capable of incorporating it into their daily life outside the hospital environment (Donovan, 1991).

Although the involvement of the hand in the rheumatoid process can be very disabling and the deformities extremely dramatic, the hand therapist must always view the treatment of the rheumatoid hand in the context of the overall management of an individual with a chronic disease.

TREATMENT

Treatment is aimed at:

1. Relieving pain
2. Maintaining/increasing joint mobility
3. Maintaining/increasing muscle strength and endurance
4. Preventing deformity
5. Assisting with the emotional adjustment to disability
6. Educating the patient and their family about the condition
7. Maintaining/increasing functional abilities.

All of these aims are relevant to the prevention of hand deformities as well as the maintenance of hand function. They are achieved by specific treatment techniques. Some techniques are more appropriate during particular phases of the disease, and are chosen to achieve a specific outcome. There is however considerable overlap regarding the timing and effects of particular treatments, and none should be viewed in isolation but rather as part of an integrated approach to the management of the patient with rheumatoid arthritis.

TREATMENT TECHNIQUES

Hand assessment

Health Assessment Questionnaires (HAQs; Kirwan and Reeback, 1986) or the Arthritis Impact Measurement Scale (AIMS; Meenan et al., 1992) are frequently used to measure global function in arthritis. It is important to supplement these with a detailed hand assessment. This should include evaluation of symptoms, assessment of function and a physical examination. Hand assessment aims to identify the extent and detail of limitations, and to provide a baseline for treatment. It is also used to set, evaluate and modify treatment goals and to provide a tool for research and audit (David and Lloyd, 1998).

Objective tests

These include measurement of:

- pain
- range of movement
- grip strength
- oedema
- activities of daily living (ADL)
- function.

It is important that assessment methods and equipment are standardized so that comparisons of sequential recordings can be made and used in therapeutic decision making.

Pain relief

The perception of pain and how it is dealt with varies from individual to individual. It is influenced by employment and social situations, family and peers, education and culture, and prior experience (Gifford, 1998). Pain management must recognize all of these factors and address them if it is to be truly effective. Pain relief is at the core of many therapeutic interventions for sufferers of rheumatoid arthritis. Joint protection techniques, patient education and the provision of aids and splints, in addition to having specific objectives, attempt to minimize the pain experienced on a day-to-day basis.

Pain in rheumatoid arthritis can be variable and unpredictable. In the acutely inflamed joint, pain tends to be constant and described as 'aching'. The joint that is no longer inflamed and has suffered severe erosive changes may be pain-free all of the time, or painful only with particular movements and activities. Pain-relieving techniques must reflect this pain spectrum.

Ice

Cold has a long history of medical use, and has been applied to relieve pain for thousands of years (Licht, 1984). Today ice is the commonest method for the application of cold to the body, and is frequently used in both the hospital environment (flaked ice) and home (pack of frozen peas). The two physiological effects produced by cold that have the greatest effect on pain are first the effect on the local circulation, and secondly the effect of cold on the nervous system. Local cooling of an affected joint produces alternating vasoconstriction and vasodilation; this removes substances produced as a result of inflammation from the area and thus reduces pain. The application of ice to normally innervated skin produces a very powerful stimulus and this has been shown to be useful in relieving muscle spasm associated with inflammation; eliminating spasm allows previously compressed blood vessels to carry blood through the muscle (Palastanga, 1994). This technique is particularly appropriate when joints are acutely inflamed, where it can be used twice a day if necessary. The contraindications to the use of ice in rheumatoid arthritis are vasculitis and Raynaud's phenomenon.

Heat

The application of heat to an acutely inflamed joint is contraindicated since it may increase inflammation. The use of heat is however useful during remission and for chronic inflammation. Its effects are to relieve pain associated with muscle spasm and to have a sedative effect on sensory nerve endings (Low and Reed, 1990). Heat is often used in rheumatoid arthritis prior to exercise, as increased collagen extensibility occurs at elevated temperatures (Lehmann et al., 1970). Heat can be applied in a variety of ways. At home it can be applied via a hot water bottle or a commercially available hot pack; in the hospital environment it is often applied via an infrared lamp, wax baths or electrically heated pads.

Transcutaneous electrical nerve stimulation

TENS can be used to relieve acute and chronic pain. For rheumatoid arthritis, its use in the acute situation is often confined to postoperative pain. Many individuals suffer chronic pain or movement-initiated pain, and for some the need for regular high doses of analgesia to control pain produces unacceptable levels of toxicity. TENS can be a viable substitute. It is particularly appropriate for chronic back, leg or neck pain (Frampton, 1994).

Exercise

In the rheumatoid hand exercise is used to maintain joint range, prevent contracture and minimize the development of deformity, as well as to reduce pain and thus improve function.

The ethos of exercise therapy is to maintain overall hand function, but the amount of exercise performed to achieve this will vary according to disease activity:

1. During the acute phase the aim of exercise is to maintain range of movement, and minimal repetitions only are required.

2. During the sub-acute phase the number of repetitions is increased and light resistance is introduced to compensate for decreased grip strength brought about by pain and disuse during the acute phase.

3. During the chronic phase functional exercise and an increase in specific exercise is indicated.

Exercise must never produce pain during or after performance, and should be reduced or ceased if this occurs.

The most commonly taught exercises include:

- fist formation (finger curl involving MCP, PIP and DIP joints)
- full extension of the MCP, PIP and DIP joints (finger lift)
- intrinsic strengthening (bridging of the hand with the digits straight)
- radial deviation exercises for the MCP joints with emphasis on finger extension followed by radial deviation (finger walking).

Exercise is also performed at the wrist so that range of movement and strength are preserved for power grip; specifically this consists of wrist flexion and extension as well as radial and ulnar deviation.

Joint protection and energy conservation

Joint protection and energy conservation techniques aim to:

- maintain joint integrity
- maintain muscle strength
- reduce pain
- reduce fatigue

so that patients can continue to function at their optimal level of independence.

Cordery's (1965) article outlined the principles of joint protection and energy conservation. Since then, many therapists have used these techniques to form the basis for education programmes. Cordery describes the principles of joint protection as:

> **Clinically** joint protection is the instruction of the client on how to perform daily activities with a minimal amount of stress to the involved joints in order to reduce pain, preserve joint structures and conserve physical resources (energy). **Theoretically** joint protection is the integration of the implications of pathology, anatomy and kinesiology with the client's way of life and his daily activities so that physical status and functional ability can be best preserved.

Since the publication of this article many therapists have taken these principles and incorporated them into their education and treatment programmes for patients with rheumatic diseases. In order to incorporate joint protection techniques in everyday activities the patient requires knowledge of how articular functions can be maintained and improved, and therefore the teaching of joint protection should form part of a long-term education programme. It is often necessary to provide additional input and reinforce joint protection principles at critical times, for instance during a flare-up of disease activity when joints are particularly vulnerable and energy limited, and particularly following reconstructive surgery of the upper limbs so that soft-tissue reconstructions and joint arthroplasties can be protected from excessive strain and their effective life prolonged.

For patients to change the way in which an activity is performed and incorporate this into their lifestyle, even on a 'good day', requires not only an understanding of the benefit that can be gained from it but also the motivation to do it. Throughout the course of their lives patients with rheumatoid arthritis experience a wide range of emotions, many of which make them unreceptive to education and treatment. It is not until patients have recognized and accepted the fact that they have a chronic disease that they will be motivated to incorporate joint protection techniques into their daily routine, and many patients will require counselling, information and time before they are receptive.

The use of joint protection techniques for preserving joint structures and improving function in the upper limb are particularly relevant, as the hand is the tool that is used to explore and manipulate the environment.

The principles of joint protection

The principles of joint protection most commonly taught are to:

1. Respect pain
2. Balance rest and work
3. Maintain muscle strength and joint range
4. Reduce effort
5. Avoid positions of deformity
6. Spread the strain over several joints or one large joint
7. Avoid a static position
8. Use assistive equipment and splinting.

Respect pain The patient needs to know the source of joint pain and how to monitor activity appropriately. Activity should be carried out only to the point of fatigue or discomfort and stopped before pain begins. Time or effort spent on activity should be reduced if pain occurs. It is essential to review activities that are commonly overdone – gardening, housework and knitting, to name but a few (Cordery, 1965; Melvin, 1982).

Balance rest and work Rest helps the body to combat systemic disease and improves overall endurance for activity and for specific muscle groups, so its value should not be underestimated.

Resting for a short period during the course of an activity, before pain or fatigue is experienced, will also significantly improve overall endurance for that activity (Melvin, 1982; Furst *et al.*, 1987).

Maintain muscle strength and joint range This can be achieved through functional activity and specific exercise; both are appropriate during periods of disease remission. During periods of active inflammation activity is contraindicated, and maintenance of joint range through passive or gentle assisted exercise is sufficient (Melvin, 1982; Trombly, 1983).

Reduce effort Most tasks can be simplified so that less effort is required, resulting in less pain in the joints and strain upon them. The introduction of a suitable gadget at the appropriate time can reduce the effort required to perform an activity, as can the use of adapted techniques and work simplification methods. Patients should be encouraged to develop behavioural awareness and problem-solving skills and apply them to the home and work situation (Cordery, 1965; Brattstrom, 1987; Furst *et al.*, 1987).

Avoid positions of deformity Internal and external stress and its direction influence the development of deformities in joints, and so patients are taught to avoid using their joints in positions that are thought to exacerbate deformity. How this actually applies in the hand can be illustrated by reference to the MCP joints. There are many factors that lead to the development of ulnar drift and volar subluxation at the MCP joints; one of them is the functional use of the hand. All functional activities that involve MCP joint flexion, especially power pinch and grasp, increase the ulnar forces across the MCP joints. The force applied between the tip of the index finger and the thumb during pinch is magnified three times as it crosses the MCP joint. This stress is compounded by two factors:

1. As the flexor tendon sheath becomes damaged by the effects of synovitis, the flexor tendon is allowed to pull across the MCP joint in an exaggerated volar/ulnar direction during pinch and grasp activities.
2. The ulnar interossei demonstrate a power dominance over radial interossei during functional use.

This 'internal' stress, which arises out of the compressive forces of the muscles and traction from tendons, is a significant deforming force to the inflamed MCP joints and should not be exaggerated by excessive 'external' force. The use of large handles on tools and cutlery, using potentially less deforming grips, and paying attention to the position of the joints during work, leisure and rest are all important considerations that can help to avoid 'external' stress and therefore minimize 'internal' stress. External forces can stress MCP joint implants and cause them to fracture; it is therefore necessary to avoid positions of deformity and external stress following reconstructive surgery of the hand.

To protect other hand structures Cordery also advises that:

• the range of movement at the shoulder, elbow and wrist should be maintained, as hand positioning depends on these joints
• strain on the collateral ligaments should be avoided by enlarging handles
• co-ordination and balance between intrinsic and extrinsic muscles should be maintained
• radial pressure at the interphalangeal joints should be avoided
• abduction of the thumb MCP and IP joints should be minimized.

(Cordery, 1965; Ellison *et al.*, 1971; Melvin, 1982; Brattsrom 1987.)

Spread the strain over several joints or one large joint Large joints are protected by stronger muscles and are better able to tolerate stress. The use of stronger and larger joints includes the use of the pelvis rather than the hands to open heavy doors, lifting with the forearms and trunk rather than the hands, and the use of the palms rather than the fingers to lift and push. This advice is designed to avoid the pain experienced during activity and to avoid joint damage in the longer term (Cordery, 1965; Mody *et al.*, 1989).

Avoid a static position Muscles fatigue in a static position, and thus transmit positional stress to the underlying ligaments and joints. Sustained joint compression can lead to damaged articular cartilage. The position of the joints should be changed every 20–30 minutes, and the patient should move frequently enough to avoid the stiffness and pain associated with prolonged static positioning (Cordery, 1965; Melvin, 1982; Brattstrom, 1987).

Use assistive equipment and splinting Consideration should be given to the use of assistive equipment, particularly that which increases leverage and enlarges the diameter of grip, and to the introduction of adaptations to furniture and home prior to the presence of deformity and not only as a compensation for it. The use of splints for selected activities is also worthy of consideration. (Ellis, 1984; Brattstrom, 1987; see also Chapter 16).

Splinting

(See also Chapter 16.)

Recent advances in the manufacture of low temperature thermoplastic materials, coupled with increased therapeutic knowledge and skill surrounding the fabrication of custom-made splints, makes the provision of hand splints for the patient with rheumatoid arthritis a realistic treatment alternative. Much has been written concerning the biomechanics of hand splinting and the care and precautions that must be observed during the fabrication and use of splints. Splinting is a potentially damaging technique if due consideration is not given to design, application and use, and never was this more true than in the rheumatoid hand with its multiple joint instabilities, stiffness, fragile skin and already greatly diminished function.

Before providing any splint, the therapist must establish sound reasons for it and be prepared to review its effectiveness and usefulness on a regular basis. Since many problems coexist in the rheumatoid hand, it is necessary to place these problems in order of priority. Sometimes this involves *not* providing a splint that you know would be of benefit for a particular activity/deformity, because its issue would damage the patient's morale, interfere with function or exacerbate other problems.

Melvin (1989) refers to splinting for the rheumatoid hand in four groups:

1. Therapeutic
2. Prophylactic
3. Functional
4. Post-operative.

This is a very useful categorization for the therapist involved with the prescription of splints for the patient with rheumatoid arthritis.

Therapeutic splinting

Therapeutic splinting is commonly used to immobilize joints and thus reduce inflammation. If an inflamed joint is supported, the muscles surrounding the joint relax and the pain associated with movement is eliminated, and thus there is a local reduction in inflammation (Gault and Spyker, 1969). A splint frequently prescribed for this purpose is the wrist/hand resting splint. This splint is used during periods of acute disease activity, when many joints are inflamed, and is worn continuously except for essential functions and the maintenance of joint range of movement. Immobilization of the wrist and small joints of the hand will break the cycle of movement > pain > reflex muscle spasm > increased joint pressure > inflammation. Immobilization of joints in their optimal position for function also discourages the effect of deforming forces. The position in which the wrist and hand are immobilized is vitally important, as it aims to eliminate the development of the most frequently encountered rheumatoid hand deformities that result from inflammation of the joint and soft-tissue structures. Correct positioning discourages radial deviation and subluxation of the wrist, and supports the metacarpophalangeal joints against subluxation and aligns them. This eliminates ulnar deforming forces such as the pull of the flexor tendons and the ulnar interossei and encourages PIP joint flexion to minimize the development of swan-neck deformities, which result from the pull of the flexor tendons on the lateral bands. The thumb is positioned so as to maintain pulp-to-pulp opposition and prevent the development of adduction contractures associated with CMC joint subluxation. During periods of reduced inflammation or remission this splint can be worn at night to prevent contractures and reduce pain (Johnson *et al.*, 1992), but it must be reviewed periodically to establish its continued appropriateness. For those patients who have less aggressive disease with one or two joints inflamed rather than several, a satisfactory therapeutic effect can often be achieved by immobilization of only the affected joints.

Another application of therapeutic splinting is when serial splinting is used to correct contractures through the application of prolonged slight traction to the involved joints. This technique was described by Brand (1992), and is particularly appropriate for the correction of fixed flexion contractures of the PIP joints. In the extreme form fixed flexion contractures are very limiting to function, resulting in the inability to open out the hand to pick up or let go of objects, and can also make skin hygiene in the palm of the hand difficult to perform. Opening out the joint will not necessarily restore active extension to the joint – this will depend on the condition of the extensor mechanism – but achieving passive mobility will improve the patient's ability to handle large objects and clean the hand. This is essential before reconstructive surgery is attempted.

Prophylactic splinting

Prophylactic splinting aims to prevent the development of deformities by maintaining optimal joint alignment for function; to date, no empirical evidence is available to support or refute this view. Prophylactic splinting, although it may not eliminate fibrosis, can prevent contractures from developing in a non-functional position. Clinical observations indicate that prophylactic splinting is worthy of consideration since it does maintain anatomical alignment between structures and it is known that disorganization of one joint can have a 'knock-on' effect on adjacent joints.

An example of a prophylactic splint is the wrist support. Worn for activity and work during periods of less disease activity or remission, it will maintain the alignment of extensor carpi ulnaris and thus prevent supination of the carpus. In this way it minimizes the effects of radially deforming forces at the wrist joint, which in turn gives a degree of protection against the development of ulnar deviation of the MCP joints.

Functional splinting

Functional splinting aims to stabilize the joints and minimize pain, thus effecting an improvement in hand function as well as protecting joints from the mechanical stresses generated during forceful activities such as turning a tap. Pain and instability of joints are both major contributors to diminished hand function. Reflex muscle inhibition, secondary to pain, limits the force that can be transmitted through a joint. Supporting a painful joint will diminish the amount of pain experienced and allow greater power to be transmitted through the joint. Unstable joints collapse when any significant force is applied to them; supporting the joint will stop this collapse and allow power to be transmitted across it. Functional splinting is often used for the wrist where joint destruction frequently produces pain and instability. The use of a well-fitting splint that immobilizes the wrist but allows full range of movement at other joints can significantly improve hand function (Mercer and Davis, 1995), and many patients with moderate or severe wrist joint involvement have successfully made wrist splints part of their daily routine.

Post-operative splinting

Post-operative splinting has three main aims:

1. To maintain surgically achieved mobility and alignment
2. To assist post-operative strengthening
3. To prevent or minimize post-surgical adhesions.

The variety in construction and design of post-operative splints is extensive; this is to be expected, since each splint is made to suit the individual's needs and particular surgical programme. There is, however, some pattern to post-operative splinting:

- some splints are designed to immobilize, for instance following a wrist arthroplasty or arthrodesis
- some are designed to allow movement in a prescribed arc or plane, for instance following joint arthroplasty or soft tissue reconstruction of the MCP joints
- some are designed to facilitate movement at a particular joint, for instance following flexor-tenosynovectomy, when it is often necessary to direct movement towards stiff PIP joints rather than the more mobile MCP joints.

The purpose of any post-operative splint must be carefully explained to patients, and the splint must be monitored regularly for fit and effectiveness. If patients discard the splint prematurely because they do not understand its importance or because it is ineffective or uncomfortable, the results of surgery will be compromised.

AIDS AND ADAPTATIONS

The introduction of technicians and designers into the manufacture of aids for the disabled and the increasing awareness that home and work environments should be accessible to able-bodied and disabled alike, plus advances in technology, offer the sufferers of rheumatic disease a far greater opportunity for independence and normality than ever before. For many, aids to daily living and environment modification mean not only the difference between dependence and independence, but also a means of reducing pain and preserving joint integrity. With regard to hand function, it is ideally better not to use an aid at all but to utilize a suitably designed piece of 'normal' equipment. However, if none is available and an aid is necessary, most needs can be met by the application of a few basic principles – make the tool bigger, longer, lighter, more sensitive.

1. Enlarging the diameter of a handle allows the 'tool' to be gripped more effectively and with less force
2. Using a longer lever arm means that more leverage is available and less force is required
3. Using lightweight equipment or dividing a load into smaller segments enables weak hands and wrists to lift and carry with comfort and safety
4. Choosing equipment that requires only a light touch to operate it or is operated by remote control compensates for joint instability, weakness and loss of movement, and also reduces the pain experienced through activity.

This is a very simplistic approach, but when the most frequently used aids are analysed they invariably fall into one of these categories.

Before any aid is prescribed, the therapist and the patient must be sure that it is necessary, that the patient can use it, and that it is affordable. Some patients will require few aids and others quite a lot; some will only be needed in times of crisis and others used all of the time. Periodic review should form an integral part of ADL assessment. Areas worthy of close scrutiny for the provision of aids and adaptations designed to assist upper limb function are work, home, self-care, mobility and leisure.

Work

Increased awareness by the employer and employee, supported in some cases by legislation, has improved work place accessibility as well as equipment safety and design. This makes it easier and safer for everyone, including the individual with rheumatoid arthritis, to achieve gainful employment. Job evaluation is still in its infancy in the UK, but as it continues its momentum it will be possible to evaluate the exact content of most jobs and match jobs to individual abilities and disabilities. In addition, the changing picture of available employment, away from manual work and light industry towards information technology and its spin-off industries (call centres, telesales etc.), makes the individual with rheumatoid arthritis potentially employable. The therapist can assist patients in acquiring the right skills for this and encourage them in their attempts.

Home

In today's competitive market emphasis is placed on good design, and much of this assists the individual with diminished hand function. Whenever possible, 'normal' equipment should be used in the home – difficult taps can be replaced by levers, and sharp knives, food processors, convenience food and microwave ovens can all be useful in food preparation. Often all that is necessary to improve function is reorganization of the kitchen environment and work simplification. Shopping has never been easier; assistance with packing groceries, home delivery services, mail order and internet shopping are services that the disabled should be encouraged to use.

Self-care

Choosing clothing that is lightweight and comfortable greatly assists in getting dressed; there is a wide range of suitable sports wear available that often has the added advantage of elasticated waists and front zip fastenings. Even if this type of clothing is not worn all of the time, it does allow individuals the ability to dress independently some of the time and reserve asking for assistance only when it is absolutely necessary.

Large-handled combs and brushes are invaluable, as is an easy to manage hairstyle. A toothpaste dispenser is also a valuable asset.

Mobility

The ability to attend work and social events independently is important to most people. Often all that is necessary for the individual to drive a car is an enlarged steering-wheel grip. Some patients will find their pain is considerably reduced by the use of power-assisted steering and/or an automatic gear shift. For those with multiple problems, assessment at a mobility centre is usually appropriate and rewarding. For those who need to use a walking stick to assist with mobility, a Fischer stick considerably reduces the force transmitted through the MCP joints. If the patient has limited outdoor mobility without sticks, then the provision of an attendant-propelled wheelchair is appropriate.

Leisure

The importance of leisure should not be underestimated. Often individuals can continue with their chosen leisure activity if they just approach it a different way or modify the equipment required. If this is not possible, they should be supported in exploring different leisure pursuits. It is important to encourage patients to make time and save energy for leisure, even if this involves using aids and adapted methods in other areas in order to do this.

EDUCATION

Education of patients, partners and carers is an essential element in the overall management of rheumatoid arthritis. It aims not only to prevent illness but also to minimize the physical, social and psychological effects on the individual.

To be effective, education programmes must do more than just deliver information; they should also bring about behavioural change. This requires assisting individuals to increase their self-efficacy (Bandura, 1977, 1986). Education must be sensitive to the factors that influence self-efficacy. The content, format and length of education programmes also has an impact on how much information is retained and incorporated into behaviour.

Since patient education is such an important element in rheumatology, those involved with running education programmes should very carefully consider what is necessary for it to be effective and review their current practice if appropriate (Hammond, 1997).

REFERENCES

Ahlmen, M., Sullivan, M. and Bjelle, A. (1988). Team versus non-team outpatient care in rheumatoid arthritis. *Arthr. Rheum.*, **31**, 471–9.

Bandura, A. (1977). Self-efficacy: toward a unifying theory of behavioural change. *Psychol. Rev.*, **84**, 191–215.

Bandura, A. (1986). *Social Foundations of Thought and Action: A Social Cognitive Theory.* Prentice-Hall.

Brand, P. W. and Hollister, A. (1992) *Clinical Mechanics of the Hand,* 2nd edn, pp. 92–128. Mosby.

Brattstrom, M. (1987). *Joint Protection – Rehabilitation in Chronic Rheumatic Disorders.* Wolfe Medical Publications.

Cordery, J. C. (1965). Joint protection: a responsibility of the occupational therapist. *Am. J. Occup. Ther.*, **19(5)**, 285–94.

David, C. and Lloyd, J. (1998). The hand in rheumatology. *Rheumatological Physiotherapy,* pp. 173–91. C. V. Mosby.

Donovan, J. (1991). Patient education and the consultation: the importance of lay beliefs. *Ann. Rheum. Dis.*, **50**, 418–21.

Ellis, M. (1984). Splinting the rheumatoid hand. In: *Clinics in Rheumatic Diseases, The Hand* (C. B. Wynn Parry, ed.), **10(3)**, pp. 673–95. W. B. Saunders.

Ellison, M. R, Flatt, A. E. and Kelly, K. J. (1971). Ulnar drift of the fingers in rheumatoid disease. *J Bone Joint Surg.*, **53A**, 1061–82.

Emery, P. (1994). The optimal management of early rheumatoid disease: the key to preventing disability. *Br. J. Rheum.*, **33**, 765–8.

Frampton, V. (1994). Transcutaneous Nerve stimulation and chronic pain. In: *Pain, Management By Physiotherapy.* 2nd edn. Butterworth Heinemann

Furst, G. P., Gerber, L. H., Smith, C. C. *et al.* (1987). A programme for improving energy conservation behaviours in adults with RA. *Am. J. Occup. Ther.*, **41(2)**, 102–11.

Gault, S. and Spyker, J. (1969). Beneficial effects of immobilisation of joints in the rheumatoid and related arthritides: a splint study using sequential analysis. *Arthr. Rheum.*, **12**, 34–44.

Gifford, L. (1998). Pain, the tissues and the nervous system: a conceptual model, *Physiotherapy*, **84**, 27–36.

Hammond, A. (1997). Joint protection education: what are we doing? *Br. J. Occup. Ther.*, **60(9)**, 401–6.

Johnson, P. M., Sandkvist, G., Ederhardt, K. *et al.* (1992) The usefulness of nocturnal resting splints in the treatment of ulnar deviation of the rheumatoid hand. *Clin. Rheumatol.*, **11**, 72–5.

Kirwan, J. R. and Reeback, J. S. (1986). Stanford health assessment questionnaire modified to assess disability in British patients with rheumatoid arthritis. *Br. J. Rheum.*, **25**, 206–9.

Lehmann, J. F., Masock, A. J., Warren, C. G. *et al.* (1970). Effect of therapeutic temperatures on tendon extensibility. *Arch. Phys. Med. Rehabil.*, **51**, 481.

Licht, S. (1984). History of therapeutic heat and cold. In: *Therapeutic Heat and Cold,* 3rd edn (J. Lehmann, ed.). Williams & Wilkins.

Low, J. and Reed, A. (1990). *Electrotherapy Explained: Principles and Practice.* Butterworth-Heinemann.

Meenan, R. F., Mason, J. H., Anderson, J. J. *et al.* (1992). AIMS2: the content and properties of a revised and expanded Arthritis Impact Measurement Scale health status questionnaire. *Arthr. Rheum.*, **35(1)**, 1–10.

Melvin, J. L. (1982). Joint protection and energy conservation in rheumatic disease. In: *Occupational Therapy and Rehabilitation,* pp. 351–71. F. A. Davis.

Melvin, J. L. (1989). *Rheumatic Diseases in the Adult and Child.* F. A. Davis.

Mercer, C. and Davis, M. (1995). A survey of the uses and benefits of prefabricated wrist and thumb supports. *Br. J. Ther. Rehabil.*, **2**, 599–603.

Mody, G. M., Meyers, O. L. and Reinach, S. (1989). Handedness and deformities, radiographic changes and function of the hand in RA. *Ann. Rheum. Dis.*, **48**, 104–7.

Palastanga, N. P. (1994). Heat and cold. In: *Pain, Management by Physiotherapy,* 2nd edn. (P. E. Wells, V. Frampton, D. Bowsher, eds). Butterworth-Heinemann.

Roche, P. A. and Klestov, A. C. (1995). Anxiety, depression and the sense of helplessness: their relationship to pain from rheumatoid arthritis. In: *Moving on in Pain* (M. O. Shacklock, ed.), pp. 60–90. Butterworth-Heinemann.

Taal, E., Rasker, J. J. and Wiegman, O. (1996). Patient education in the rheumatic diseases: a self-efficacy approach. *Arthr. Care Res.*, **9**, 229–37.

Trombly, C. A. (1983). *Occupational Therapy for Physical Dysfunction,* 2nd edn. Williams & Wilkins.

Tucker, M. and Kirwan, J. R. (1991). Does patient education in rheumatoid arthritis have therapeutic potential? *Ann. Rheum. Dis.*, **50,** 422–8.

Vliet Vieland, T. P. M., Zwinderman, A. H., Vanden-brouke, J. P. *et al.* (1996). A randomised clinical trial of inpatient multidisciplinary treatment versus routine outpatient treatment care in active rheumatoid arthritis. *Br. J. Rheumatol.*, **33,** 475–82.

Wells, K. B., Stewart, A., Hays, R. D. *et al.* (1989). The functioning and well-being of depressed patients: results from Medical Outcome Study. *JAMA*, **262,** 914–19.

FURTHER READING

Frank, A. O. and Maguire, G. P. (1998). *Disabling Diseases: Physical, Environmental and Psychological Management.* Heinemann Medical Books

Newman, S. P. and Revenson, T. A. (1993). Coping with rheumatoid arthritis. *Bailli'eres Clin. Rheumatol.*, **7,** 259–80.

Palmer, P. and Simmons, J. (1991). Joint protection: a critical review. *Br. J. Occup. Ther.*, **54(12),** 435–58.

15 The rheumatoid hand: a surgical approach

Ann Birch and Lynda Gwilliam

The resulting pain, instability/stiffness and deformity that accompany involvement of joints and soft tissue structures in the disease process all contribute to functional deficit. Eliminating pain, restoring stability, minimizing stiffness and correcting deformity should bring about improvement in function, assuming that treatment is appropriately targeted. When many joints are involved it can be difficult to establish exactly which is or are the prime contributors to functional deficit. For this reason careful pre-operative assessment is sometimes necessary, both to highlight the most problematic joints and to determine which surgical procedure will best resolve the problems and so bring about functional improvement. As well as functional considerations there are medical and mechanical factors that must also be considered when setting priorities.

SURGICAL PRIORITIES IN RHEUMATOID ARTHRITIS

Intact tendon mechanisms and the motor power to use them are essential for hand function. Preserving the integrity of nerves and tendons is therefore a high surgical priority. Nerve compression can lead to permanent loss of sensation and motor power, so if there is evidence of significant nerve compression that has not responded to conservative management, this must be dealt with as a matter of urgency, even if the patient perceives that other problems are more pressing.

Tenosynovitis, resulting in compression of tendons by excessive synovium, can lead to multiple tendon rupture. Decompression of tendons and preservation of their integrity is therefore a very high priority.

When considering joint surgery the priorities are much more dependent on the needs of the individual, but there are some guidelines that are useful with complex deformities and multiple joint involvement:

1. As a general rule, lower limb surgery (such as hip or knee replacement) should be carried out first because weight bearing through the upper limbs in the rehabilitation phase can damage delicate hand surgery. The only exception to this is a wrist arthrodesis, which, if performed prior to lower limb surgery, can improve rehabilitation by enabling the patient to transmit power through a stable, pain-free wrist and thus through a walking aid.

2. As far as the upper limb is concerned, if the elbow and shoulder are so painful that they inhibit use of the hand then they should be treated first. It is pointless to carry out a series of operations on the hand to improve function if that function is limited by pain in the shoulder or elbow.

3. Moving distally, it is advisable to correct wrist deformity and pain before tackling hand joints since a painful and/or unstable wrist will inhibit hand function (Mannerfelt, 1987).

When it comes to considering the order of surgery regarding metacarpophalangeal (MCP) and proximal interphalangeal (PIP) joints, this is dependent on the nature of the deformity (for a detailed description of the deformities see Chapter 13).

1. *Subluxed MCP joints and swan-neck PIP joints.* In this combination the MCP joint deformity should be corrected first. If the swan-neck deformity is corrected first it will recur, since the volar subluxation at the MCP joint, one of the causative factors of swan-neck deformity, remains uncorrected.

2. *MCP disease in combination with gross PIP flexion deformity.* In this combination the flexion deformity of the PIP joints should be corrected first. Boutonni'ere deformities in particular predispose toward hyperextension of the MCP joint, and this makes achieving a good range of flexion at the MCP joint in the post-operative period very difficult. In some instances the two problems can be resolved together by manipulating and temporarily wiring the PIP joints into the maximum possible extension.

3. *Extensor tendon disease in combination with MCP disease.* Extensor tenosynovectomy of intact tendons can be performed in combination with MCP joint surgery. However, when the extensor tendons have ruptured in the presence of gross MCP disease it is better to replace the joints first, so that when the tendons are subsequently repaired the tension can be accurate and the tendons glide over stable joints (Nalebuff, 1984). In the interval between these two procedures the patient can use a dynamic splint to substitute for the action of the ruptured tendons.

4. *Flexor tendon disease in combination with MCP joint disease.* If the flexor tendons are at risk of rupture from synovitis, or if they are tethered in the sheath preventing active flexion, preservation of the tendons should always take priority, even with the knowledge that the tendons will not achieve full range of movement in the presence of subluxed MCP joints. This situation can either be accepted or, alternatively, flexor tenosynovectomy and MCP joint replacement can be performed at the same time. This does mean that the patient is subjected to surgery on both palmar and dorsal surfaces of the hand and to a complex and difficult post-operative regime,

with possibly disappointing results from both procedures, but sometimes it is the best solution to this problem. Another option, instead of replacing the joints, is to stabilize the MCPs with Kirschner wires and simply perform a flexor tenosynovectomy. In this way the patient will achieve good excursion of the tendons, but this must be followed up by MCP joint surgery within 2 months if the benefits are not to be lost. Similarly, in the case of ruptured flexor tendons a flexor tendon graft is performed first, with the MCP joints stabilized by K-wires, followed as quickly as possible by MCP joint replacements.

Thumb surgery is often performed at the same time as other surgery, but if this is not possible the finger deformities should be corrected first so that the thumb can be accurately placed in opposition to the fingers. Sometimes in a very complex situation where all three joints of the thumb are involved, the only realistic option in order to improve function may be to arthrodese one of the joints. This can improve the function of the hand immensely; in fact, fusion of the MCP or interphalangeal (IP) joint of the thumb has been referred to as a 'best buy' operation.

Summary

Careful assessment is essential before surgery is embarked upon. For the individual patient with multiple joint involvement, identification of the joints or soft tissue structures contributing most to the functional deficit is necessary so that surgery can be appropriately targeted. Once this is done the anatomical problems must be prioritized in order to protect and preserve vital structures, and an order of surgery constructed so that the best possible result can be obtained from each surgical procedure:

1. Nerves take priority, closely followed by tendons
2. Lower limbs are operated on before the upper, except for a wrist fusion
3. Painful proximal joints are operated on before the hand
4. The wrist is operated on before the hand
5. MCP versus PIP surgery depends on the type of PIP deformity
6. MCP joints are operated on before ruptured extensor tendons
7. MCP joints and flexor tendons – careful thought is required before deciding upon the order of surgery
8. Fingers are operated on before thumb if there has to be a choice, although sometimes the thumb alone is treated.

Having chosen the appropriate procedure(s), it is now important to consider the post-operative management.

SURGICAL PROCEDURES FOR THE RHEUMATOID UPPER LIMB AND THEIR POST-OPERATIVE MANAGEMENT

Although some procedures do have 'routine' post-operative rehabilitation programmes, it is frequently necessary to modify them to suit the individual. All therapy for the rheumatoid hand must recognize the continued existence of disease and its effect on other soft tissue structures.

Flexor and extensor tenosynovectomy

Persistent synovitis on either surface of the hand or wrist can compromise the integrity of the tendon mechanisms, and will ultimately result in tendon rupture (Bengsten and Schutt, 1994). To prevent this from happening, a tenosynovectomy is a commonly performed surgical procedure. This involves removing the diseased synovium from around the tendons and ensuring that the tendons glide sufficiently to perform their action.

The aims of treatment are to:

1. Maintain tendon glide
2. Maintain the range of movement in the joints.

Treatment programme
The treatment of choice is early active movement of the small joints of the hand and the wrist. This begins on the first post-operative day, and must be continued for a minimum of 6 weeks to prevent the formation of adhesions. For patients who have no fixed deformity, the necessity for 'hands on' treatment is minimal; patients are taught appropriate full range of movement and tendon gliding exercises and checked regularly to ensure that they are achieving their maximum potential. Heavy activity should be avoided for at least 6 weeks to minimize the risk of tendon rupture.

Unfortunately there are situations when following this simple programme is not possible and treatment becomes more complicated.

Factors complicating the treatment of extensor tenosynovectomy
1. *Deformities of the MCP joints.* Subluxation of these joints results in the inability to perform active extension. When this is the case it is necessary to fit the patient with an extension assist splint, usually an outrigger, to assist MCP joint extension and thus maintain maximum tendon excursion. The patient is instructed to regularly perform active flexion of the MCP joints and allow the elastic recoil of the dynamic splint to assist with extension of the subluxed MCP joints. During the night the lively splint is removed and replaced with a static splint, which holds the MCP joints in their maximum comfortable extension.
2. *Poor tendon quality.* The surgeon, who has observed the tendon quality, should commu-

nicate this information to the therapist prior to the commencement of treatment. If the tendons appear ischaemic, then unrestrained active movement in the immediate post-operative phase could result in tendon rupture. However, this is not a complete contraindication to movement. The risk of rupture can be minimized by restricting wrist flexion and fitting the patient with an extension assist splint; these measures will ensure adequate excursion of the tendons while minimizing the risk of rupture. During the night the patient wears a static extension splint to maintain the MCP joints in extension and reduce the strain on the extensor tendons. As the tendons increase their strength, free active movement can be introduced.

3. *Associated surgery.* Wrist surgery is frequently performed at the same time as extensor tenosynovectomy, since involvement of extensor tendons is often a result of severe wrist disease, and the post-operative therapy programme must take account of this associated surgery. Most surgical procedures on the wrist require immobilization of the wrist in the immediate post-operative period and great care must be taken that the cast or splint used to achieve this does not impede MCP joint movements, as the MCP joints must be free to flex and extend in order to obtain maximum excursion of the extensor tendons. Post-operative swelling and pain also need to be well controlled so that they do not inhibit movement.

Factors complicating the treatment of flexor tenosynovectomy

The extent of flexor tenosynovectomy is determined by the extent of the synovitis and the density of adhesions. Surgery can range from a simple flexor tenosynovectomy confined to the palm of the hand and sometimes extending into the digits, to a much more complex procedure involving not only synovectomy of the tendons but also tenolysis and manipulation of the stiff interphalangeal joints that accompany this density of synovitis and adhesions. The post-operative therapy regime must consider these factors and take account of the tendon quality; this is important because the tendon itself may have been invaded and weakened by the synovium.

For the purpose of clarity it is useful to think of the differing post-operative regimes in relation to disease phases, since they often correspond.

Acute phase Acute flexor tenosynovitis that persists for more than 3 months becomes a surgical priority, and a flexor tenosynovectomy is indicated. At this stage of the disease tendon quality is still good, there is a minimum of adhesions between the tendons and the sheath, and the joints are usually still mobile. Post-operative therapy in this situation is as described earlier – the therapist acting as educator and ensuring that the patients carry out their home

therapy programme faithfully and for a long enough period. To reduce the frequency of exercise sessions or to discontinue them too soon, i.e. within 6 weeks of surgery, will result in adhesion formation and loss of range of movement.

Sub-acute phase Flexor tenosynovitis is not always acute and dramatic; frequently it is a slow and insidious process that happens over many years. For the inexperienced therapist it can be difficult to recognize, since the stiff joints in which it ultimately results are easily attributed to intra-articular problems rather than to pathology of the tendons. This is understandable, as rheumatoid arthritis is often mistakenly thought of in terms of damage to joints alone. Persistent tenosynovitis leads to tendon infiltration and adhesion formation, which in turn leads to stiff joints. Flexor tenosynovectomy alone is not going to resolve this problem; it must be accompanied by tenolysis between the tendons and their sheaths as well as between the flexor digitorum profundus (FDP) and flexor digitorum superficialis (FDS), plus gentle manipulation of the IP joints. This is a much more demanding procedure for surgeon, therapist and patient than that of 'simple' flexor tenosynovectomy. Post-operative therapy is directed towards:

- relieving pain
- reducing oedema
- maintaining/increasing the range of movement at the proximal and distal joints
- obtaining tendon excursion
- maintaining differential glide between FDS and FDP
- re-educating of the pattern of digital flexion ('roll-up') – whilst the fingers have been stiff patients will have become accustomed to flexing the MCP joints with their fingers straight; after surgery they must learn to flex at each joint.

Before the therapy programme begins the therapist requires operative details from the surgeon so that the programme can be tailored to the individual patient.

It is essential for the therapist to know:

- the quality of the tendons, since this will dictate the treatment method
- the quantity, location and type of adhesions
- the amount of tendon glide obtained
- the potential ROM in the joints.

If the quality of the tendons is poor, then the treatment programme must take account of this. Poor quality tendons must be allowed time to re-establish their nutritional source; to embark on an intensive therapy programme that includes unrestricted active movement before this is accomplished substantially increases the risk of tendon rupture. Strickland (1989) describes a therapy programme called 'The frayed tendon programme'. This was originally described for the post-operative management of ischaemic tendons following tenolysis, but it can equally be applied to ischaemic rheumatoid flexor tendons following flexor tenosynovectomy. This programme is also referred to as 'place and hold'.

The wrist and MCP joints are protected against full extension by a dorsal splint, with the wrist held in neutral and MCP joints in 40° of flexion. The patient is taught to passively flex the PIP and DIP joints. When maximum passive flexion is obtained, the patient initiates active flexion to hold the digit in this flexed position. Active extension returns the digit to its resting position. This has the effect of obtaining tendon glide without unduly stressing the tendon. It is necessary to protect the tendon in this way for 6 weeks, and to avoid resistance for a further 6 weeks.

If the quality of the tendons is good, then the post-operative management of this procedure can be very intensive and should begin immediately following surgery. Patients attend regularly for a minimum of 6 weeks, and are also given a home therapy programme. To achieve the treatment objectives it is often necessary to use several treatment modalities. Those commonly employed include:

1. *Elevation*. This reduces swelling and pain and thus facilitates movement.
2. *Transcutaneous nerve stimulation* (TENS). Therapy is frequently a painful procedure, particularly if the joints have been manipulated, therefore pain control is essential if maximum movement and patient compliance are to be obtained.
3. *Constant passive motion* (CPM). Passive movement should not replace active movement, but it can supplement it. The use of the CPM seems to have a pain relieving effect that facilitates active movement; it also maintains maximum ROM in the joints.
4. *MCP block*. The pattern of digital flexion prior to surgery is often concentrated at the mobile MCP joints, with the PIP and DIP joints remaining stiff because of poor flexor tendon pull through. This pattern of movement often persists after surgery. In order to re-educate the more normal pattern of grasp and direct movement towards the less mobile interphalangeal joints, the MCP joints must be prevented from moving. This can be achieved by the use of a small blocking splint worn during exercise sessions. This splint can be made from a conforming thermoplastic material, moulded round the hand to limit MCP joint movement but allowing PIP and DIP joint movement.
5. *Neuromuscular stimulation*. This can be useful to re-educate muscles when they have been inhibited from proper use by flexor tendon problems.

Chronic phase During the chronic phase of rheumatoid arthritis therapists are frequently faced either

with this situation of stiff joints and adherent tendons or with ruptured tendons in addition to the other deformities associated with established disease. When the flexor tendons have ruptured there is usually no alternative but to carry out tendon grafting, since primary repair of the tendon is not possible due to the insidious nature of the rupture and poor tendon quality. Grafting of flexor tendons in an attempt to restore some function to the hand should be viewed as a salvage procedure, and the preservation of flexor tendon integrity should therefore have a high priority to avoid this situation.

The management of flexor tendon grafts in the rheumatoid patient

Flexor tendon grafting is a technically demanding procedure for the surgeon. In addition to this, there may be problems identifying sufficient donor sites if multiple ruptures are present. The challenge for the therapist is to obtain maximum tendon excursion and thus limit adhesion formation in the presence of associated unstable or stiff joints. One of the most difficult problems to overcome is that of ulnar deviated unstable MCP joints. This is a very common end-stage rheumatoid hand deformity that often coexists with ruptured flexor tendons. Particular attention must be paid to realigning and stabilizing the MCP joints by post-operative splintage so that maximum tendon excursion can be achieved. Stiff IP joints can also present difficulties in the post-operative management of flexor tendon grafts. If it is possible to obtain passive movement in the IP joints prior to surgery then this is obviously the course of action to follow, but frequently the amount of articular damage present prevents little more than limited movement. Since the amount of joint movement dictates the amount of tendon excursion it follows that this will not be full, but it should be adequate to achieve a functional range and a stable finger.

The two most commonly applied methods of post-operative management of flexor tendon grafts are the regime described by Kleinert (van Strien, 1990), which is elastic band traction into flexion with active extension, or the regime of early active movement, which is controlled active flexion and extension within a protective dorsal splint (Small *et al.*, 1989). The choice of method is dictated by the patient's compliance and ability to understand the treatment regime and by the surgeon's judgement having seen the actual tendon quality. During healing rheumatoid tissue reaches maturity at a much slower rate than healthy tissue; therefore it is often necessary to protect the tendon graft from unrestrained active movement and to discourage resisted flexion and forced extension for longer than is usual for 'normal' tissue. Despite the difficulties and variable outcomes associated with flexor tendon grafting in the rheumatoid hand it is still a worthwhile procedure, since it can restore adequate function to what is often a very disabled hand. The ideal, however, is to prevent flexor tendon ruptures from occurring by early medical, therapeutic and surgical measures.

The management of extensor tendon repairs in the rheumatoid patient

Once an extensor tendon has ruptured, it is very unlikely that an end-to-end repair can be performed. This is because the proximal end of the tendon recoils, making it difficult to locate, and the tendon itself is also often of very poor quality. If the rupture was very recent it is very occasionally possible to perform a direct repair, but usually it is necessary to perform a side-to-side anastomosis to an adjacent tendon (Bengston and Schutt, 1994). Since many extensor tendon ruptures result from attrition against a bony prominence, this must be removed to prevent recurrence. It may even be necessary to perform a more extensive wrist stabilizing procedure at the same time as the extensor tendon repair, since wrist joint disease and extensor tendon problems are closely associated. Extensor tenosynovectomy of intact tendons also routinely accompanies this procedure.

The aims of treatment are to:

1. Protect the tendon repair
2. Maintain tendon glide
3. Maintain joint range of movement.

There are three possible treatment regimes in the initial post-operative period. The choice of method is arrived at after discussion with the surgeon and is dictated by:

- the quality of the tendons
- the quality of the repair
- the condition of the bed on which the tendons lie.

Method 1– good quality tendons/good repair/bed may be scarred or smooth The post-operative dressing is removed on the first day following surgery, taking care to hold the MCP joints in extension during the dressing change to protect the repair. A dynamic extension splint is fitted to the hand; this supports the MCP joints in extension whilst allowing active flexion. It is essential to include all four digits in the splint, since the extensor tendons have a common muscle belly and the repair is usually to an adjacent tendon. The tension of the recoil of the elastic bands (or springs) should allow full active flexion of the MCP joints but be sufficient to return the joints to neutral alignment without the action of the extensor tendons. Whenever possible the wrist joint should be positioned in slight extension to minimize the tension on the tendon repairs, but this is not always possible to achieve due to pre-existing deformity or surgery.

The patient is instructed to wear this dynamic extension splint all day and to perform regular exercise sessions to achieve tendon excursion and prevent joint stiffness – 10 repetitions per hour of active MCP joint flexion with passive extension from the recoil of the splint is sufficient to achieve this. Since most functional activities require sustained grip these are prohibited, even with the splint on. At night the patient may choose to remain in the dynamic splint, or may be more comfortable in a resting splint that supports the MCP joints at neutral and the wrist in its desired position. Rheumatoid tissue and the medications used to control the disease result in slow tissue maturation, so it is essential to adhere to this regime for 6 weeks. During this period therapeutic measures are aimed at education and supervision, with particular attention being paid to preventing stiffness in the other joints of the limb, especially the interphalangeal joints. The use of the lively extension splint can be discontinued at 6 weeks post-operation and light functional activity resumed, but sustained strong flexion must be avoided for a further 6 weeks. Night splinting with the MCP joints in extension is also continued for a further 6 weeks.

Method 2 – questionable quality tendons and/or repair/tendon bed scarred The dilemma in this situation is to protect the repair whilst minimizing tendon adhesions. This is achieved by resting the MCP joints at neutral with the wrist in slight extension for an initial 3 weeks, and then proceeding as with Method 1 for a further 3 weeks. There is no need to immobilize the IP joints, since the long extensors play no part in their action, and attention should be directed towards maintaining full range of movement in these joints as they very quickly become stiff. Once commenced this method should be adhered to and no attempt made to shorten the initial immobilization period, as the repair is at its weakest point around 10 days post-operatively and any movement (even protected movement) at this time will increase the risk of rupture.

Method 3 – very poor quality tendon The wrist and MCP joints are immobilized for 6 weeks in order to allow the repair to heal. This is obviously not the preferred method of treatment, and is only subscribed to when the quality of the tendons is so poor that mobilization (even protected mobilization) would cause rupture. It is inevitable using this method that the MCP joints will become stiff and the tendons adherent. For this group of patients it is unlikely that full range of MCP joint movement will be regained. By obtaining some improvement in extension, the patient is likely to lose some flexion. The consequences of any likely gains and losses should be considered prior to surgery, and considerable therapeutic skill is needed to identify those patients who will benefit from surgery.

The shoulder

The shoulder is very often affected in RA, and it can be extremely painful and functionally disabling. Surgical intervention is often seen as a last resort and only considered when the shoulder is so badly destroyed that salvage surgery is the only option. However, with the introduction of arthroscopic surgery earlier intervention is now more frequently considered. Arthroscopic synovectomy can dramatically reduce pain and restore lost range of movement in the short term, although its long-term effects are as yet unknown. Arthroscopic subacromial decompression is another procedure that can be considered to preserve the rotator cuff. If the articular surfaces of the shoulder are damaged, then total or hemi-arthroplasty is indicated. With the advent of the Neer procedure in the 1970s (Neer et al., 1982) shoulder replacement became a much more popular procedure, but the glenoid component still presents something of a problem, particularly in the rheumatoid patient with bone loss. The search continues for a glenoid that can restore the subacromial space and be reliably fixed, and consequently many surgeons perform a hemi-arthroplasty using a humeral component only.

If the arthroplasty is carried out when the rotator cuff muscles are still intact the results can be very good, both in terms of pain relief and increased range of movement. When the rotator cuff is already damaged the pain relief element is good but active range of movement will be limited, though it will be adequate for self-care.

The post-operative course is determined by the status of the rotator cuff. If this is healthy and fully intact, mobilization is begun on the first post-operative day. The patient begins with passive movement, at first helped by the therapist, but rapidly progresses to auto-assisted movement using a pulley and an exercise stick to gain maximum range of movement. Surgical techniques vary, so it is wise to check with the surgeon as to which structures need to be protected; this determines the precise details of the post-operative programme. The delto-pectoral approach is the one most commonly used; this involves dividing the subscapularis, so it is this that needs to be protected. Lateral rotation is limited to 30° from neutral until 6 weeks post-operation, and abduction combined with lateral rotation for the same length of time. Apart from this the patients are allowed to progress as quickly as they are able, from passive to assisted active and then to active movement. How quickly they progress is dependent on the pre-operative condition of the muscles.

If the cuff is badly destroyed and surgical repair is excluded, then a similar regime to the above is followed; however, the results in terms of active movement will not be as good. If the cuff is repaired at surgery, mobilization is delayed for between 3 and 6 weeks and the arm is rested in an abduction splint. In these cases, progression from passive to active movement is much slower.

The elbow

The elbow, in conjunction with the shoulder, allows the hand to be moved towards or away from the body. Even a well-preserved and dextrous hand cannot be utilized if it cannot be positioned adequately. Elbow involvement, like the shoulder, tends to be very painful. There are basically two operations performed on the elbow once conservative measures have stopped being helpful: synovectomy, with or without radial head excision, or total arthroplasty.

Elbow synovectomy and radial head excision
Individuals with moderate joint destruction often benefit from these procedures, either separately or in combination, since they aim to relieve pain and restore movement. The treatment following surgery is simple. Gentle mobilizing exercises are encouraged, flexion and extension as well as forearm rotation. These are commenced within 1–2 days of surgery, to minimize the formation of post-operative adhesions. In addition the patient is encouraged to rest the arm in either a sling or resting splint between exercise sessions to allow pain and oedema to subside. The patient should be encouraged to regain full functional movement within 6 weeks of surgery. If range of movement is slow to return, more specific treatment may be needed to improve mobility.

Elbow replacement arthroplasty
When the joint is severely damaged, replacement arthroplasty is usually the operation of choice. Excisional arthroplasty may also be considered, but this leaves a very unstable arm, often with incomplete pain relief, and should only be considered when all other options have been exhausted.

Total elbow arthroplasty has evolved from a fully-constrained hinge prosthesis with a very high incidence of loosening (68 per cent) to the present semi- and non-constrained implants with a much lower associated incidence of loosening (12 per cent). The unacceptably high incidence of loosening associated with the first generation of implants appeared to result primarily from forces generated during activity. The present generation of implants considers the elbow to be a weight-bearing joint for the purpose of implant design, and this has undoubtedly had a dramatic effect on reducing the incidence of loosening. However, many clinicians and engineers consider that activity may still be a factor associated with loosening of the prosthesis. It is therefore essential that a pre-operative assessment of the patient's functional status is carried out when a total elbow replacement is being considered; not to exclude an individual from the procedure, but to help them to benefit from it in both the short and the long term. It is important for the patient fully to understand the limitations and implications of this operation – that it is very good at providing pain relief and a functional range of movement, but that it must never be considered to be a weight-bearing joint. Many patients with rheumatoid arthritis have lower limb problems and need to use their arms to assist them when rising from a bed or chair; this, together with regular use of walking aids, is still suspected as contributing to loosening of the prosthesis. For most people pain relief following this procedure is good, and this alone can be a reason for considering the operation, but in addition although the range of movement post-operatively is rarely full it is more than adequate for self care and is often an improvement on the pre-operative range

A typical post-operative regime, following a procedure with no intra-operative complications and intact collateral ligaments, is outlined below. It may be necessary to alter the period and position of immobilization in the presence of epicondylar fractures or ligament repairs.

In the theatre, the elbow is immobilized in maximum extension in a plaster of Paris (POP) posterior slab. For the first 5 days the arm is rested in elevation and shoulder and hand movements are encouraged. Elevation is best achieved using pillows rather than a roller towel or Bradford sling because it is important to avoid pressure on the olecranon process, as ischaemia of the overlying skin can occur as a post-operative complication. The olecranon should be inspected regularly to monitor the tissue viability.

From the fifth day until 3 weeks post-operatively, the patient wears two different splints – a night splint with the elbow held in maximum extension, and a day splint with the elbow positioned at 90° flexion. The patient is instructed to remove the splint, initially four times a day and progressing to eight, in order to perform active exercise to achieve the optimum range of movement.

At 3 weeks the day splint is discarded and the patient can commence light activities such as feeding, washing and dressing. The night splint is retained for a further 3 weeks, and should be remoulded regularly in order to gain maximum extension.

After 6 weeks the patient may gradually increase the level of activity; it is at this stage that he or she should once again be reminded of joint protection principles and given assistance to adopt activity patterns that do not subject the arthroplasty to high forces. The actual 'hands on' therapy following total elbow arthroplasty is actually quite small; the therapist's role is directed more towards education and encouragement.

The wrist

A pain-free and stable wrist is essential for the hand to function adequately. Treatment for the wrist depends on the degree of destruction caused by the disease process.

When synovitis is the major problem, with no bony changes, the initial treatment is rest combined with splintage in a position of function, in either slight extension or neutral.

Surgical synovectomy
If synovitis persists, a surgical synovectomy is performed in order to preserve the structures of the wrist. During this procedure the extensor tendons are brought outside the extensor retinaculum in order to protect them from any subsequent damage from recurrent synovial proliferation. It is usual for a small strip of retinaculum to be placed over the tendons to prevent bow-stringing.

Darrach's procedure
When the distal radio-ulnar joint (DRUJ) is affected a Darrach procedure is frequently performed (Darrach, 1913), which can improve pronation and supination and provide pain relief. The technique involves removing a part of the ulnar head and stabilizing the distal ulna. Surgeons nowadays limit the amount of bone removed to 12 mm because extensive bone resection destabilizes the distal ulna, with resulting pain and instability on rotation of the forearm. Similarly, an important part of this procedure is the relocation of the extensor carpi ulnaris tendon onto the dorsum of the wrist, where it should stabilize the ulna stump. Rotation of the forearm in the immediate post-operative period is very painful for the patient; it is also undesirable because early movement inhibits formation of the scar tissue around the ulna, which is needed to increase the stability of the joint. For these reasons the wrist, forearm and elbow are immobilized in a splint to prevent pronation and supination for a period of at least 6 weeks. This prolonged immobilization does not result in long-term limitation of movement, and most individuals achieve full, pain-free rotation within a couple of weeks of commencing mobilizing exercises, without instability of the distal ulna.

Frequently the effects of the disease process are not confined to the DRUJ alone but also involve the carpus. For those individuals who show evidence of early translation of the carpus, performing a Darrach procedure in isolation has the effect of further destabilizing the wrist, and ulnar carpal shift occurs (Bieber *et al.*, 1988). This can, in time, cause the carpus to collapse. To prevent carpal shift in predisposed individuals, the ulna head should not be removed unless a procedure to stabilize the carpus is also performed. This may take the form of a partial wrist arthrodesis, a replacement arthroplasty, or a full carpal arthrodesis.

Radio-lunate fusion

For those patients with ulna carpal translation but who have a relatively undamaged mid-carpal joint, a 'Chamay' or radio-lunate fusion can resolve the problem. In this procedure, the wrist is relocated and the translation eliminated by bringing the lunate back into contact with the radius and fusing it in place using a plug of bone from either the resected head of the ulna or the radius. The position is held with Kirschner wires, and a wrist immobilization splint is applied until fusion is seen to be taking place. When the wires and the splint are removed, routine mobilizing and strengthening exercises are carried out, bearing in mind that the movement is now taking place at the mid-carpal joint and is only likely to be about half of normal range (Terrono *et al.*, 1995).

When all the carpal joints are affected partial arthrodesis is no longer an option, and complete arthrodesis or replacement arthroplasty should be considered if the wrist is painful or presents functional difficulties. The decision as to which procedure is most appropriate for a given individual is often made on functional grounds. A wrist arthroplasty provides some mobility but must not be considered as a weight-bearing joint, whereas a wrist fusion is suitable for weight bearing but deprives the individual of all wrist motion. Therefore the status of the ipsilateral joints as well as the condition of the contralateral upper limb and the lower limbs must be taken into account. It is also important to consider the particular tasks that patients need to perform – for example, they may need to retain some wrist mobility to carry out personal hygiene or continue with a much loved hobby such as drawing or embroidery, or they may need the strength provided by a wrist fusion to use walking aids and assist with transfers. In a patient with bilateral problems, it may be preferable to have one fused wrist for strength and weight bearing and one replaced wrist for dexterity. The choice of procedure, replacement or fusion, and whether it should be right or left, will depend on individual needs and not on any predetermined rule.

Replacement arthroplasty

There are a variety of commercially available wrist implants, and two are described here. The silicone elastomer implant designed by Swanson acts as inert flexible spacer after excisional arthroplasty of the joint. The implant is quickly surrounded by a synovial-like layer of tissue, which remains in contact with the implant, and surrounding this a stronger capsule develops (Swanson, 1969). A vital part of the surgery is the careful alignment of tendons and ligaments to allow for balanced movement in the post-operative phase. The bi-axial wrist arthroplasty is an example of a two-part replacement articulation. The implant is an ellipsoid device with convex–concave articulating surfaces,

and was developed between 1978 and 1982 (Tyson *et al.*, 1996).

Post-operative management is similar with either type of prosthesis, and aims to provide a stable, pain-free wrist with a useful arc of movement.

The optimum range of movement following arthroplasty is 30° flexion, 30° extension, 10° ulnar deviation and 5° radial deviation. Excessive movement predisposes to fracture of the Swanson silicone implant, and loosening of the cement around the stem of the bi-axial prosthesis.

The wrist is initially immobilized in a cast for 3 weeks, at which stage the cast is removed and the range of movements are gently assessed. If the wrist moves easily to the optimum range, it is immobilized again for a further 3 weeks. However, if the wrist is extremely stiff mobilization is commenced. The patient is provided with a removable splint and taught gentle mobilizing exercises, with the splint being worn between exercise sessions and for all functional activities. By 6 weeks all patients will have commenced mobilization, and all will retain splints for functional activities until such time as the wrist extensors have regained sufficient strength to support the wrist at neutral against light resistance. For long-term protection, patients are advised never to lift a weight unless the wrist extensors are strong enough to support the wrist in neutral while holding it. All patients are warned that this is not a weight-bearing joint and that they should wear a strong work splint if they are forced to do any heavy manual work.

Wrist arthrodesis

When bony erosion and ligament damage is extensive and the wrist collapsed, a wrist arthroplasty may not be possible or appropriate and the whole wrist joint may need to be fused. Wrist arthrodesis on the authors' unit is carried out using a Stanley pin; this is a modified Steinman pin that is countersunk into the third metacarpal, through the carpus and into the radius. The fusion is completed by use of bone graft taken from the excised head of the ulna. This method of fusion dictates that the wrist position must be neutral, which allows the patient adequate grip and is a suitable position for many functional activities including feeding and personal hygiene. The post-operative management following wrist arthrodesis is directed towards protection of the wrist while bony union takes place, as well as maintenance of movement in adjacent joints.

The above are the most commonly performed surgical procedures for the rheumatoid wrist, but there are other procedures that can provide further individual options.

The metacarpophalangeal joint

The goal of surgery at the MCP joints is to maintain or improve function, and this is achieved by relieving pain and preserving joint structures or, in more severe cases, correcting deformity and stabilizing the joint.

Synovectomy

When the joint surfaces are preserved, the operation of choice is synovectomy of the joint and correction of soft tissue deformities. When the joint surfaces have been eroded this is not sufficient to correct the problem, and in this situation MCP joint arthroplasty is indicated.

MCP joint arthroplasty

Various implant designs and materials have been used to reconstruct the MCP joint, ranging from simple metal hinges to more complex metal and ceramic designs (Niebaeur et al., 1968; Flatt and Ellison, 1972; Nicole and Calnan, 1972). These have largely passed out of use, leaving the silicone implant designed by Alfred B. Swanson in the early 1960s as the implant of choice (Swanson and Swanson, 1982). At present various modifications using different materials and slightly different shapes are being used, but none has as yet emerged as pre-eminent.

The MCP joint implant acts as a flexible spacer in the same fashion as the Swanson wrist implants previously described. The physiological process is the same; the implant becomes encapsulated and collagen is formed around it. Similarly, the post-operative management is aimed at achieving a useful arc of movement whilst protecting the soft tissue repairs. Some surgeons perform a crossed intrinsic transfer at the same time as MCP joint arthroplasties; this involves transferring the ulnar intrinsic tendon to the radial side of the adjacent finger and attaching it to the radial collateral ligament. This helps to reinforce the radial collateral ligament and provides some dynamic correction against the tendency towards ulnar deviation, which still exists despite surgery. Whether synovectomy, soft tissue reconstruction or joint replacement is performed, the post-operative management is the same.

The aims of treatment following MCP joint arthroplasty are the same as those following Swanson wrist arthroplasty – to provide a useful arc of movement and protect soft tissue repairs. This is achieved by early controlled movement, which stimulates the formation of a strong but flexible capsule around the implant whilst protecting soft tissue repairs. The current authors' unit subscribes to the method described by Swanson (Swanson and Swanson, 1990), which is early movement controlled by the use of a dynamic splint. There are other methods of treatment (Stothard et al., 1991) that do not use dynamic splints, but no long-term results are available to support these protocols.

Five days post-operatively the patient is fitted with this splint, which is then worn all day before changing to a resting splint at night.

The aims and purpose of the outrigger are to:

1. Maintain the alignment achieved by surgery
2. Protect the soft tissue repairs
3. Correct any residual deformity
4. Provide controlled movement in the plane of flexion/extension, i.e. limiting movement in an ulnar direction
5. Assist extension.

The patient is taught from the earliest possible moment, usually when the resting splint is fitted, to contract the first dorsal interosseous muscle and abduct the index finger, as this is necessary for the re-education of pulp-to-pulp pinch. When the outrigger splint is fitted, the patient continues with this exercise. The patient is now taught to flex the MCP joints. The forearm is placed on a flat table with the fingers free to move over the edge and the MCP joints are then flexed, stretching the elastic bands. Only when they have reached their maximum movement is the patient allowed to flex the interphalangeal joints to attempt to make a fist. This has to be taught very carefully, or the patient will be exercising ineffectively. All joints must be flexed simultaneously at the end of the movement in order to prevent tightness of the extensor tissues.

At all times it must be remembered that the patient has a systemic disease and that other joints are affected. The final total active movement will be affected by the status of all the joints. Some patients, particularly those who have good range of movement at the IP joints, find it very difficult to isolate flexion at the MCP joints. If repeated education and demonstration with assisted active movement do not solve this problem, it may be that the patient's intrinsic muscles are too weak to be able to perform the action. This can be overcome by fitting the patient with removable finger tubes to block movement at the IP joints. The effect of this is twofold; it teaches the patient the required action and it concentrates the power of the long flexors on the MCP joints. These patients should alternate between exercising with the IP blocking splints and without them to maintain as much range of movement as possible in all the joints. When wearing the outrigger splint, the patient is encouraged to practice radial movement of all the fingers to strengthen the radial deviation muscles and is also taught to practice pulp-to-pulp pinch of the index finger to the thumb but without applying pressure.

After 3 weeks the patient still wears the outrigger for most of the time but may remove it three or four times a day to progress the exercise programme, although functional activities are still contraindicated for the affected hand. On removing the outrigger, the patient is taught to lay the hand on a flat table and gently massage the scars (assuming the wound is soundly healed). 'Finger walking' is then performed. This involves moving each finger in turn in a radial direction, starting with the index finger.

The whole hand is then lifted off the table to allow the fingers to relax, and the process started again, thus working the radial intrinsics only. This exercise becomes easier as active extension improves. For the second exercise, the hand is held on its side with the little finger resting on the table and the wrist in slight extension. Starting with the movement at the MCP joints, the fingers are flexed and extended.

At this stage, if flexion is not increasing some stretching force is applied. This can be done by applying manual pressure or by fitting the patient with flexor loops, which they can wear for periods of up to half an hour three times a day. The loop is applied over the proximal phalanx and attached to Velcro on the volar wrist support of the outrigger splint. If the stiffness is extreme, an extension may need to be added to the splint in order to obtain a more satisfactory angle of pull.

The patient continues in the outrigger splint until 6 weeks post-operatively, when an assessment is made. If there is still a tendency to ulnar drift or if the patient has severe disease necessitating the use of immunosuppressive drugs (which alter the rate of collagen maturation), the outrigger may be retained for another 2–3 weeks. If the joints are stable and correction is good, it may be discarded at this stage and some other type of ulnar drift splint provided. Progressive strengthening of the hand by squeezing sponges or using graded therapeutic putty may now begin. The patient is encouraged to begin light functional activities and is taught specific joint protection techniques, which should be practised long term. Patients should already be aware of general principles, but MCP joint specifics need to be reinforced, for example:

- ensure that pulp-to-pulp and tripod pinch grips are used – not key or lateral pinch grips
- *do not* push out of a chair using the fingers – use the forearms wherever possible.
- avoid sustained grip – build up pan handles if necessary to avoid stress on the joints.
- write or knit for short periods only and then rest the hand.

This list is not exhaustive. Once the patient is made aware of the principles, alternative ways of functioning are evident. During 'at risk' activities, patients continue to wear ulnar protection splints.

At the end of the treatment period it is hoped that the patient will have gained a functional grasp, the ability to open the hand wide enough to hold items such as jars and glasses, and the ability to manipulate small objects such as coins or buttons with pulp-to-pulp pinch. Whilst of academic interest, the actual range of movement gained is not as important as the patient's functional achievements.

Proximal interphalangeal joint surgery

The PIP joint is the most difficult joint in the hand to treat. To restore a functional range of movement once injury or disease has attacked it is extremely difficult.

In rheumatoid arthritis, the PIP joint can be affected in a number of ways:

1. The joint surfaces can be destroyed but the joint remains stable, and no complex deformity develops
2. The joint can become unstable laterally, but again with no complex deformity
3. A swan-neck deformity can occur, with or without joint destruction
4. A boutonnière deformity can occur, again with or without joint destruction.

Surgery for the stiff stable joint or laterally unstable joint

For stiff joints, the options are arthrodesis or arthroplasty. If the finger affected is the index or middle finger, the choice is likely to be an arthroplasty with the joint in enough flexion to allow pinch. This is because these two fingers are liable to lateral stresses and there is a high risk of collateral ligament failure if silastic implants are used. For ring and little finger problems, a replacement arthroplasty of the Swanson type can be performed. For joints with lateral instability the same options apply, except that the ability to replace the joint will depend on the possibility or not of satisfactorily repairing the damaged collateral ligament.

PIP joint replacement arthroplasty

As with the MCP joint implants, the PIP implant is a flexible spacer and post-operative management is directed towards the care of the soft tissues involved. Thus the management of Swanson replacements depends on the pre-existing deformity. In the case of the stiff joint, the treatment is directed towards protection of the structures that have been divided in order to gain access to the joint and to protect the collateral ligaments in the healing phase. If the surgeon is confident that the repair of cut structures is sound and the collateral ligaments are stable, early active movement may be started using an MCP blocker splint to localize movement. The patient also has a paddle splint between exercise sessions. However, in practice it has been found that most joints have a tendency towards collateral instability in an ulnar direction, and it is therefore wiser to begin movement within the constraints of an outrigger to prevent the development of deformity. The outrigger splint used is a low profile type, with the dorsal slab extending over the proximal phalanx and the direction of pull at 90° to the middle phalanx. The splint is used for a minimum of 3 weeks, at which time stability is assessed.

When the joint is laterally unstable to begin with and one of the collateral ligaments has to be repaired, it is of paramount importance that this is well protected. In this case the joint is immobilized for 3 weeks. This may be done at surgery with

Kirschner wires. After this period movement can begin, but is controlled by a splint that provides stability in the radial direction.

PIP joint arthrodesis

This is carried out using Kirschner wires, which are retained for around 6 weeks. Usually the joint is arthrodesed in approximately 30° of flexion, and post-operative management is directed at maintaining movement where possible in adjacent joints and helping the patient to re-educate function once the pins are removed.

Swan-neck deformities The treatment of Swan-neck deformities depends on their severity. In early swan-neck deformity where the joint surfaces are not affected and the joint is mobile, tenodesis is suitable. There are a number of tenodesis procedures. The principle is to prevent the joint from fully extending so that the flexor tendons are able to act normally and flex the PIP joint. Whichever technique is chosen, the post-operative management is very similar. When the immediate post-operative dressing is reduced, the hand is placed in a dorsal splint with the wrist in neutral, the MCP joints in about 40° flexion and the PIP joints in 30–40° flexion. The splint is strapped in such a way as to immobilize the MCPs in this position so that the proximal phalanges are held against the splint, thus preventing full extension at the PIP joints. The patient is encouraged to flex the PIP joints and extend them as far as the splint allows. Because of the nature of the deformity it may be that the DIP joint tends to flex first, and in this case a small splint can be taped to the DIP joint to concentrate movement at the PIP joint. In between exercise sessions, the fingers are supported with a wide padded strap.

To maintain movement at the MCP joints, the patient is taught to flex the PIP joints, hold them in flexion, loosen the MCP strap and gently mobilize the MCP joints. If the patient does not fully understand this manoueuvre or is unable to manage it adequately for any other reason, then it must be done by the therapist. It is vital to the success of the operation that the PIP joints are not fully extended until the repaired tissues have had time to heal. The above regime should be followed for 6 weeks. At the end of that time the dorsal splint may be discarded, but the patient may be fitted with ring splints in order to prevent full extension of the joints.

More severe swan-neck deformities, where the integrity of the joint has been damaged and the deformity is becoming fixed, need to be treated by either arthrodesis or arthroplasty.

The management for replacement arthroplasties in the presence of swan-neck deformities is as for tenodesis, and given in detail above.

Boutonnière deformity Early mobile boutonnière deformities can be treated by repairing the central slip of the tendon and thus restoring active extension to the PIP joint. Post-operative treatment depends on the quality of the tissues and the surgeon's judgement regarding the stability of the repair. The choice is between:

- resting the fingers in extension at the PIP joints with the DIPs free for 3 weeks and then mobilizing in a PIP outrigger
- mobilizing after 3–4 days in a outrigger.

Whichever one of these is chosen, the fingers should either be protected in extension or have assisted extension for a minimum of 6 weeks.

Because of the nature of the boutonnière deformity, it is important to mobilize the DIP joints into flexion as soon as possible. Some surgeons carry out a tenotomy of the distal tendon, known as a Dolphin procedure, to release the hyperextension at the DIP joint.

Late stage boutonnière deformities, where the joint surfaces are destroyed and contractures have formed, are difficult to treat successfully. The choices are once again fusion or replacement, and the choice between these depends on the possibility of restoring first passive then active extension, and on which finger is involved.

If the index or middle fingers are affected, arthrodesis may be the operation of choice in the interests of stability, as explained above. The ring and little fingers can have replacement performed, assuming that the collateral ligaments are intact and it is possible to repair the extensor mechanism.

The post-operative management of Swanson arthroplasties for boutonni'ere deformities is directed towards the protection of the repaired extensor mechanism. This is the same as for the repair of a boutonnière deformity as described above.

Surgery to the thumb

When planning a surgical programme for the thumb, all the complex factors mentioned earlier must be taken into consideration. Rheumatoid arthritis affects multiple joints and is also progressive, this may be stating the obvious after all that has gone before in these chapters, but it is particularly relevant when considering surgery to the thumb. Surgery taking place now should not compromise function, and nor should it limit future options. For example, arthrodesis of the CMC joint may seem a viable option if the other two joints are healthy, but function will be severely limited if at a later date the IP or MCP joints become unstable and require arthrodesis. It is much better to replace the CMC joint and preserve some movement in it, however limited.

Correction of the 'boutonnière' deformity of the thumb

This deformity normally originates at the MCP joint, so correction starts here as well. The most usual treatment is to arthrodese this joint in a neutral position. If the deformity is not severe, the IP joint will automatically correct when the MCP joint is stable. If this does not occur, it may be necessary to perform either replacement arthroplasty or tenodesis of this joint to correct or prevent recurrence of the hyperextension. Rupture of the FPL tendon can mimic this deformity. This should be treated either by grafting of the tendon or by arthrodesis of the IP joint. Tendon grafting is preferable if the IP joint is intact, as it restores power to pulp-to-pulp pinch.

Correction of 'swan-neck' deformity of the thumb

This deformity usually originates at the CMC joint, and so correction begins here. As explained above, it is essential to retain or restore movement at this joint to preserve the unique function of the thumb.

CMC arthroplasty

There are a number of different techniques available for replacing or excising this joint. They are all aimed at correcting the adduction deformity and restoring some movement at the CMC joint. The hyperextension at the MCP joint must be corrected at the same time, otherwise the deformity will recur. This can be done by tenodesis, replacement or fusion, depending on the condition of the joint.

The post-operative management following all the techniques for replacing the CMC joint is very similar.

The thumb is immobilized in a scaphoid-type plaster extending from above the wrist to the IP joint of the thumb for 3–6 weeks. When this is removed the patient is fitted with a thermoplastic splint, which is removed several times a day to carry out mobilizing exercises.

At this stage, the aims of treatment are to:

1. Restore movement in the CMC joint, particularly abduction and opposition
2. Restore movement to the MCP joint of the thumb
3. Mobilize the scar – an adherent scar can restrict movement and cause tension on the terminal branch of the radial nerve.

No surgery for the rheumatoid patient can return normal function once the disease has done its worst. The real solution lies in finding a way of preventing the tissue damage in the first place, by discovering a medical means of curing or preventing the disease itself. Until this happens, surgery and the all-important post-operative therapy will continue to play a vital part in maintaining and improving the patients' quality of life.

REFERENCES

Bengston, K. A. and Schutt, A. H. (1994). Rehabilitation of the rheumatoid hand. *Physical Medicine & Rehab. Clinics of N. America*, **5(4)**, 729–45.

Bieber, E. J., Linscheid, R. L., Dobyns, J. H. and Beckenbaugh, R. D. (1988). Failed distal ulna resections. *J. Hand Surg.* **13A(2)**, 193–200.

Darrach, W. (1913). Partial excision of the distal end of the ulna for deformity following Colles fracture. *Ann. Surg.*, **57**, 764–5.

Flatt, A. E. and Elison, M. R. (1972). Restoration of Rheumatoid Finger Function III. *J. Bone and Joint Surg.*, **54A**, 1317–22.

Mannerfelt, L. G. (1987). Timing in surgery of the rheumatoid hand. *Rheumatology an Annual Review*, **11**, 3–5.

Nalebuff, E. A. (1984). The rheumatoid hand: reflections on metacarpophalangeal arthroplasty. *Clinical Orthopaedics and Related Research*, **182**, 150–9.

Neer, C. S., Watson, K. C. and Stanton, F. J. (1982). Recent experience in total shoulder replacement. *J. Bone and Joint Surg.*, **64A(3)**, 319–37.

Nicole, F. V. and Calnan, J. S. (1972). A new design of finger joint prosthesis for the rheumatoid hand. *The Hand*, **4**, 135–46.

Niebauer, J. J., Shaw, J. L. and Doren, W. W. (1968). The silicone dacron hinge prosthesis. *J. Bone and Joint Surg.*, **50A**, 634.

Small, J. O., Brennan, M. D. and Colville, J. (1989). Early active mobilisation following flexor tendon repair in zone 2. *J .Hand Surg.*, **14B**, 383–91.

Stothard, J., Thompson A. E. and Sherris, D. (1991). Correction of ulnar drift during silastic metacarpophalangeal joint arthroplasty, *J. Hand Surg.*, **16B(1)**, 61–5.

Strickland, J. W. (1989). Flexor tendon surgery part 2 free tendon grafts and tenolysis. *J. Hand Surg.*, **14B**, 368–82.

Souter, W. A. (1979) Planning the treatment of the rheumatoid hand. *The Hand*, **1(1)**, 3–16.

Swanson, A. B. (1969). Finger joint replacement by silicone rubber implants and the concept of implant fixation by encapsulation. *Ann. Rheum. Dis.*, **28(5)**, Suppl, 47–55.

Swanson, A. B., Swanson, G. and de Groot, Leonard J. (1982). Joint replacement in the rheumatoid metacarpophalangeal joint. In: *Inglis AAOS Symposium on Total Joint Replacement of the Upper Extremity*, pp. 217–37. Mosby.

Swanson, A. B., Swanson, G., de Groot, Leonard, J. and Boozer, J. (1990). Postoperative rehabilitation programmes in flexible implant arthroplasty of the digits. In: *Rehabilitation of the Hand*, 3rd edn. Hunter Schneider Mackin and Callahan (eds.), pp. 912–28. C. V. Mosby.

Terrono, A. L., Feldon, P. G., Hills, W., Millender L. H. and Nalebuff, E. A. (1995). Evaluation and treatment of the rheumatoid wrist, *J. Bone and Joint Surg.*, **77A(7)**, 1116–26.

Tyson, K., Beckenbaugh, R. D. and Rochester (1996). Biaxial total-wrist arthroplasty. *J. Hand Surg.*, **21A(6)**, 1011–21.

Van Strien, G. (1990). Postoperative management of flexor tendon injuries. In: *Rehabilitation of the Hand*, 3rd edn. Hunter Schneider Mackin and Callahan (eds), pp. 390–409. C. V. Mosby.

16 Upper limb splinting for rheumatoid arthritis

Sheila Lawton

The management of rheumatoid arthritis (RA) is complex and includes many types of treatment that have to be fitted into a patient's lifestyle so they can continue functioning with a good quality of life.

ROLE OF SPLINTING

Splinting is just one aspect of treatment which plays a vital role in maintaining joint position and function, and it must be tailored individually according to the changing needs of the patient throughout the many years of disease.

With modern treatment, splinting plays a less dominant role than in the past because:

- synovitis is controlled more quickly by effective drugs and local corticosteroid injections, which prevents the long-term stretching of soft tissues round joints that leads to poor control of joint posture
- the role of active physiotherapy at the onset of disease is recognized, with specific precise hand exercises taught to counteract deformity
- joint protection techniques are taught early to limit stress while functioning
- appropriate surgery is undertaken early while joints and soft tissues are mobile.

Essentially, splints for the rheumatoid arthritic should be few in number and as simple as possible, and patients should be given a say in what they need and when they will be worn. Splints should if possible be supplied early in the course of the disease, before deformities are seen. Pain, soft tissue swelling and joint instability are the main indications for splinting, as they cause weakness and poor joint posture, which then endangers other distal joints.

AIMS OF SPLINTING FOR RA

The aims of splinting for rheumatoid arthritis are to:

1. Rest a joint where there is active synovitis and/or pain
2. Support a joint when muscles are weak or the joint is unstable, in order to reduce pain and improve function in adjacent joints and general stamina
3. Prevent or reduce the rate of deformities occurring, by splinting early and maintaining the correct length of soft tissues through very careful positioning of each joint
4. Counteract existing deformity to enhance function while the splint is worn
5. Mobilize a joint by providing lateral stability or controlled resistance to movement to encourage increased range of movement, usually following surgery.

PRINCIPLES OF SPLINTING FOR RA

- Always bear in mind the normal progression of deformities that are likely to occur, and splint early.
- Static splints are not worn continuously for 24 hours. They are removed for exercise and often alternated with other splints. Post-surgery is occasionally the exception.
- A corrective moulding technique should always be used when making a splint.
- The splint must maintain or correct alignment as well as control the flexion or extension of every joint.
- Metacarpophalangeal (MCP) joints should normally be splinted in extension and the proximal interphalangeal (PIP) joints slightly flexed to provide an opportunity for stretched collateral ligaments to shrink.
- Subluxation of the wrist and MCP joints must be counteracted by definite support under the carpus and proximal phalanges, with an opposing force supplied by straps over the distal end of forearm and dorsum of metacarpals. A strap must never be placed over the carpus as it could cause subluxation.
- Thumb lateral instability at the MCP and interphalangeal (IP) joints is common, so splints should not apply lateral forces to the medial aspect of the thumb. Correct splint patterns are essential.
- The thumb should be splinted abducted and in opposition to the index finger to prevent the common metacarpal adduction deformity and also maintain the ability to pinch.
- If possible, straps should not be applied over painful joints or the ulnar styloid.

POSITIONING OF THE RHEUMATOID PATIENT WHEN SPLINTING

- Sit the patient in a supportive chair to aid comfort and relaxation.
- Support the forearm and hand at a comfortable height for the patient, and at right angles to his or her body.
- Place a soft pad under a painful elbow or when forearm nodules are present.
- Work with the arm pronated, never supinated, as this twisted position will give incorrect splint

conformity and alignment of the limb cannot be seen.

• The therapist must work in front of the patient, looking down the forearm. This enables correct alignment of the limb to be seen throughout the splinting process.

SUITABILITY OF MATERIALS

• Materials must be strong enough to control the position and prevent the contracting forces. Reinforcement under the wrist or individual fingers may be necessary.
• Materials must be long lasting, washable and capable of regular alteration to accommodate fluctuations in the joint state.
• Materials must be as lightweight as possible because of weakness.
• Enclosed splints require a material that will spring open easily, i.e.1.5 mm Vitrathene; 1.5 mm Orfit or X-Lite (maximum two layers).
• Draping materials are difficult to use, as they distort when applying pressure to correct the posture. The material thins under the pressure, and therefore becomes weak in the place where strength is required. Smoothing materials while warm by stroking to get a good finish is not good technique, as it requires releasing the grip on the patient, which may cause pain and loss of the original corrected position.
• Padding may be required for bony prominences or nodules, although normally the splint material should be stretched sufficiently to relieve pressure.
• Linings to splints are occasionally needed for friable steroid skin that bruises easily, and to relieve sweating or irritation. Unless the lining is as thin as paper, it should be applied before moulding the splint to ensure that splint conformity is not distorted.

Suppliers of materials are listed in Appendix A.

TYPES OF SPLINTS

There are four main types of splint:

1. Static splints are most commonly used either as a slab or an enclosed splint.
2. Dynamic splints without resistance in the direction of movement, usually hinged.
3. Dynamic splints with resisted movement achieved by pulling against elastic or spring steel wire. These splints are contraindicated for joints with active synovitis, as the resistance will increase joint swelling, and are normally used post-surgery.
4. Custom-made splints are most commonly used, as the rheumatoid has abnormal posture of joints and specialized requirements.

Prefabricated splints

Remember that arthritis causes distortion and hands are therefore not normal in shape, so great care needs to be taken in correct selection, size and fitting of prefabricated splints. Prefabricated splints can be categorized into five groups:

1. Wrist braces in extension. There are various types of these, which can be used in the early stages of disease where only a little support is required (Ball and Penton, 1994). Most are elastic with a metal bar on the palmar surface, which must be bent to fit the patient correctly. Ensure that MCP joint flexion is not restricted. Neoprene wrist braces are softer and weaker, but can be cut to the required shape round the thumb and at the MCP level.
2. Swan-neck ring splints for day wear, made of silver or other metal. These are not suitable for pronounced deformity.
3. Boutonnière ring splints. These are only usable where the PIP joint is easily passively extended.
4. MCP joint ulnar drift splints. There are various types such as in the Rolyan and North Coast range: wrist braces with soft lateral finger support allowing some flexion and extension; static splints in Wire–foam which realign the MCP joints only; and hinged MCP joint hand splints to allow flexion and extension.
5. Hand rest splints, static, with fingers separated by spacers correcting MCP joint ulnar drift. Selection of the correct thumb support is essential.

SPLINT FASTENINGS

• Buckles, stiff materials and press studs are contraindicated.
• Velcro is ideal. The top piece of Velcro must be longer then the base piece so the patient can grip it to pull open. A loop can be sewn onto the end of the Velcro to enable a finger to be slotted through and eliminate pinch.
• Where a strap needs to be done up tightly or to close an enclosed splint, use a rectangular loop so the Velcro can be threaded through and folded back on itself. An ideal loop is the Zytel nylon D-shaped type, which stands up while being threaded.
• Soft foam strapping is available, i.e. SoftStrap, for use on sensitive areas and after surgery where oedema is present.

HANDLING THE RHEUMATOID ARTHRITIC PATIENT

Remember that this is a painful condition, and the skin may be fragile and the patient easily bruised.

Always handle patients very gently and do not touch them unnecessarily. Do not press on the joints or make any sudden movements. A slow sustained stretch can be given, but never release this quickly. Joints should be slowly moved in one plane and then corrected into alignment, and never twisted. When the desired position has been achieved this must not be released until the splint has hardened, otherwise the patient will experience discomfort and positioning may be lost.

EXAMINATION AND ASSESSMENT

This comprises four aspects; observe, examine, ask and test.

1. Observe for:
   - colour, type of skin and bruises
   - obvious swellings at the joints, dorsal sheath and carpal tunnel areas
   - thickened palms and loss of the palmar arch
   - subluxation of the ulnar styloid, carpus and MCP joints
   - deformities, both flexion and extension and alignment
   - bony enlargement of joints
   - nodules on the forearm or hands
   - vasculitic lesions around the finger nails
   - muscle wasting.
2. Examine:
   - all joints for swelling, minimal or pronounced
   - palms – soft or firm; skin mobile or tight
   - for flexor tendon involvement, firm proximal phalangeal pulps; for flexor tendon nodules, locking of finger joint and lateral laxity due to tendon slippage
   - for subluxation, including springing ulnar styloid
   - for lax collateral ligaments – i.e. the finger will move sideways when MCP joint is held flexed
   - for intrinsic tightness – i.e. inability to flex the PIP joints when the MCP joints are held in extension
   - for shortened ulnar intrinsics – i.e. an inability to flex the PIP joints when the MCP joints are held with ulnar drift corrected
   - for partial or total rupture of a tendon, particularly the extensor tendon – the test for a ruptured extensor pollicis longus is an inability to flex the IP joint when the thumb is held abducted
   - the ability of the patient to relax the muscles.
3. Ask the patient:
   - to move all the joints in turn through the full range, starting with the shoulder
   - about pain – in which joints it occurs, and if it is made worse by certain positions, functions or time (i.e. morning stiffness)
   - about weakness
   - about numbness or pins and needles. Consider nerve compression at carpal tunnel, elbow or neck
   - what function is inhibited and why
   - what he/she wants from splinting.
4. Test:
   - practical items of function, and note any instability, incorrect posture, limitation of range or increase in deformities when the joints are loaded; listen to the patient regarding pain and weakness
   - grip strength if liked, though results can vary enormously from day to day and morning to afternoon
   - joint ranges, and record the outcomes – this is important if the splint to be made is designed to improve range of movement.

DECIDING ON APPROPRIATE SPLINTING FOR THE RHEUMATOID ARTHRITIC

The patient should have:

1. A long-term static prophylactic splint for involved joints to wear at night if:
   - the patient has been started on a disease-modifying drug, indicating aggressive disease and a sero-positive rheumatoid factor
   - there is obvious joint swelling, particularly of wrist and/or MCP joints, as deformity is likely to occur when the swelling subsides and leaves the surrounding tissues lax; continuing the splint after subsidence is therefore vital
   - deformity is present, to prevent the soft tissues tightening further and the deformity increasing; splints can often be serialized over months or years to increase joint range or improve alignment.
2. A static splint to support an individual joint during the day if:
   - joint pain and/or muscle weakness are inhibiting function, particularly in the wrist
   - a joint that is essential for function is unstable – i.e. thumb MCP joint
   - there is nerve compression at the carpal tunnel – the wrist should be extended
   - surgery is planned, in order to maintain function.
3. A dynamic splint without resistance to an individual joint for day wear if:
   - there is loss of elbow function due to a painful, unstable and destroyed joint
   - MCP joint ulnar drift is inhibiting function and surgery is contraindicated, but the patient is motivated to use the hand

- a swan-neck deformity is snapping or starting to stick in hyperextension, or causing excess pain when functioning.
4. A dynamic splint with resistance for:
   - an extensor tendon which has become stretched, to provide assisted extension for at least 6 weeks
   - post-surgery cases, particularly MCP joint arthroplasties.

All the day splints in points 2 and 3 above should be worn according to patients' needs, and removed when not necessary.

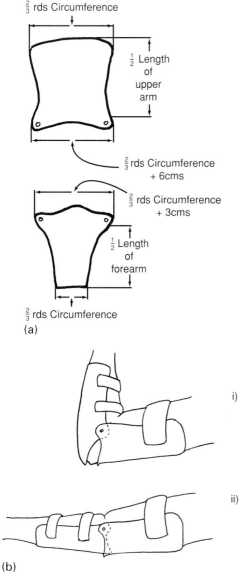

$\frac{2}{3}$ rds Circumference

$\frac{1}{2}$ Length of upper arm

$\frac{2}{3}$ rds Circumference + 6cms

$\frac{2}{3}$ rds Circumference + 3cms

$\frac{1}{2}$ Length of forearm

$\frac{2}{3}$ rds Circumference
(a)

i)

ii)

(b)

Figure 16.1 (a) Pattern for hinged elbow splint. (b) Hinged elbow splint: (i) flexed, (ii) extended. Note that the forearm section provides protection to the tip of the olecranon process.

ELBOW SPLINTS FOR RA

Elastic splints

Prefabricated supports can be useful if the elbow joint is markedly swollen. The Arthropad, being padded with gentle pressure, provides good comfort, while an elastic splint will provide more support. Ideally this should be the type with straps so that it is not pulled onto the arm. These splints should only be worn intermittently because of the pressure.

Static splints

These splints are only appropriate for night wear, and should be in the position of comfort, usually about 90° flexion and in mid-pronation/supination.

Hinged elbow splints

These splints are used for painful destroyed joints, and usually give exceptional reduction of pain and provide lateral stability without any restriction in range of movement. Function of the arm is immediately improved. The splint should be worn as much as the patient feels necessary, as it can do no harm. Patients normally only remove it for washing. The splint is made out of 1.5 mm Vitrathene with 3 mm Plastazote lining; this makes it very light, durable and capable of accommodating various thickness' of garments.

The splint comprises two short backslabs hinged together at the elbow with plastic rivets (Figure 16.1). The forearm slab supports the elbow to the tip of the olecranon process when the elbow is flexed to 90°, thus providing protection to the joint, and should slide under the lipped distal end of the humeral slab to allow full elbow extension. The forearm section is moulded first in the neutral position. The rivets must be directly opposite each other and positioned midway between the epicondyle and end of the elbow crease.

Check that:

- flexion, extension, pronation and supination are not restricted
- there is no pressure on the humeral condyles or forearm nodules
- wrist movements are not inhibited.

A wrist splint can be worn in conjunction with the elbow splint, and it should be moulded to fit over the elbow forearm slab.

HAND RESTING SPLINT

This is worn at night and during daytime rest periods. Usually only one splint is worn at a time so the patient is not too restricted (Figure 16.2).

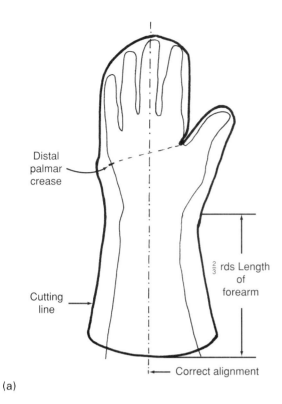

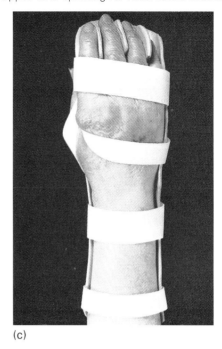

(c)

(a)

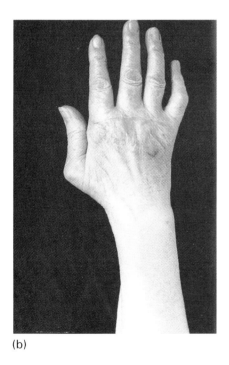

(b)

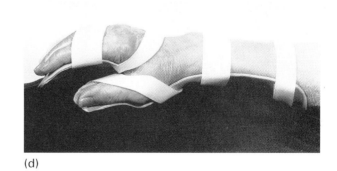

(d)

Figure 16.2 (a) Pattern for hand rest splint. Note that the slot at thumb web is essential to allow thumb to be placed in opposition and for a strap to correct alignment. (b) Hand showing Z thumb deformity and early recurrence of third MCP joint ulnar drift 6 years after Swanson's arthroplasty. (c) Hand rest splint showing diagonal thumb strapping to hold metacarpal in abduction and extend MCP joint. Finger alignment is corrected by finger spacers, with counteracting force from strap originating in thumb web. (d) Hand rest splint showing thumb abduction and good extension of finger MCP joints to stretch the flexor soft tissues and prevent subluxation.

The aims of the splint are:

1. To rest the joints in correct alignment
2. To prevent soft tissues contracting in the long term.

Positioning

Wrist

- The wrist is in a comfortable position of neutral or slight extension with radial drift corrected.
- The carpus is supported and its arch maintained.
- The strap presses down on the distal end of the radius and ulna, and never over the carpus, which could sublux.
- The strap originating from the thumb web maintains wrist alignment.

Palm The palmar arch is supported. To achieve this, sufficient space must be allowed for the thenar eminence.

MCP joints

- These are in comfortable maximum extension to neutral, to stretch the palmar soft tissues and counteract any tendency to subluxation.
- Ulnar drift is corrected to the maximum tolerated, and the position is maintained by providing support to the ulnar border of each finger and not just to the fifth. The fingers should not be squashed together, as fingers normally separate as the MCP joints extend.
- The strap originating from the thumb web and passing over the metacarpals is essential to maintain the finger alignment and MCP joint extension.

PIP joints

- These are flexed to 25–30°.
- Lateral drift, if present, is corrected with finger spacers.
- If there is swan-neck deformity, the PIP joints are flexed to 45° and a strap is applied to press down over the middle and distal phalanges.
- If there is Boutonnière deformity, the PIP joints are extended to the maximum tolerated and a strap applied to press down over the proximal phalanges. Ensure that the distal interphalangeal (DIP) joint is not hyperextended.

DIP joints The DIP joints are in a neutral or slightly flexed position.

Thumb

- The thumb is in the functional position, with the metacarpal abducted and in opposition.

- The thumb is supported on the palmar aspect (Figure 16.2). Do not apply medial pressure to the MCP joint or IP joint, as this can increase the likelihood of lateral instability.
- The MCP and IP joints are correctly aligned, and this position is supported along the lateral border.
- Care must be taken to mould carefully around the thenar eminence, otherwise pressure on this will reduce palmar arch support.
- If a Z deformity is present (i.e. MCP joint flexed and IP joint hyperextended), the position is corrected and held with a diagonal strap pressing down over the first metacarpal (Figure 16.2).

Options

1. Exclude the thumb if it is not a problem. This enables both splints to be worn at night as it allows some function.
2. Leave the fingers free from the PIP joints.
3. Exclude the forearm if the wrist is not a problem.
4. Isotoner gloves are useful for reducing swelling. They allow movement of all joints, but do not control their position, and only apply one pressure. Purpose-made pressure gloves by Jobst in England can provide two grades of pressure (Ellis, 1984).

Problems

1. If the ulnar styloid is painful, place the strap proximal or use diagonal strapping.
2. If there are nodules, stretch the splint to relieve the pressure or pad the strap with a cut-away section for the nodule.
3. If skin is fragile, use a soft lining on the splint when moulding and soft foam strapping.
4. If sweating is a problem, use alternative material such as X-Lite or Fractomed, which breathes, or supply cotton stockinette to use between the splint and skin.
5. If there are deformed fingers in different positions, cut the splint between each finger and then mould it to each finger in the best possible position and alignment.
6. If there are tight intrinsics and subluxed MCP joints, the patient will tend to lift off the palm and move distally up the splint. Ensure that this is prevented by the dorsal metacarpal hand strap originating from the thumb web.
7. If there is insufficient rigidity, reinforce the splint under the wrist and fingers.

The resting splint should be viewed as an essential long-term prophylactic splint, where comfort, accurate fit and corrective positioning are paramount. Patients must be seen regularly for checking and modifications; every 6 months, or earlier if their condition changes.

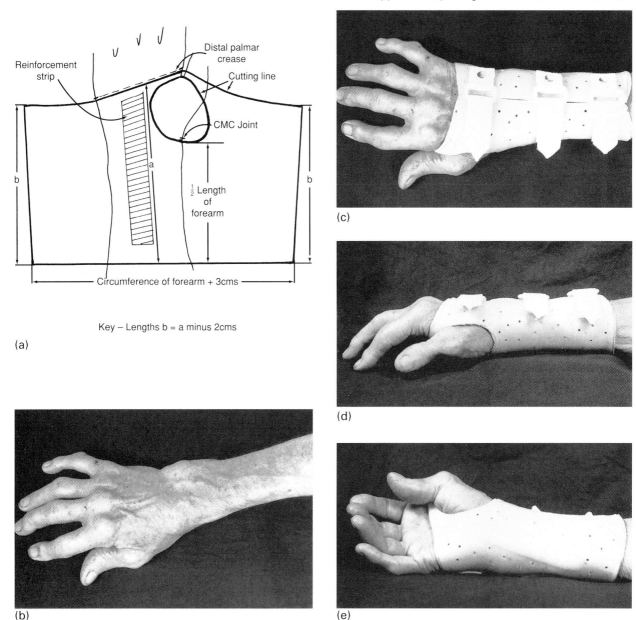

Figure 16.3 (a) Pattern for enclosed wrist splint made in 1.5 mm Vitrathene and 3 mm Plastazote. (b) Hand showing swelling at wrist and ulnar styloid with obvious forearm muscle wasting. (c) Enclosed wrist day splint showing the careful shaping over the ulnar styloid and looped straps to close the splint edges. Note that the splint finishes proximal to the MCP joints. (d) Lateral view showing wrist extension and splint lipped out at proximal palmar edge. (e) Accurate fit on palm maintains arch while allowing full finger flexion, and thumb movement from the carpometacarpal joint.

WRIST SPLINT

This is a static splint to be worn during the day when working to relieve pain, support the wrist and improve grip strength and stamina (Figure 16.3). It is particularly suitable for patients in the later stage with joint erosions, subluxation, poor alignment or instability, as it supplies exceptional

control of posture if made correctly and remarkable comfort (Lawton, 1974).

The splint should be removed for light activities to maintain wrist movement and muscle power. It can be worn at night to relieve pain on the alternate hand to the resting splint.

The splint should totally enclose the wrist to maintain correct position, prevent flexion when functioning and yet be comfortable by distributing pressure. Keep the splint small; the maximum length is half the length of the forearm. The most suitable material is 1.5 mm Vitrathene with 3 mm perforated Plastazote lining.

Positioning

- The wrist is in comfortable extension, maximum 30°. To maintain wrist extension, pressure should be down on the forearm and not on the carpus or ulnar styloid.
- Radial drift is corrected to neutral alignment.
- The carpus is supported and its arch maintained.
- The palmar arch is supported.
- The thenar eminence is completely free to allow full opposition and extension of the thumb.
- The MCP joints are completely free to fully flex and extend. The splint must end 0.5 cm proximal to the distal palmar crease, and proximal to the metacarpal heads on the dorsum.
- The section in the thumb web must be kept narrow and accurately shaped to the second metacarpal to allow free thumb and index movements.

Options

1. A palmar wrist extension slab splint may be used, although this is not normally comfortable enough for the rheumatoid patient.
2. An elastic prefabricated wrist brace is only suitable in the early stages of the disease. The type with D-ring fastening and extra padding can provide good comfort with moderate support. The metal bar must be bent to fit the patient correctly.
3. A dorsal slab splint with a wide 5-cm strap under the carpus will provide support, and a shaped palm bar will maintain the palmar arch.

Problems

1. If the palm is covered and the splint interferes with function, make the splint with ulnar reinforcement and cut a hole away in the palm, leaving a thin arched bar at the distal end. Alternatively, try the dorsal slab splint.
2. If there is ulnar styloid pressure when supinating, stretch the splint on the lateral aspect to relieve the pressure. Never add extra padding, as this will increase the pressure.
3. If there is variable swelling, use the adjustable straps and enlarge the thumb hole on the dorsum.
4. If the patient's work situation causes excessive heat or the need to sterilize the splint, use Vitrathene and supply a second splint and two sets of removable straps.
5. If there is breakage at the thumb web area due to using the splint with a walking stick, reinforce

this area when making the splint or replace the section with a piece of leather riveted in position.

MCP JOINT ULNAR DRIFT CORRECTION SPLINTS

Normally the night rest splint should be sufficient to maintain length of soft tissues and alignment. Most patients also require wrist day splints as a priority to enhance function, so day splinting to the MCP joints in the early stages is usually not feasible. However soft prefabricated types can be tried (see p. 294).

When wrist splints are not needed, a small hand splint with a hinged bar to correct the ulnar drift can be used if the patient particularly feels the need due to pain, and if subluxation of the MCP joints has not occurred (Houchin and Cheshire, 1971). The patient should be referred for a surgical opinion.

Static palmar ulnar drift correction splint

This is a useful splint in the later stages of disease when MCP subluxation has occurred, the joint movement is limited, and when finger contact with thumb is difficult (Figure 16.4). Other indications include:

- marked pain in the MCP joints
- the fourth and fifth fingers becoming knocked or caught in items during function
- a patient who is not a candidate for surgery.

Positioning

- The ulnar drift is corrected to the maximum possible by supporting the proximal phalanges on the ulnar side with a counteracting pressure at the first dorsal interrosseus.
- The MCP joints are flexed.
- The palmar arch is maintained.
- There is no restriction to flexion of the PIP joints.
- Active MCP joint extension is possible by making the finger supports straight.

This splint is quick to make, robust, easy for the patient to apply and remove, and has good comfort and acceptability. Keep the palm section as small as possible, and ensure the edges between the fingers are perfectly smooth.

Options

1. Only include the fingers causing a problem.
2. Use a dorsal splint of the same design, but this will restrict extension.
3. Use a soft prefabricated type (Goldsmith, 1996).

Problems

If there is pressure on the second MCP joint or second metacarpal, lip the splint out at the joint and mould with padding over the metacarpal.

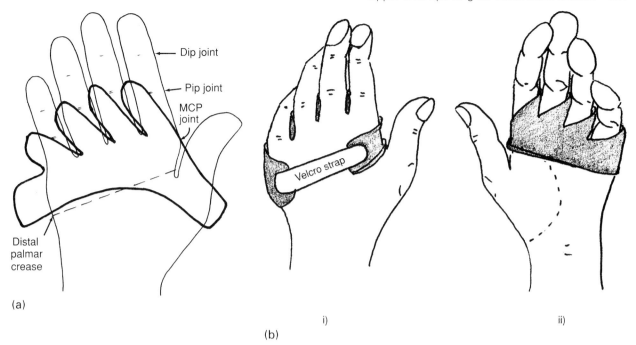

Figure 16.4 (a) Pattern for static palmar finger ulnar drift correction splint. (b) Static palmar finger ulnar drift splint: (i) dorsal view showing fingers realigned, (ii) palmar view showing no restriction to thumb or PIP joints.

SWAN-NECK CORRECTION SPLINTS

At night the hand rest splint should be used with the PIP joints flexed to 45° and a distal finger strap placed over the PIP joints. Ensure the MCP joints are supported in maximum extension.

The day splint allows full flexion without resistance, but prevents hyperextension of the PIP joint (Figure 16.5). Use thin material, preferably 1.5 mm Orfit, which will remain strong despite being stretched. The finger is pushed through the holes in the order indicated in the pattern.

Indications include:

- finger snapping from extension to flexion at the PIP joint and causing pain
- the PIP joint starting to lock in extension, although flexion is possible.

These splints are not suitable for the advanced case with rigidity and no active flexion.

Positioning
- The PIP joint is flexed to 15°.
- The palmar bar is positioned at the PIP joint or slightly proximal. If it is placed distal to the joint, the splint will tend to slip off.
- The splint sides must be flattened and not rub on adjacent fingers, or catch an adjacent splint.

Options
- Make a figure-of-eight splint, crossing under the PIP joint, using a 0.5 cm wide strip of thermoplastic.

- Use a static dorsal gutter splint with a strap only round the proximal phalanx; this will then allow flexion.
- Use silver rings (see page 294).

Problems
1. If the extension push is too strong, use a thicker material or use the figure-of-eight method.
2. If an enlarged bony PIP joint prevents the splint being pushed onto the finger, widening the splint may cause the splint to become loose and allow extension. The dorsal gutter splint can be tried.

BOUTONNIÈRE CORRECTION SPLINTS

Use the night rest splint to hold the PIP joint in maximum extension, or a single finger gutter can be used and gradually serialized over months. Day splints are not normally applicable, as they prevent grip and function. Occasionally a gentle dynamic spring wire splint (e.g. Capener) can be used if there is no active synovitis at the PIP joint.

THUMB DAY SPLINTS

MCP joint splint

This splint (Figure 16.6) is used to:

- counteract a Z deformity Nalebuff type 1 (MCP flexion and IP hyperextension) to facilitate a power pinch

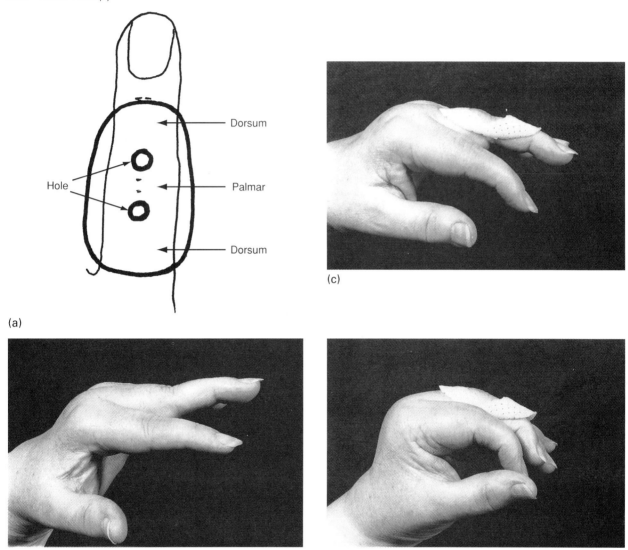

Figure 16.5 (a) Pattern for swan-neck splint. (b) Swan neck deformity of middle finger in patient with long-standing active disease and limited flexion. (c) Swan-neck splint correcting hyperextension. (d) Flexion of PIP joint not restricted by splint.

- provide lateral support to MCP joint that is unstable.

It is made from 1.5 mm thermoplastic, preferably Orfit.

Position
- The MCP joint is in maximum comfortable extension, up to 5°of flexion.
- Lateral drift is corrected into alignment and supported by deep sides to the phalanx gutter, and the splint extended round the thenar eminence (Figure 16.6a).
- A strap round the wrist maintains the splint in position.

- The thumb is threaded through the hole so the proximal phalanx is supported on the palmar surface, and the sides of the splint are bent dorsally.

Options
Fully enclose the proximal phalanx. This splint may be difficult for the patient to apply if the IP joint is swollen, and widening the opening will reduce correction of MCP joint.

Never use a splint that goes round the back of the hand in a C-shape to the hypothenar eminence for a rheumatoid patient, as this will restrict the carpometacarpal joint movement and increase the likelihood of metacarpal adduction deformity.

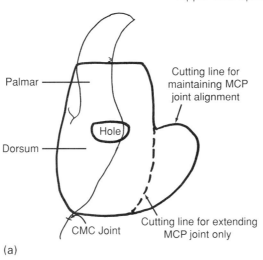

(a)

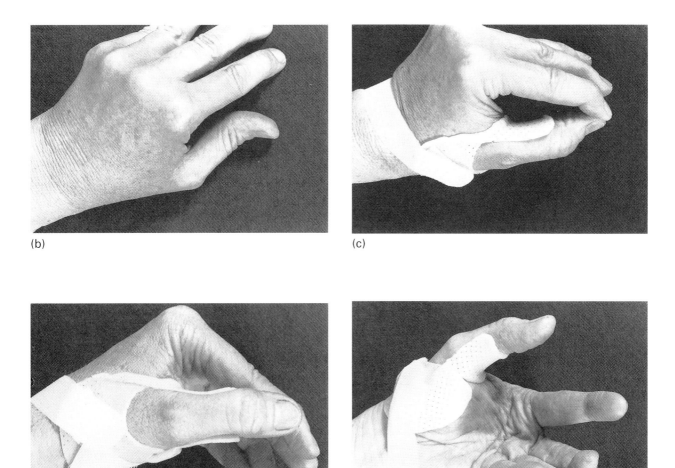

(b)

(c)

(d)

(e)

Figure 16.6 (a) Pattern for thumb MCP joint splint. (b) Z deformity of thumb, Nalebuff Type 1. (c) Thumb MCP joint flexion corrected and strength of pinch improved. (d) Dorsal view showing lateral support to proximal phalanx. (e) Palmar view showing splint over thenar eminence in order to hold alignment of the MCP joint and prevent the splint slipping dorsally.

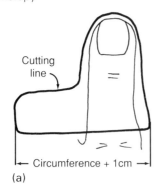

Cutting line

Circumference + 1cm

(a)

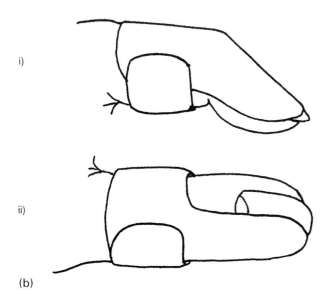

i)

ii)

(b)

Figure 16.7 (a) Pattern to support thumb IP joint. (b) Thumb IP joint support splint: (i) positioned dorsally to prevent hyperextension, (ii) positioned laterally to prevent lateral drift.

Thumb IP joint splint

This is used when the IP joint is laterally unstable and/or hyperextends excessively when pinching, so power is markedly reduced (Figure 16.7).

It is made from 1.5 mm thermoplastic.

Positioning
- The alignment is corrected and maintained with lateral support. The splint is placed on the lateral border when moulding.
- The IP joint is flexed 15° and maintained with the splint placed dorsally when moulding.

The enclosed proximal phalanx design eliminates the need for a strap, which reduces bulk. If the ends are overlapped but not sealed, it can be sprung over an enlarged IP joint. This splint must allow full IP flexion and leave the thumb pulp completely free for pinching.

DYNAMIC SPLINTS

These can be of various designs; high or low profile, and fixed to a dorsal slab, a palmar slab or an enclosed wrist splint with an ulnar opening. The latter is the most comfortable for the patient, and this should be considered when the splint is required for long-term use. The palmar splint is preferable to the dorsal as it supports the carpus and palmar arch and provides a firm base to flex the fingers down against, thus aiding mobilization of the MCP joints.

Stretched extensor tendons

Tendons can become thin and fragile due to the rheumatic disease and to rubbing against uneven bone. This causes one or more fingers to drop down, and if the tendon is still intact and not ruptured, prophylactic dynamic splinting should be tried so that surgery may be avoided.

The fingers must all be supported as soon as possible to prevent further tendon stretching or complete rupture. Ensure that the patient has a night hand rest splint with the finger fully supported and the MCP joint extended to neutral.

Dynamic day splint

Select the type of wrist support, preferably enclosed. Dynamic extension must be supplied to all the fingers to hold the MCP joints in neutral when relaxed. All the extensor tendons will be weak and vulnerable and must therefore be safeguarded.

The overhead bar or spring steel wire providing the finger elevation can be fixed on with rivets and caps to the splint base, so that the pull is at right angles to the MCP joint.

The splint should be worn all the day for at least 6 weeks. Often active extension is then regained and surgery is no longer indicated. In this case, the splint is gradually weaned off over a further 3–6 weeks.

Post-MCP joint arthroplasty splint

Usually all four finger MCP joints will be replaced at the same time, but even if only one joint is replaced the splint is normally the same.

The regime following MCP joint arthroplasty will be governed by the surgeon's preferences, but normally a dynamic MCP joint extension splint is applied within 1 week of surgery and continued for 6 weeks to allow healing of the joint capsule.

A night rest splint should also be supplied, with the fingers fully corrected into alignment and the MCP joints extended to neutral. Care must be taken to ensure that the fifth MCP joint is not hyperextended.

Select the type of wrist support, preferably palmar slab, which will then require high profile extension. Surgery is performed to correct MCP joint ulnar drift and subluxation, so the ulnar and palmar soft tissues need stretching post-surgery to prevent recurrence.

Position
- The MCP joints are extended to neutral and pulled in a radial direction to a maximum angle of 45°.
- The elastic pull must be sufficiently weak to allow full MCP joint flexion. The fifth finger needs a very gentle pull, as flexion of this joint is difficult to regain.
- The overhead support is placed above the proximal phalanges. If placed distal, the tension on the elastic will increase significantly during flexion.
- Finger loops support the proximal phalanges, but if the patient tends only to flex the PIP joints during exercise rather than the required MCP flexion, then wide finger loops can be made to cross the PIP joints (Harris, 1996).
- The palmar splint ends 0.5 cm proximal to the distal palmar crease to allow full MCP joint flexion and is cut round the thenar eminence so the thumb movements are not restricted.

The patient should exercise in the splint every hour, and attend physiotherapy. After 3 weeks light activities can be started while wearing the splint, and gradually upgraded until the splint is discarded after 6 weeks, or according to the surgeon's wishes. The night resting splint must be continued indefinitely while disease is active.

REFERENCES

Ball, C. and Penton, P. (1994). A review of the different static splint designs for the thumb. *Br. J. Hand Ther.*, **1(8)**, 8–12.

Ellis, M. (1984). Splinting the rheumatoid hand. *Clin. Rheum. Dis.*, **10(3)**, 673–96.
Goldsmith, N. (1996). MUD splint. *Br. J. Hand Ther.*, **2(4)**, 10–12.
Harris, S. (1996). MCP joint replacements. The Billericay experience with silastic MCP joint replacements. *Br. J. Hand Ther.*, **2(4)**, 3.
Houchin, R. and Cheshire, L. (1971). Splintage for ulnar deviation. *Br. J. Occup. Ther.*, **34(10)**, 9–19.
Lawton, D. S. (1974). Hand splinting in rheumatoid arthritis. *Br. J. Occup. Ther.*, **37(12)**, 219–26.

FURTHER READING

Adams, J. (1996). Splinting the rheumatoid wrist and hand: evidence for its effectiveness. *Br. J. Ther. Rehabil.*, **3(11)**, 621–4.
Barr, N. R. (1975*). The Hand, Principles and Techniques of Simple Splint Making in Rehabilitation.* Butterworth-Heinemann.
Culic, D. D., Battaglia, M. C., Wickman, C. *et al.* (1979). Efficacy of compression gloves in rheumatoid arthritis. *Am. J. Phys. Med.*, **58**, 278–99.
English, C. B. and Nalebuff, E. A. (1972). Understanding the arthritic hand. *Br. J. Occup. Ther.*, **35(7)**, 473–83.
Evans, D. M. and Lawton, D. S. (1984). Assessment of hand function. *Clin. Rheum. Dis.*, **10(3)**, 697–725.
Henwood, J. (1975). Hinged working splint for the elbow. *Br. J. Occup. Ther.*, **38(12)**, 265–6.
Janssen, M., Phifersons, J., van de Velde, E. and Dijkmans, B. (1990). The prevention of hand deformities with resting splints in rheumatoid arthritis patients. A randomised single blind one-year follow up study. *Arthr. Rheum.*, **33**, 123.
McClure, P., Blackburn, L. and Dusold, C. (1994). The use of splints in the treatment of joint stiffness. Biologic rationale and an algorithm for making clinical decisions. *Phys. Ther.*, **74**, 1101–7.
Medical Devices Agency (1997). *Wrist Splints for People with Rheumatological Disease, A Comparative Evaluation.* Prosthetics & Orthotics PO1, DOH.
Stack, H. G. and Vaughan Jackson, O. J. (1971). The zig zag deformity in the rheumatoid hand. *Hand*, **3**, 67.
Tasker, J. (1996). Splinting compliance. Night resting splints and the rheumatoid arthritis patient. *Br. J. Hand Ther.*, **2(4)**, 6–9.

Appendices

Appendix A

SUPPLIERS – MATERIALS AND EQUIPMENT FOR SPLINTING

Joint Jack Company, 108 Britt Road, East Hartford, CT06118, USA. UK agent: Linn Medical Ltd., Grace Cottage, Church Lane, Lacey Green, Bucks. HP17 0QX. Fax: 01844 343276.

Neoprene: Kettering Surgical Appliances, 73 Overstone Road, Northampton NNI 3JW, UK. Fax: 01604 629689.

North Coast Medical Inc., 187 Stauffer Boulevard, San Jose, CA 95125. Fax: +01 408 283 1950.

Orfit products: Orfit Industries, Vosveld 9A, B-2110 Wijnegem, Belgium. Fax: 3-326 14 15. British agents: Promedics (address below).

Otoform K-Paste silicone moulding compound: Dreve Otoplastik GmBH, Max Planck Strasse, D-4750 Unna, Germany. Fax: 2303 82909. British agents: PC Werth Ltd, Audiology House, 45 Nightingale Lane, London, SW12 8SP, UK. Fax: 0208 675 7577.

Plastazote: Kettering Surgical Appliances (as above).

Powernet Lycra: Spentex BCA Ltd, Street 7 Thorp Arch Trading Estate, Wetherby, West Yorkshire, LS23 7BJ, UK. Fax: 01937 541237. Also: Gilbert and Mellish Ltd, Block 13, Ground Floor, Leopold Street, Long Eaton, Nottingham, NG10 4QG, UK. Fax: 0115 973 3902.

Promedics, Moorgate Street, Blackburn, Lancashire, BB2 4PB, UK. Fax: 01254 619001.

Rigilene boning/reinforcement: John Lewis, department stores and haberdashers.

Silipos (UK) Ltd, 85a Stanmore Hill, Stanmore, Middlesex, 8A7 3DZ, UK. Fax: 0181 420 7212.

Smith and Nephew Homecraft Ltd, Lowmoor Road Industrial Estate, Kirkby in Ashfield, Nottingham, NG17 7QX, UK. Fax: 01623 755585.

Spring wire/piano wire (technical description hard polish stainless steel wire also obtainable from piano/tuners' suppliers): Ormiston Wire Ltd, 1 Fleming Way, Worton Road, Isleworth, Middlesex, TW7 6EU, UK. Fax: 0208 569 8601.

Steeper RSL, Queen Mary's University Hospital, Roehampton, London, SW15 5PL, UK. Fax: 0208 788 0137.

Turbocast thermoplastic: T-TAPE Company, BV, Hogebergdreef 60, 4645 Ex Putte, The Netherlands. Fax: +31 10 47 72 430. British supplier: Athrodax Surgical Ltd, Great Western Court, Ashburton, Ross-on-Wye, Herefordshire, HR9 7DW, UK. Fax: 01989 768140.

VM wrist supports: VM Marketing, St Peters, Ubbeston, Halesworth, Suffolk, IP19 0EX, UK. Fax: 01986 798040.

Vitrathene: Kettering Surgical Appliances (as above).

X-Lite open mesh thermoplastic: Runlite SA, 9 Avenue de la Cooperation, B-4630 Micheroux, Belgium. Fax: 41 77 46 83. British supplier: Orthopaedic Systems Ltd, Unit G22, Oldgate, St Michael's Industrial Estate, Widnes, Cheshire, WA8 8TL, UK. Fax: 0151 495 2150.

Appendix B

EXAMPLES OF OCCUPATIONAL THERAPY ACTIVITIES FOR A PATIENT FOLLOWING FLEXOR TENDON REPAIRS

Early stage of treatment

Broad aims of treatment:

1. To increase active range of movement
2. To decrease oedema.

Using light activities with no resistance or power work.

Definition: In the following tables, the column 'Grading' identifies ways in which the therapist can alter the difficulty of the task, so changing the amount and type of range of movement and muscle strength required.

Jewellery making (e.g. construction of dangling earrings)
Equipment: small beads, jewellery fastenings (e.g. earring loops, pins), small electronics pliers.

Therapeutic value	*Grading*
Pulp/pulp pinch grip Lumbrical action to pick up a bead from out of a pot Fine manipulation of bead to align hole and jewellery pin Learning how to use the anaesthetic hand, using vision to compensate for loss of sensation **Note**: the patient should not use pliers in the injured hand until 6 weeks post-repair	Pour beads into saucers if the patient cannot reach into a pot Saucers could be slightly elevated within the line of sight

Basketry (e.g. construction of a tray)
Equipment: ready-made tray bases, plastic cane, two sizes (weaving and large staking), clippers, beads (optional, to form handles).

Therapeutic value	*Grading*
Stage 1: cutting out the cane stakes	
Pulp to pulp or tripod grip	The distance marks for the length of cane need not be on a table but could be on a wall or wall-elevated table, so that activity can be performed in elevation for reduction of oedema
Note: If the patient is in the early stage of treatment the clippers must not be used in the injured hand – they will provide too much resistance if used within 6 weeks from the time of repair and could lead to rupture of recently repaired tendons. The patient must use the uninjured hand with the clippers. The injured hand can be used to hold the cane to measure the stake lengths against reference marks.	
Stage 2: threading the large staking cane into the tray base and weaving the single track foot-border	
Pulp/pulp or tripod pinch grip Learning how to use an anaesthetic hand, using vision to compensate for loss of sensation Care of anaesthetized skin – this includes regular checking of skin condition Wrist flexion and extension Establishing normal patterns of movement Toughening up very soft skin	None
Stage 3: weaving the wall of the tray with three stands of weaving cane	
As for Stage 2	Can be completed from an elevated wall table for reduction of oedema
Stage 4: weaving the plaited two-rod five-stroke border	
As for stage 2 Dexterity and manipulation Concentration	No adaptation possible The patient will need a lot of help from the therapist to start and finish the plait
Note: This stage of the task can get tough and should be completed towards the middle stage of treatment	
Stage 5: trimming and finishing the edges As for stage 1	None

Typesetting (e.g. construction of headed note paper or business cards)
Equipment: Type of different styles and sizes, leads, composing stick (and blocks for it to rest on).

Therapeutic value	*Grading*
Pulp/pulp or tripod pinch grip Facilitation of flexor digitorum profundus function Manipulation to align the type face Concentration Use of anaesthetic hand	Size of type Complexity of task The fingers will get dirty with old ink, therefore do not use with open wounds; however, this also enables the therapist to check the usage of the fingers – very helpful! Sloping table to support type tray (standard traditional printing furniture) for elevation If the patient holds the composing stick in the uninjured hand, he or she is forced to use the injured hand to pick up the type In the middle stage of treatment the type can be picked up using tweezers for improving pinch grip. Different weights of tweezers will offer different amounts of resistance. The resistance can be increased by putting a coin into the fulcrum of the tweezers

Large solitaire
Equipment: large solitaire peg board, large pegs, wall table for elevation, clamps to secure the peg board to the elevated table.

Therapeutic value	*Grading*
Pulp/pulp or tripod pinch grip Finger extension with ab/adduction Wrist extension Elbow extension Shoulder flexion Reduction of oedema	Cover the pegs with elastic bands to help improve a poor grip

Tiddlywinks
Equipment: Commercial tiddlywink counters.

Therapeutic value	*Grading*
Flexor digitorum profundus function	Do not allow the patient to play tiddlywinks in the early stage of treatment as it offers too much resistance. However, tiddlywink counters can be used to adapt many other remedial games. Ensure the patient picks up the counters and does not slide them. This can be achieved by using adapted boards that have walled pockets

Halma
Equipment: commercial Halma board and pieces, two or four players.

Therapeutic value	*Grading*
Pulp/pulp pinch Finger extension and ab/adduction Use of anaesthetic hand Concentration Competition and interaction with other patients	Construct a tool that has a hole into which the Halma pieces will fit easily. This tool can be used to slide the pieces around the board. A number of handles can be made to fit onto this tool (e.g. cylinder, span). The game can then be played with a group of patients who each need a different type of grip
	In the middle stage of treatment the game can be played using clothes pegs to pick up the suitably shaped Halma pieces. This is a good activity for pinch grip. Clothes pegs can be graded for increasing resistance in the following sequence: plastic, wooden, wooden with elastic bands around the top of the peg to increase resistance

Middle stage of treatment
Broad aims of treatment:

1. To increase active range of movement
2. To begin to work against resistance for tendon strengthening
3. To increase muscle power in a gentle graded manner
4. To facilitate functional use of the hand.

Macramé (e.g. construction of hanging plant holder)
Equipment: Macramé or stool seating cord, beads, scissors, instruction book.

Therapeutic value	*Grading*
Pulp\pulp and tripod pinch grip Dexterity and manipulation – considerable amount in knotting Power and pinch grip – e.g. in construction of wrap knot Use of anaesthetic hand Toughening up skin condition and desensitization of specific areas Whole upper limb range of movement Elevation, if this is still necessary Concentration and planning Creativity	Complexity and size of project, from jewellery and belts to wall hangings and rugs

Use of scissors
Equipment: scissors, paper (e.g.. designs such as mobiles and greeting cards), cane, cord or string (e.g. basketry, stool seating and macramé), plastic (e.g. construction of stocking gutters).

Therapeutic value	*Grading*
Finger and thumb flexion and extension Pinch and power grip Wrist extension	Type of material Time

Handwriting (e.g. signing name, writing short letters, advanced colouring books)
Equipment: paper, different types of pencils and pens (e.g. felt pens, biros).

Therapeutic value	*Grading*
Tripod pinch grip Fine dexterity Pinch grip strength Encourage normal use of hand Use of anaesthetic hand Encourage functional use of hand Increase speed Begin to explore the minimum skills the patient will need for return to work Begin the psychological process of adjustment as the patient starts to plan for the future	Explore the use of adaptations to make the task easier at this stage. Hopefully, these will only be needed temporarily and the patient can be moved towards normal function as soon as possible. Permanent adaptations may need to be considered in cases of severe trauma Wherever possible enable the patient to continue to use the dominant hand, as a successful change in dominance requires considerable time, effort and practice Make the task easier by adapting the pen – e.g. by padding the handle with foam and tape, using commercial rubber pen grips, or by the choice of pen size Elastic bands wrapped around the pen will help to improve grip for a patient with sensory loss Set the patient timed tasks to improve speed Length of the task (i.e. time) Ensure overall posture is checked

Keyboard skills
Equipment: computer keyboard (typing tutor), word processing, arcade games, typewriter, electronic musical keyboard (with headphones!).

Therapeutic value	*Grading*
Finger extension and flexion Ab/adduction of fingers Thumb extension and abduction Span Dexterity and speed Strength Use of anaesthetic hand Functional use and sense of achievement and enjoyment Work assessment	Amount of resistance on keys – e.g. an old-fashioned typewriter can offer considerable resistance Time Speed and accuracy requirements – e.g. different arcade games can offer a range of skill Complexity of task Strap forearm onto a support to ensure use of the hand and wrist rather than the whole arm

Late stage of treatment

Broad aims of treatment:

1. To improve muscle strength and power grip
2. To encourage normal functional use of hand and arm
3. To assess work skills, and return to employment.

Printing (e.g. construction of headed note paper and business cards)
The patient may be printing the cards that he or she type set in the early stage of treatment, or those of another patient. The task involves blocking the type into the chase, aligning the chase in the printing press and printing the cards.
   Equipment: Printing press, chase, furniture, ink and cards.

Therapeutic value	*Grading*
Dexterity and manipulation Grip strength (e.g. use of Allen key, printing press handle) Upper limb strength and range of movement Finger flexion Wrist extension Forearm pronation and supination (e.g. positioning chase into press) Use of anaesthetic hand Problem solving Concentration	Time Adapted handles on the press handle, e.g. patient may have the hand strapped onto an extension board for PIP joint passive extension or strapped directly onto the press handle for passive finger flexion

Use of hole punch
Equipment: Hole punch, paper.

Therapeutic value	*Grading*

If the hole punch is gripped between fingers and thumb:
    Finger and thumb flexion
    Power grip
 	
If the hole punch is depressed whilst it is on a table:
    Wrist extension
    Weight bearing through the hand
	Amount and weight of paper
	Time

Magic square
Equipment: Large magic square board – about 1 m (3 ft) square with flat sliding pieces. The patient plays this game on the floor whilst kneeling on all fours, and uses the injured hand to slide the pieces around the board.

Therapeutic value	*Grading*
Passive stretch for combined finger and wrist extension Weight bearing through the injured hand and arm Improve upper limb muscle strength Slow stretch of scar tissue	Time

Sawing by hand

Therapeutic value	*Grading*
Using the injured hand to grip the saw: 　Power grip 　Finger flexion 　Whole upper limb strength 　Work assessment *Using uninjured hand to grip the saw and injured hand to stabilize the wood:* 　Finger flexion in a hook grip 　Finger extension 　Passive wrist extension 　Weight bearing through the injured hand 　Power grip and forearm supination/pronation 　to support the plank 　Work assessment	Time Size and type of wood Weight of saw Assess cold intolerance by moving the task from indoors to outdoors in stages – e.g. workshop to outside shed to the open

Barrel construction (i.e. construction of wooden barrels for plant tubs)
Equipment: Hammer and drift, wooden staves and barrel base, metal bands (large and small size, and a building band for the construction process), electric hand drill with drum sander.
　The task involves positioning the barrel staves against a building band to form the barrel in an upside-down position. A large metal band is pushed over the staves and the building band removed. The barrel is turned up the right way and the base inserted and hammered into position. The barrel is then turned upside-down again and the small band hammered into place. The edges of the barrel are then sanded.

Therapeutic value	*Grading*
Power grip Upper limb strength with bilateral power work Finger flexion Whole upper limb range of movement Dexterity and manipulation Improve upper limb circulation Use of anaesthetic hand Toughen skin condition Desensitize hand Lifting General stamina Improve confidence Work assessment	Time

Internet Websites

British Association of Hand Therapists

http://www.hea.uea.ac.uk\baht\default.html

College of Occupational Therapists

http://www.cot.co.uk

Chartered Society of Physiotherapists

www.csp.org.uk

Clinical Interest Group in Orthotics, Prosthetics and Wheelchairs (Specialist Section of the College of Occupational Therapists

http://homepages.enterprise.net/cigopw

International Hand Library
Official library of the IFSSH. This is a free resource for surgeons, hand therapists, researchers, etc.

www.handlibrary.org